Pickerill

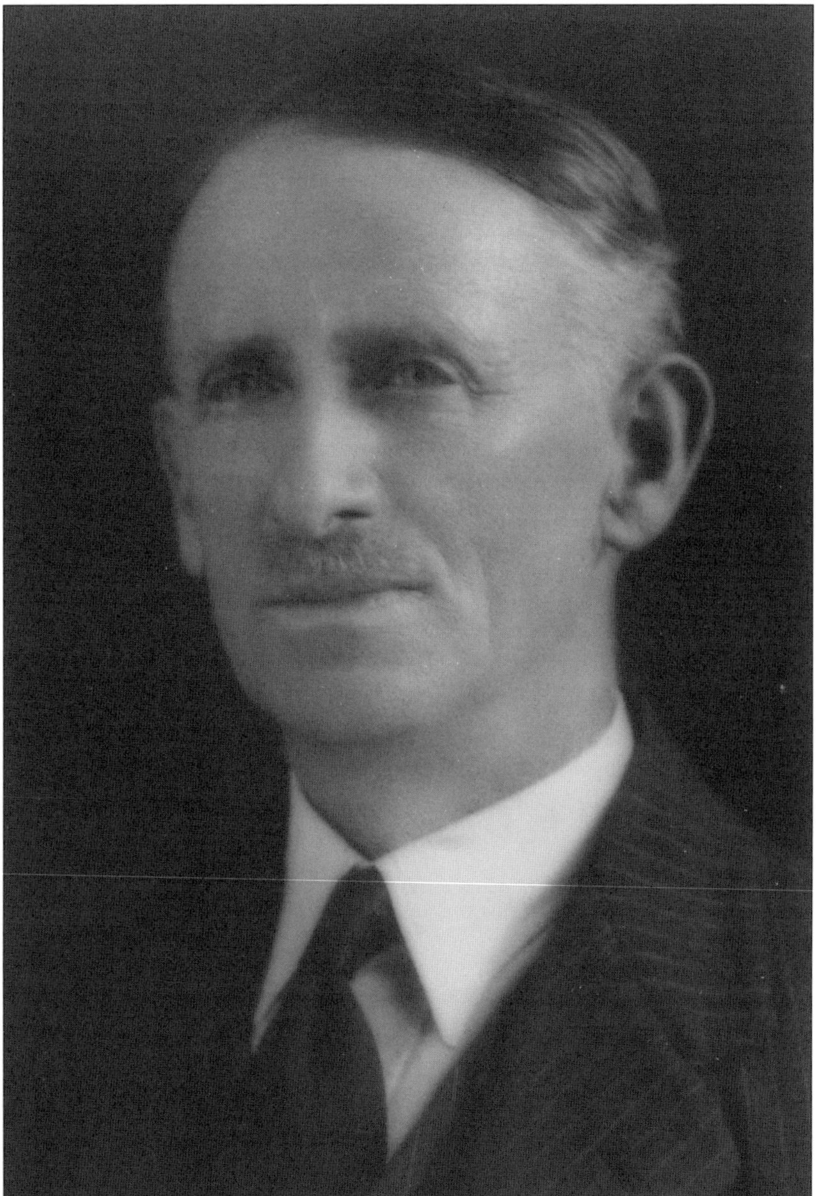

Henry Percy Pickerill, CBE, OBE, MD, MCh, MDS, BDS, MB, ChB, LDS(Eng).

Portrait by Falk, Sydney, c. 1930

Pickerill

Pioneer in Plastic Surgery, Dental Education, and Dental Research

Harvey Brown

OTAGO

Dedication

This biography of Henry Percy Pickerill is dedicated to his daughter, Mary Margaret Ann Frazer (née Pickerill), whose love and respect for her father's memory and achievements have been a constant inspiration to the author.

Published by Otago University Press 2007
PO Box 56/Level 1, 398 Cumberland Street
Dunedin, New Zealand
Fax: 64 3 479 8385, Email: university.press@.otago.ac.nz
www.otago.ac.nz/press
First published in this edition in 2007

ISBN 978 1 877372 46 9

Cover image: Portrait of H.P. Pickerill by Lois White, 1956.

Printed in Hong Kong through Condor Production.

Contents

Acknowledgements

I am very grateful to the many people who have assisted me in the preparation of this biography of Henry Percy Pickerill. It is dedicated to his younger daughter, Margaret Frazer, who has generously made available many letters, photographs, journals, articles, and other records and memorabilia of her father. These have proved invaluable, and most are now in the Pickerill Papers at the Hocken Collections in Dunedin. Without Margaret's constant support, this book may well not have been written.

I also thank Professor Tom Brooking of the Department of History, University of Otago, for his encouragement. I had the privilege of assisting Tom with his book *A History of Dentistry in New Zealand*, published in 1980 to mark the centenary of the passing of the first Dental Act in New Zealand. Since then we have shared our interests in the history of the dental profession, and his continuing guidance has been greatly appreciated.

Mr Michael Bagge, MA, has been my highly valued research assistant. Michael's professional understanding of the avenues and byways of historical research, and his knowledge of the records of the University of Otago presented me with a vast amount of information that I would have otherwise had great difficulty in accessing. I thank him for his expertise and commitment.

The employment of Michael Bagge was made possible by a grant from the New Zealand Dental Association's Dental Research Foundation, for which I am most grateful. The Board of the Foundation accepted without question that the documentation of the historical events within the life of the profession and the education of its members are legitimate areas of research, and for this I am most appreciative. I also greatly appreciate two further grants from the Foundation. A travel grant awarded in 2004 assisted with expenses in England where I accessed archives of the First World War at Queen Mary's Hospital in Sidcup, visited Pickerill relatives in Essex and, following a brief visit to Hereford, researched material at the University of Birmingham. A further grant came in 2006 toward publication expenses. This generous support from the Foundation is gratefully acknowledged.

Dr Andrew Bamji, Director of Medical Education at Queen Mary's Hospital and Archivist of the World War I records, was an excellent source of information, and freely made available the many resources held there; these included Pickerill's own surgical records held in the Macalister Archive. I thank him for his assistance and encouragement.

I am grateful to Mr John Harnden, researcher associated with the Hereford Records Office, who provided information about the Pickerill family in that city.

Mrs Vivien Jones and the late Mrs Sylvia Lamb, nieces of Henry Percy, were very helpful with information about the Pickerills' family life in Hereford. The hospitality of Vivien and Michael Jones in Chelmsford, Essex, was greatly appreciated.

Another family member who assisted greatly is Mr Gerald Fogg, grandson of Henry Percy, and son of Stanley and Kathleen Fogg (née Pickerill). He was very close to his grandmother Mabel Pickerill and provided respectful and empathetic insights into aspects of her life after the separation and divorce.

Members of the staff of the Special Collections Department in the Library of the University of Birmingham were extremely helpful. Pickerill's student days were somewhat of a mystery to family members, but during my visit a very full picture of his energetic and pioneering life as a student emerged. I am grateful for the interest and enthusiastic assistance of the Archivist, Ms Philippa Bassett, and her colleagues.

I appreciate very much the generosity of Mr Anthony Dreaver in reviewing my first hesitant steps in writing this work. Although facing deadlines in a major historical work of his own, he kindly critiqued and edited several early chapters. The outcome was not only an improved style, but also much encouragement to continue documenting the life of a person, previously unknown to him, who immediately captured his interest.

The in-depth review of the full manuscript by Associate Professor Geoffrey Rice, Head of the School of History, University of Canterbury, was especially valuable. He suggested areas that would benefit from further development, and his complimentary comments were greatly appreciated. I acknowledge with thanks his expertise and the generous gift of his time.

Several people have helped me gather illustrations. I especially thank Dr Darryl Tong and Professor Murray Meikle, both of the University of

Otago School of Dentistry; Dr Richard King, my former close colleague in the School; Mr Mel Littlejohn of SciTech Photo Services, Dunedin, for his professional expertise; and Ms Mary Lewis, of the section of Pictorial References and Reproductions in the Hocken Collections (formerly the Hocken Library) in the University of Otago.

Other members of the staff in the Hocken Collections gave much valuable assistance at various stages in my research. All were helpful and patient in my approaches to them, and I especially acknowledge the interest and help of Ms Anna Blackman, Curator of Archives and Manuscripts.

Pickerill records from the Bassam Hospital had been preserved at the Library of the Wellington School of Medicine and Health Sciences, University of Otago. I thank Ms Megan Clark, formerly Medical Librarian, for helping me access these records, which are now included in the Pickerill Papers at the Hocken Collections.

Last, but not least, I thank my wife, Janet, for her very practical support. Not only was she a very helpful and critical first reader of various drafts, she was also consistently patient when, over several years, Henry Percy Pickerill dominated our home, taking over the dining-room table when my tiny study filled to overflowing.

HARVEY BROWN
Waikanae, February 2007

Preface

In a distinguished career, Henry Percy Pickerill ventured into numerous fields that brought him national and international recognition.

His academic achievements at the University of Birmingham resulted in undergraduate and postgraduate qualifications in both medicine and dentistry. In 1907, just eighteen months after graduation in medicine, and at the age of twenty-eight, he was appointed foundation Director of the Dental School and Hospital in the University of Otago, and shortly afterwards Professor of Dentistry and Dean when the Faculty of Dentistry was created. He became a world leader in research on the nature, causes, and prevention of the major scourge of tooth decay. He was deeply involved in the affairs of the New Zealand Dental Association, serving as both Secretary and Editor of the *New Zealand Dental Journal*. His impressive military record began as co-founder and Assistant Director of what was later to become the Royal New Zealand Dental Corps; in England from 1917 to 1919 he commanded the New Zealand Facial and Jaw Section, first at the Second New Zealand General Hospital, Walton-on-Thames, and then at The Queen's Hospital, Sidcup. There he was one of the pioneering plastic surgeons specialising in the management of the dreadful facial injuries sustained by troops on the Western Front; he continued this work in Dunedin after the First World War. He was committed to State involvement in the dental care of children, but his approach eventually proved so contrary to the developing policy of the New Zealand Dental Association that a bitter fallout ensued.

After he resigned from the University in 1927, he practised plastic surgery in Sydney, Australia, for seven years before returning to New Zealand and becoming Senior Plastic Surgeon at Wellington Hospital. Subsequently, with his second wife, Cecily (later Dame Cecily) Pickerill, he laid the foundations for the Plastic Surgery Unit at Middlemore Hospital in Auckland; at Bassam, the Pickerills' private hospital in Lower Hutt, they specialised in the repair of cleft lips and palates, and introduced the revolutionary system of children being nursed by their mothers. In the final weeks of his life, he was one of those responsible for the founding of the Plastic Surgery Section of the Royal Australasian College of Surgeons.

This diversity of interests and activities confirms that Pickerill was a researcher and clinician of vast energy and enthusiasm. His searching mind and ability to identify and analyse problems led him to propose unique and innovative solutions. Such diversity creates problems for his biographer. Throughout the first half of his career, up to his resignation as Dean in 1927, these specialised areas of interest were intimately entwined. Each needs to be explored in order to reveal the extent of his achievements. In doing so, however, there is a risk of losing, at least to some extent, the ongoing thread of Pickerill's life and the way these areas of interest interacted. As a result some readers – especially those with limited interest, for example, in dental caries, the management of a dental school, or maxillofacial surgery – may find the attention given to these topics a diversion from the main story of the man. Another biographer may well have adopted a different plan, but this writer's own background in academic, clinical, and public health dentistry drew him to the conclusion that it was logical, indeed essential, to separate out the various fields of interest, and to deal with each in depth. This approach has some advantages, however, as it serves to invite critical analysis of his achievements by experts in these areas. Such a review of the pioneering contributions of Pickerill and others to the development of caries research and plastic surgery would be welcome.

In using this approach, the writer trusts that the essentials of Pickerill as a person are not completely hidden. He was a man of great intellect who attacked problems with vigour and enterprise, and who firmly defended his beliefs – at times, as shown by the bitterness of the arguments about the structure of the School Dental Service, to the point of arrogance. His private life was also full, and not without controversy and even scandal. After he left his wife and family behind in Dunedin when he resigned from the University of Otago, his former house surgeon, Cecily Clarkson, joined him in Sydney. Following the ensuing divorce, Pickerill and Clarkson subsequently formalised their surgical partnership by marriage.

The bitterness of this family breakdown is still expressed by some descendants today. The children of the first marriage are now all deceased and few written records have been found or contributed. Details of the Pickerill family's life in Dunedin are therefore sparse, but grandson Mr

Gerald Fogg has provided a number of insights. Mrs Margaret Frazer, the only child of the second marriage, believes that, in his later years, Pickerill began his autobiography, but no such writing has been found. She has, however, carefully preserved letters, documents, published articles, and other memorabilia. These she has generously donated to the University of Otago School of Dentistry, and they will be placed with the Pickerill Papers in the University of Otago's Hocken Collections in Dunedin.

Aside from his professional life, Pickerill brought an innovative approach to his farming venture. He was a dedicated trout fisherman with a great love of the New Zealand outdoors. His deep interest in the Maori is shown by his pioneering research into the dental health of the people of the Urewera during two expeditions, and by the observations he recorded on their diet and customs. But despite this immersion in New Zealand life, it is hard to escape the impression that, to a large extent, he remained an English gentleman, loyally devoted to things British and to his *alma mater*, the University of Birmingham.

He was indeed a complex person, with many interests and many achievements, albeit tempered by some missteps. But his achievements far outweigh any such faltering, and a full account of his rich and vigorous life is long overdue.

1

Growing up in Hereford

Henry Percy Pickerill, known as Percy, was born in Hereford, England, on 3 August 1879, the eldest child and only surviving son of Mary Ann and Thomas Pickerill. Thomas was born in Hereford in 1855; grandfather John Pickerill was born in Nottingham in 1815, but is recorded as living in Hereford at the time of his marriage to Mary Ann Todd Collins. John Pickerill was a 'currier', a vocation in the leather trade that involved dressing and colouring tanned leather.

Thomas Pickerill, Percy's father, was employed in the Lugwardine Tile Works of W.H. Godwin, a company that made ornate porcelain tiles. The firm advertised itself as 'Godwin's Encaustic Tiles, Tesselated Pavements etc. For Churches, Entrance Halls etc. May be seen in Worcester Cathedral, Gloucester, Hereford, St. David's Exeter, Chichester, Rochester, Salisbury & Carlisle Cathedrals. Also Windsor Castle'. The use of the company's tiles in Christchurch Cathedral was an early but incidental connection with New Zealand. Thomas was a loyal servant of the company for about forty years. His marriage certificate shows he was the 'Accountant'; on Percy's birth certificate he is 'Commercial Clerk'; and on Percy's marriage certificate, he is shown as 'Managing Director'.

Percy's mother, Mary Ann Pickerill (née Gurney), was the daughter of William Gurney, shown as an ironmonger on her marriage certificate. The Gurney family was prominent in the life of Hereford, for Alfred Gurney, Mary Ann's uncle, was mayor in 1895, and a cousin, Edwyn Gurney JP, was mayor in 1905.[1] Mary Ann and Thomas married at the Registrar's Office in Hereford on 15 August 1878. At the time of Percy's birth, they were living in 34 Harold Street. Hereford's streets were renumbered in the 1930s and 1940s, and 34 Harold Street in 1881 was one of a long row of terraced houses. When Percy was nine, the family moved to a new home, No.1 Montrose Villas, at 13 Harold Street.

No. 1 Montrose Villas is a substantial semi-detached residence that suggests its occupants were comfortably off. According to the 1901 Census, No. 2 Montrose Villas was occupied by Francis Dallow, the Deputy Chief Constable of Herefordshire, and his wife, Susan. The Pickerills and the Dallows were related, as Susan was a sister of Thomas. On the night of the Census, John Pickerill, Percy's grandfather, then aged eighty-five, was staying with his daughter and son-in-law at No. 2.

Mary Ann and Thomas also had six daughters who survived infancy – Frances M. (May), Mary Gertrude (Gertie), Ethel (Tottie), Grace (Kitty), Edith M. (Maud), and Hilda Doris. Doris was born in 1898, when Percy was aged nineteen. Four other children did not survive infancy – Thomas Cecil (died 28 December 1881, aged eight months), John Collins (died 23 March 1886, aged ten months), Cyril (died 17 December 1886, aged four days), and Daisy (died 11 August 1893, aged four days).[2] The 1901 Census does not mention any live-in domestic help, but family tradition names Potter Green as a loyal and devoted servant. The 1881 Census records Harriet Davenport, aged thirteen, as a servant at 34 Harold Street.

An insight into the family's financial circumstances in 1912, by which time Percy had left England for New Zealand, comes from a summary of bankruptcy proceedings against Thomas's employer, then known as William Godwin and Son.[3] In September 1906, Thomas Pickerill, then manager of the works, and A.F. Godwin, the grandson of the founder, were taken into partnership. The firm was already in financial difficulties, and Thomas advanced it £300. He retired in 1908, but when the firm was wound up in 1912, he was owed £1,179.8s. Thomas had been receiving a salary of £250 per annum prior to his retirement, in those days a substantial sum that would have allowed the family to live comfortably if modestly.

The only information available on the family and its lifestyle has come from Percy's reminiscences to his daughter Margaret Frazer, and from nieces Sylvia Lamb and Vivien Jones, daughters of Kitty (Bullar), who recalled snippets of family history as told by their mother and aunts. It was a close-knit and very happy family, and the sisters looked up to and worshipped their brother. Picnics on the River Wye, especially at the nearby village of Holme Lacy, were summer highlights, and winter activities included skating on the River Lugg, a tributary of the Wye, with Percy leading the way and his sisters hanging onto his coat-tails. Thomas was considered an expert salmon fisherman; Percy shared this interest and would row his father to favourite spots on the beautiful River Wye. Percy was subsequently to take his skills to New Zealand, where he enjoyed recreational fishing for trout and salmon.

At the time of their marriage in the Registry Office, Mary Ann and Thomas worshipped with the Society of Friends, but later attended the Baptist Church. Percy was married in the Parish Church, Birmingham, and remained a staunch member of the Church of England until his death.

Percy was educated at the Chandos School and then at the Hereford County College. Unfortunately no records of either establishment exist, but Chandos House was the Collegiate School of Hereford, situated at the Gatehouse. It was one of several excellent private schools of the day.[4] Percy's senior years were spent at the County College, where he received a book prize for distinction in scripture in 1894, and another book prize in 1895 when he was in the lower sixth form.

Family members believed Percy studied at the University of Oxford before going to Birmingham, and Percy himself stated in his application for the Dunedin position that he received his scientific training at the Universities of Oxford and Birmingham. The Oxford archives, however, have no record of him attending the University or taking the matriculation examination. He did, however, receive a book prize from the University of Oxford 'In connection with a course of 6 lectures on Workingmen, Inventors and Discovery', which were given in Hereford in January–March 1899, and he received another prize later that year. His Oxford connection was therefore confined to extension lectures. Neither are the records clear on where he matriculated. The Birmingham Regulations of 1900–01 recognised a number of options in lieu of its own Matriculation – 'Responsions of the University of Oxford',[5] matriculation of any other university in the United Kingdom, Oxford or Cambridge Junior Local Examinations (First or Second Class Honours), the Higher Leaving Certificate of the Oxford and Cambridge Boards, and the Oxford and Cambridge Senior Local Examination (Honours). Percy's Birmingham records show that, at twenty-one, he was exempt from the Preliminary Examination, and that he was granted 'Honorary Matriculation'. Margaret Frazer believes Percy's father wanted him to study law at the University of London, but Percy had other ideas and soon returned to Hereford. A brief stay in London might explain a note in records of the University of Birmingham suggesting he matriculated through the University of London.

Percy's sisters did not have the privilege of a university education, but whether this was due to the family's inability to support more than one child at university or from inclination is not known. However, the girls' education was not neglected – Kitty attended art college and became a teacher, and Tottie and Doris also taught; Maud worked in a shop, and Gertie remained at home.

Mary Ann Pickerill died in 1914, and Thomas died in Wilton, Wiltshire, in 1925.

What led Percy into medicine and dentistry is uncertain. Margaret Frazer believes her father wanted a career in medicine, but the family was not able to afford this; dentistry was seen as a less expensive training that could later lead into medicine. At that time, the training for dentistry included a minimum of two years' apprenticeship in a dental practice, attendance at a recognised medical school and hospital for courses in anatomy, physiology, medicine, and surgery, and attendance at a recognised dental hospital or dental department of a general hospital for courses in specific dental subjects. The qualification required for registration was the Licentiate in Dental Surgery of the Royal College of Surgeons of England – the possibility of qualification by university degree was imminent, but was probably not known to the young Pickerill at that time. He entered the practice of Mr A.G. Levason, a prominent Hereford dentist, as an apprentice, presumably after his brief flirtation with studying law. After the completion of the apprenticeship, he enrolled at Guy's Hospital in London. But just then, as he recalled many years later, 'Joseph Chamberlain's dream of a great new Midland University had come to fruition, so I changed over to Birmingham … If I had stayed at Guys no dental degrees would have been possible because [the University of] London did not grant them and was one of the last to do so'.[6]

He enrolled at the Mason University College in September 1900 as a candidate for the Licentiate in Dental Surgery and for the medical qualification of Member of the Royal College of Surgeons. A month after his twenty-first birthday, he left the family home in Hereford and became an undergraduate student at what was shortly to become the University of Birmingham.

2

Birmingham: from student days to marriage

Percy Pickerill's undergraduate career at the University of Birmingham was a lively combination of academic achievement, immersion in student politics and social affairs, and service in the territorial forces. His enrolment in 1900 virtually coincided with the founding of the University itself and with Birmingham becoming the first university in the Empire to establish a fully university-based programme leading to the degree of Bachelor of Dental Surgery (BDS). Pickerill was to be the first product of this pioneering development.

The University of Birmingham grew from Sir Joseph Mason's Science College, which opened in 1880. In 1882, medical students from the Queen's College in Birmingham started attending the Mason College for some of their science subjects, and in 1892 the Medical Faculty of Queen's College, with its 250 students, transferred fully to the Mason College. In 1900, by Royal Charter, Mason College became the University of Birmingham.[1]

Birmingham has also had a long involvement in formal education in dentistry.[2] The Birmingham Dental Dispensary opened in 1858, and in 1860 'offered opportunities to students to become practically acquainted with the various operations in connection with dental surgery'. Lectures were offered in dental physiology and surgery. In 1871 it moved to new premises and became the Birmingham Dental Hospital. In 1880 it was recognised by the Royal College of Surgeons for the purposes of dental education, and became known as the Birmingham Dental School. The educational components of the Hospital were incorporated into the University of Birmingham as part of the Medical Faculty in 1900.

One of the men instrumental in founding the University, and one of

Pickerill's lecturers and subsequently a colleague and supervisor, was prominent dentist John Humphreys, who was Secretary of the Dental School. Joseph Chamberlain was one of his patients, and to Chamberlain goes much of the credit for Birmingham becoming the first British university to grant degrees in dentistry. Chamberlain was the University's first Chancellor and, as the British Colonial Secretary at the time, a man of great influence.

The move to establish full university degree courses in dentistry was not widely welcomed – in London, the Royal College of Surgeons, which awarded the Licentiate in Dental Surgery (LDS), felt that its status as the controlling body for qualification would suffer. The Birmingham BDS was, however, stoutly defended by Humphreys, F.E. Huxley, and Sir Bertram Windle, the Dean of the Medical School, who maintained that 'University Degrees could not fail to enhance the prestige of dentistry, and such was their pertinacity and charm that degrees were in fact instituted'.[3]

The University moved quickly to make the degrees a reality, for Humphreys and Huxley were honoured by bestowal of the Master of Dental Surgery degrees in 1901. The first to be awarded the BDS degree were John Dencer Whittles (admitted to the degree as an 'Associate') and Harold Round. The latter gained his BDS under regulations allowing dentists who had completed the LDS qualification, while students of the Birmingham Dental School, to be examined for the BDS without completing the formal course.[4] In 1903, Arthur Hughes Parrott and Alfred William Wellings, past students of the Birmingham School, graduated BDS under the same regulations.[5] This introduction of what could be perceived as a 'short-cut' to gaining a full university qualification in dentistry would have cemented the BDS as a legitimate educational pathway: the University now had a degree course, and here were the first graduates to prove it. This approach would later be promoted by Pickerill himself as Dean of the Faculty of Dentistry at the University of Otago when, faced with a shortage of students and opposition to qualification being solely by the University course, he encouraged practising dentists to take the final examinations and gain the BDS(NZ) degree.

The *Calendar* of 1899–1900[6] shows, under Dentistry, only the Diploma in Dental Surgery of the Royal College of Surgeons of England, whereas the 1901–02 *Calendar*[7] includes the BDS and MDS degrees. Pickerill's enrolment at Birmingham thus came at the very time when the University itself came into being, and when dental education was first formalised as a full university discipline within the new Faculty of Medicine. The first BDS degrees having been awarded under special regulations, the University now needed to prove its worth by producing BDS graduates who had completed the full course of studies. Pickerill was the 'test' student, pioneering the new development. He passed the test with distinction, becoming the first in the British Empire to hold the BDS fully by course work. He thus set the path for others to follow.

Pickerill began his studies at the University on 9 September 1900. The Dean's Register of Students shows that Pickerill, Henry Percy, of 1 Montrose Villas, Hereford, age twenty-one years, was exempted from taking the Preliminary Examination because of his 'Honorary Matriculation'. His studies were recorded as leading to the Licentiate in Dental Surgery of the Royal College of Surgeons of England (LDS), and Membership of the Royal College of Surgeons of England (MRCS). He had already completed the two years' apprenticeship necessary for admission to the course leading to the LDS. 'BDS' was subsequently pencilled in under the heading 'Degree or Qualification', presumably when the Mason College became the University of Birmingham and the BDS degree was formalised. His results make no further mention of the MRCS, only the Bachelor of Medicine (MB) and, in his fifth and final year, the Bachelor of Surgery (ChB). The change in his status offered by the new degree programmes would have been an exciting prospect for the newly enrolled student. He had the opportunity of becoming the very first dentist under this new system. As his subsequent career shows, he could not resist a challenge – this one would have been irresistible.

The medical and dental courses had common subjects that greatly facilitated students to qualify in both fields. In the first year, for example, the subjects chemistry, practical chemistry, physics, practical physics, comparative anatomy, anatomy, practical anatomy (dissections), and physiology and practical physiology were all joint courses. The dental students also had dental metallurgy and dental mechanics. His second year covered further anatomy dissections, physiology, physiology practical, dental anatomy and physiology, dental histology, dissections physiology, *materia medica* (pharmacology), medicine and surgery, and diseases of the mouth. The third year covered medicine, surgery, pathology, hygiene, dental surgery, and dental bacteriology. Gaining the LDS (England) continued to be a requirement, perhaps even as an insurance against the possibility that the BDS degree might prove an unacceptable qualification for registration as a dentist; he completed this qualification in May 1903. He was now able to go on, according to the regulations of the time, to complete the BDS degree. His fourth-year subjects were medicine, surgery, therapeutics, midwifery, gynaecology, forensic medicine and toxicology, and mental diseases.

In June 1904 he completed all the requirements for his BDS. He was the only BDS graduate at the Congregation on 9 July 1904.[8] The Pickerill entry in the University's Register of Graduates is notable for his bold, seemingly triumphant signature. There was one BDS graduate in 1907, Reginald

Hudson Ashbury, who had enrolled a year earlier than Pickerill. Pickerill fulfilled all the requirements for the MB, ChB degrees during his fifth-year courses, which included medicine, operative surgery, and ophthalmology, and completed all examinations for these degrees in June 1905. He graduated at the Congregation on 8 July 1905.[9]

The Dean's Register lists examination results, some of them showing position in the class. He was eleventh equal (out of 27) in junior anatomy in the session 1900–01, but improved to second equal (out of 17) in the winter term of 1901, when he was third (out of 10) in physiology. In the spring term of 1903 he was first (out of 11) in dental surgery, and second (of 9) in practical dental surgery. In the winter term of 1903 he was third (of 29) in surgery. In other subjects, as far as can be judged, he performed consistently well, although his results were not spectacular.

The Dean's Register does not show him winning any prizes, but he did gain prizes in dentistry. He listed in his application for the Dunedin position the award of the Charles Green Medal for Proficiency in Anaesthesia, and the Ash Prize for the best essay on a given topic. His entry for the latter prize, was submitted under the pseudonym 'Aesculapius' in 1902.[10] Apparently his entry did not conform to the expected style, for he included a 'Note to the Examiners':

> Somewhat departing from custom, the writer of this essay has adopted a 'book' form in which to send it in, solely with view of rendering it more compact. Also with the same effect the illustrations have been placed on the opposite page from the written matter, and therefore it is hoped that these innovations will cause no disfavour.

This two-volume essay reveals a deep understanding of the process of tooth decay, its aetiology and significance in young children, and its effects on the developing permanent teeth. His views on the prevention of caries by means of a fibrous diet to promote chewing and natural cleansing, greatly reduced intake of sweets and sugar generally, and effective use of the toothbrush were to be continued in his later research and writing that would bring him international recognition. The treatment methods he described reflect the materials available at the time and are now well outdated; but his logical development of the topic, the presentation and clarity of the writing, and the quality of the illustrations, including radiographs, suggest the strength of his conviction that dental caries is a serious and very common condition that must be defeated; its causes, although still not fully understood, are related to diet, nutrition, and lifestyle; and prevention is the key to its management. This belief motivated the direction of his subsequent research. The essay is a remarkable document for a student in either his second or third year of studies; even though there may have been few entrants, the award of the prize appears fully justified. Pickerill also stated in his Otago application that he was awarded the Senior Prize for Operative Work, and a Special Prize for a paper read before the University Students' Society on 'The Effects of Civilization on the Teeth', the latter a topic he would also later pursue in New Zealand.

The Queen's College Medical Society

The Queen's College, the predecessor of the Mason College for medical training and hence of the Medical Faculty of the University, was remembered in the form of a study group that became incorporated into the University of Birmingham Medical Society. It met fortnightly in the evenings in the Professors' Common Room. Pickerill presented at least two papers. The first mention of his attendance was at the meeting of 11 February 1904, in his final year of dental studies, and at that meeting 'Mr Pickerill showed specimens of "Bilateral Fibromata of the Jaw", discussed by Messrs Emanuel, Billington and Nuthall'.[11] He is recorded as attending several other meetings, but his next presentation was not until 29 November 1905, after completion of his studies. He then gave a paper entitled 'Salivary Calculi from Submaxillary Gland'.

The Medical Society was a forum where he displayed his understanding of oral pathology before an audience that no doubt included senior members of staff. Throughout his career he was recognised as an accomplished and confident speaker in national and international scientific forums; these presentations, before a critical and knowledgeable audience, would have been valuable learning experiences.

Pickerill and student politics

The Charter of the newly established University of Birmingham called for there to be a Guild of Undergraduates, which would elect three representatives to the Court of Governors. This was a very worthy intention, but student politics in these early years of the University were tumultuous, and marked by heated controversy. Pickerill was to play a constructive role that helped bring order out of chaos.

Shortly after the University received its Charter, Oliver (later Sir Oliver) Lodge, Principal of the University, had called a meeting to advance the formation of the Guild. Its stormy early days were recorded in the *University of Birmingham Magazine*, a journal published by the Students' Representative

Council, another student body. An early issue of the *Magazine*[12] reported that the Guild was having difficulty settling on an acceptable constitution and, early in 1902,[13] described the meeting to elect the Guild's officers as a farce – although an organisation of undergraduates, it elected two graduates to office. Later that year, the *Magazine* reported: 'Yet the Guild is at present dormant. Few students know anything about it; fewer still exhibit the slightest interest in it.'[14] The same issue of the *Magazine* recorded that the Guild was still having problems electing a president: 150 votes were recorded, but only 113 persons were present. A subsequent meeting, early in 1903, was reported to be more orderly.

Whether Pickerill had any role in the Guild in these early days is not recorded, but when he was elected President in October 1904[15] the atmosphere was much calmer. The minutes at this time are confusing, for they record he was also elected President in October 1905,[16] although by this time he was no longer an undergraduate student. More confusion occurs where the minutes record that a further presidential election followed just a month after Pickerill's reported second election. Despite this confusion, and probable errors in the minutes, Pickerill was the President of the Guild for the year 1904–05. At a special meeting in December 1905, Pickerill, by then the Immediate Past President, presented to the University Club, on behalf of the Guild, portraits of the Warden of the Guild, the Earl of Halsbury, and the Vice-Chancellor, Alderman C.G. Beale.

At this meeting he also presented a major paper 'The Guild of Undergraduates: Its Present and Future'.[17] He began with a report on the Inter-University Congress of Students he had attended in London earlier in the year, noting sarcastically that Oxford and Cambridge had not deigned to be represented. He then made an impassioned plea for the students to unite as an *esprit de corps* would be needed if they were to host the next Congress. If there should be more 'school-boyish amusements' there would be no Congress, and Birmingham would be ridiculed and made a laughing stock. He stated that the Guild of Students was at present:

> on a firm and solid basis – capable of becoming a strong and powerful organisation, capable of organising, reforming, and controlling student affairs in the best possible manner … [the Guild] should be recognised by all as THE official body of students … we should foster that unanimity of thought and action, that feeling of good fellowship which have been in the past so conspicuous by their absence, and yet which are so absolutely necessary if we are to hold our own with other Universities – if we are to develop into a real living University in the true sense of the word, instead of remaining a conglomeration of individuals and cliques.

The reaction of his audience to these challenging words was not recorded, but they suggest past disorganisation and a frivolous attitude toward the Guild. Also not recorded is whether Pickerill actually had a mandate to invite the Congress to hold its next meeting at Birmingham – quite possibly he did this without authority, but no doubt with the best of intentions of establishing Birmingham firmly on the map of student politics.

Although he served as President of the Guild, he was not a student representative on the Court of Governors during his term of office – the representatives for 1904–05 were Mr P.J. Thompson and Lord Avebury. He was, however, the representative of the Guild of Graduates from 1 January 1906 until 24 October 1907. He did not complete this full term as he arrived in New Zealand in September 1907.

The Presidency of the Guild would have involved him in many events bringing him into social contact with University administrators, civic dignitaries, and politicians. An indication of one such event is a letter from the Secretary of Mr Austen Chamberlain, the eldest son of the University's Chancellor, Joseph Chamberlain, and at the time Chancellor of the Exchequer, acknowledging an invitation for Mr Chamberlain to be present at a guild event in Birmingham on 13 May 1905.[18]

Pickerill was also involved in the other major student body, the Students' Representative Council (SRC). In contrast to the Guild of Undergraduates, which was a corporate body of the University under the Charter, the SRC was a student-welfare organisation drawing its membership from all students. It was involved in the social affairs of the University – for example, sponsoring the hockey, tennis, and athletic clubs, and encouraging the formation of a Women's Athletic Club. It administered the Student Union, where students could be entertained by musical evenings and visiting speakers. Its journal, the *Magazine*, seemed to delight in the travails of the Guild, and there was considerable friction between the two bodies.

At the Council's meeting in February 1903, Pickerill moved a resolution:

> That this Representative Council of Students desires to bring to the notice of the Council [of the University, one of the University's three governing bodies] the extremely unsatisfactory state of the present social conditions in the University; that the Students' Representative Council also considers that the time has arrived when some form of Social Club is absolutely necessary to the well-being of the students, and it desires to know what steps the Council of the University is prepared to take in this direction.[19]

He urged immediate action on the grounds that suitable rooms in the neighbourhood would shortly become vacant; he thought the Council would look favourably on such a scheme 'at this present juncture'. A subsequent speaker thought it a 'vague request', that the Council would require a more detailed proposal, and that a small committee should be formed. By this time the meeting had lost its quorum – Pickerill's appeal for action was held over for three weeks, but this proved too late for the next meeting of the University Council. (The minutes also record that the Principal wanted to know if smoking had been going on in the writing room, a practice obviously frowned upon by the authorities.)

Like the Guild, the SRC also had its problems, for in May 1903 the committee resigned because of friction over grant funds. The final issue of the *Magazine*, June 1903, recorded the demise of the SRC and that its 'exit was far less imposing than its entrance 2 years ago.' The Guild of Students was the body that would fulfil the requirements of communication. The subsequent publication, *The Mermaid,* confirmed in its first issue that the two groups had been at cross-purposes.[20]

Pickerill seems to have had a constructive role in both bodies, serving as President of the Guild, and making positive proposals for the welfare of students through the SRC. It would all have given him the experience in University administration on which he would build in his subsequent career at Otago. The value of his contribution was recognised by the administration: the Principal, Sir Oliver Lodge, wrote in his testimonial supporting Pickerill's Otago application that:

> While a student he achieved the position of President of the Undergraduates' Guild, always a testimony to force of character and personal influence.
>
> In that position he came into contact with the Chancellor and other dignitories [sic] of the University, and took a leading part in important meetings, invariably conducting himself with dignity and effectiveness.[21]

In addition to his wider role in student politics, Pickerill was also active in the Dental Students' Society. He was the Secretary in 1902–03, and he was a member of a group that drew up a list of grievances presented to the Dean of the Dental Hospital. These grievances are not recorded, but 'eventually some reforms were carried out'. He also opened a debate on the subject 'That mechanical work is derogatory to, and is not an integral part of the dental procedure'.[22] This took place at a time when the need for a university degree in dentistry was being vigorously debated within the British Dental Association, with the proponents claiming that 'the best training for a student is not that which is chiefly directed to an impossibly perfect efficiency at the date of qualification, but that which lays the best foundation upon which more finished and elaborate structure of the professional man's capabilities in later life may be built.'[23] Opponents claimed dentistry was a practical discipline that could be learnt best as an apprentice. In view of his subsequent research career, one can imagine Pickerill's contribution to the debate having a formative influence on his strongly held philosophy that diagnosis and treatment in the healing professions must be firmly based in science, and that technical prowess alone is inadequate.

He provided an unusual insight into the student political activities of the day in a letter written many years later:

> Lloyd George Riot
>
> *Problem of the Pants*
>
> 'I was very interested to read Mr. P. Doyle's reminiscence of the above riot, for I also was there that night but on the opposite side of the square through which P.C. Doyle escorted "P.C." Lloyd George,' writes Dr. H.P. Pickerill.
>
> 'The time was the Boer War and Joseph Chamberlain, the greatest of Colonial Secretaries and originator of the Imperial conferences, was running the war for Great Britain. The whole of Birmingham was indignant that the little Welsh solicitor, the pro-Boer, should have the audacity to come and speak in the centre of Chamberlain's stronghold.
>
> 'I was a medical student at the time, and we so resented this (as we thought then) insult to our Chancellor that we, student-like, hatched a plan to kidnap L.G. We had, however, no chance to put it into execution, for the great square all round the Town Hall was packed with thousands of angry men, determined to get at Lloyd George.
>
> 'Nearly all the windows in the Town Hall were smashed, and all the doors being locked on the inside, a scaffold pole was obtained from somewhere, and with about 50 men handling it as a battering ram, the main doors were beaten in, but at this moment, unknown to the mob P.C. Lloyd George walked out at the other end.
>
> *'Riot Act and Batons*
>
> 'The Lord Mayor read the Riot Act. The police made a baton charge, and I perforce was one of those who had to run for it, and during which I witnessed one of the fatalities which occurred on that wild night long ago.
>
> 'But would Mr Doyle please inform us on a matter which intrigued us as students at the time and to which I have not yet heard the answer? What happened to the policeman who gave up his uniform to L.G.? Did he have to go home in his shirt and trouserless – for he certainly could not have got in Lloyd George's clothes?
>
> 'But it all played into L.G.'s hand, it gave him what he wanted – notoriety. It has been said with some truth that Lloyd George climbed to fame on Chamberlain's back – a political trick not unknown in these days.'[24]

Had the students' kidnap plan succeeded, dentistry in New Zealand might have followed a different course – a convicted kidnapper would undoubtedly not have appealed to the Council of the University of Otago.

Military service

According to his New Zealand military record, Pickerill was for five years a private in the University Company of the First Volunteer Brigade of the Royal Warwickshire Regiment. He was subsequently to serve with distinction in the New Zealand Army, and his experience with the Regiment gave him a solid preparation for military life. Service in the University Company included an annual camp, one of which was fully described in the first issue of *The Mermaid*.[25] It involved early reveille, long marches, joint exercises with another battalion of the Royal Warwicks and battalions of the Worcestershire Regiment, and enduring a severe storm that wrecked the camp and left no tents standing. An aim of the company was to give students the opportunity for volunteer work and social meetings, and to allow freshmen to be brought into touch with past and present students. Although the level of his involvement is not known, Pickerill would no doubt have been an enthusiastic participant in the activities.

Entering practice

His undergraduate career ended with his graduation MB, ChB in July 1905, although he was active in student affairs until the end of the year. His later application for a position in Dunedin suggests that, following his pre-university apprenticeship, he 'acquired familiarity with more modern mechanical methods, such as bridge, crown and porcelain work in the practice of Mr Breward Neale, Birmingham'. Whether this was during his student days or after graduation is not known. He also held a position at the Birmingham Dental Hospital and worked 'in my own practice', although nothing about the latter is known.

In April 1906, the University Council approved the recommendation of the Senate for his appointment as Lecturer in Dental Histology and Pathology in the Faculty of Medicine.[26] He was required 'to deliver a course of at least 10 lectures, and to conduct practical classes under the supervision of the Professors of Physiology and Pathology. The stipend [was] calculated on the basis of £1.11.6 per lecture personally delivered; the maximum payment not to exceed £15.15.0'. This part-time position would have allowed him to work as a demonstrator at the Dental Hospital and also in private practice. One of the conditions of appointment was that he could resign 'on giving three months notice in writing, which notice shall end at the expiration of one of the University Terms', although he could resign 'on the 30th of September of any year, by giving notice in writing at any time during the preceding months of July or August'. This clause was one of the reasons preventing him meeting the unreasonable time requirements for taking up the position in New Zealand – understandably, he was not prepared to sacrifice his reputation and his loyalty to Birmingham by breaking his contract to meet the demands of the Council of the University of Otago. In 1907 he was promoted from Demonstrator to Assistant Dental Surgeon at the Dental Hospital.

His immediate postgraduate employment seemed to be solely in dentistry, no references to him practising medicine being found. His commitment to dentistry is further confirmed by his holding office in the British Dental Association – he wrote in his Dunedin application that he was 'a member of the Council of the Central Counties Branch of the British Dental Association and Hon. Sec. of the Law & Ethics Committee'.

Romance and marriage

A fellow student and a firm friend in the dental course was John (Jack) Robertson Knott, and one of Jack's sisters, Mabel Louise, was an attraction. During their studies, according to granddaughter Sue Brookland, Pickerill would go to the Knott home 'and in the midst of her [Mabel's] noisy four brothers and six sisters, he would put his head between his hands at the table and swot flat out. His concentration was such that nothing would disturb him'. His career was to bear witness to these powers of concentration and dedication, but he still found time to court Mabel, who was five years older. They married in the Birmingham Parish Church on 19 June 1906 and their first child, John Percival, was born almost a year later, on 17 June. John Knott was his best man, and Kate Claire Knott was a bridesmaid. Place of residence is shown on the marriage certificate as 7 Newhall Street; at the time of Pickerill's application for the Dunedin post, the couple were living at Stoneleigh, Hazelwell, Birmingham.

The next recorded event in the Pickerill story was his sighting of the advertisement for a position in Dunedin, New Zealand. In that country, the dental profession and the University of Otago had combined in a remarkable way, not only to establish a dental school and hospital, but also to have in place its own fully university-based course leading to the BDS degree. In an appropriate complement to Birmingham's pioneering direction, its first graduate was to develop the same pathway in a far country. In New Zealand, the profession eagerly awaited his arrival.

3

An expectant profession

Percy, Mabel, and baby John Percival (Val) Pickerill arrived in Wellington on the *Corinthic* in September 1907. His arrival was greeted with delight by the members of the New Zealand Dental Association and by the University of Otago. A brand new school and dental hospital awaited him as Director, and the curriculum for the Bachelor of Dental Surgery degree had already been approved by Britain's General Medical Council. The New Zealand Dental Association was a vigorous fledgling body that, despite much heartache and frustration, had achieved a great deal in its two years of existence. The arrival of this young and energetic person, qualified in both dentistry and medicine, was seen as a major step toward elevating dentistry to a new level of professionalism and service to and respect from the whole nation.

A summary of the events leading up to this stage of development of the profession introduces the major players, many of whom became associates of Pickerill in education and in the New Zealand Dental Association. Essential to the story is the founding of the University of Otago within the University of New Zealand. The University of Otago Ordinance was enacted in 1869, and the first appointments to chairs were made in 1870.[1] In 1873, a Professor of Anatomy and Physiology was appointed, an early move in the foundation of the Medical School in Dunedin. This person's replacement, in 1877, was Professor John Halliday Scott, who became Dean of the Medical School in 1890. A remarkable servant of the University, and a powerful figure in medicine, Scott had a major role in the development of dental training and the subsequent founding of the Dental School.

The first legislation regulating dentistry was The Dentists Act, 1880. Its passage was not altogether smooth – supporters considered it essential to ensure the protection of the public, but opponents thought it 'offensive' and accused the dentists of wanting to set up a 'close guild'.[2] This latter sentiment, in one form or another, continued to echo whenever changes to dental legislation have been proposed, even to the present day.

At that time, practising dentists had a variety of training, qualifications, and experience. Basically anyone could set up practice and use the description 'dentist'. The Act provided for the registration of all who were currently practising, and prohibited the use of the title 'Dentist' by anyone not registered. Responsibility for future admission to the Register of Dentists was assigned to the Senate of the University of New Zealand.

An amendment to the Act in 1881 tidied up matters related to apprentices, allowing them to register provided they passed examinations set by a board of examiners within one year of completion of their three-year apprenticeship with a registered dentist. The Senate wanted to limit admission to apprenticeship to those who had passed 'an examination in general knowledge, equivalent to that known in our schools as the "sixth standard"', but the Registrar-General overruled this request.[3] The educational level of those wanting to begin training, and of those wanting to register their qualifications, became matters of heated debate for many years. Pickerill's very strong views were subsequently to feature prominently in these arguments.

At that time, the Board of Examiners was based in Dunedin at the University of Otago; Professor Scott was a member, and later became Chairman. Thus was established the University of Otago's involvement in the training of dentists, even though at this time its role was limited to examining.

In 1885 the Board made a further attempt to ensure those entering apprenticeship in dentistry had received an adequate preliminary education. The Senate went further and wanted an amendment to the Act so that candidates for the Certificate in Dental Surgery would be required to pass the First Professional Examination for the Bachelor of Medicine degree, but this did not eventuate. The Board persisted, however, and in 1890, Professor Scott, still Chairman of the Board and by now Dean of the Medical School, proposed to the Trustees of the Dunedin Hospital:

> to make compulsory, in addition to the pupilage now required under the Dentists Act, a short course of systematic practical instruction, such as is given in all Dental Schools. Most of the required subjects are taught in the Medical School here, and these I believe will be made use of, but Dentistry proper is not taught. The Senate is quite willing to make the required regulations on condition that some satisfactory arrangement is made for teaching this last subject. Fortunately all that is required can be very easily arranged for if you will assist by instituting a Dental Department in conjunction with the Hospital.

> This would be under the superintendence of some duly qualified dentist, who appointed by yourselves would treat cases and teach students.[4]

Professor Scott was advocating the first steps for a school of dentistry that would rely on the expertise of the Medical School and the facilities of the Dunedin Hospital. He was 'clearly ready to accept dentistry beneath the sheltering wing of his new medical faculty and the Senate of the University were also happy to accept the proposed new arrangements'.[5]

These efforts were in vain at that time. Scott and his Board were strongly opposed by others wanting to make it easier to qualify and register, and the Board was criticised because of its distance from the larger centres of population, its refusal to accept evidence related to eligibility of some candidates to take the examination, and the high standards set in the examination, resulting in what was considered an unsatisfactory failure rate.

The establishment of the first New Zealand Dental Association was another development at this time, but its existence was short-lived. The inaugural meeting was held in July 1889 in Wellington, and its first and only conference and annual meeting was in Dunedin in 1890. A letter from Alfred Boot, President of that Association, to the Chancellor of the University of New Zealand reveals the profession's concern about education. Seventeen years later, Pickerill was to be thrown into the same turmoil:

> Sir, – The New Zealand Dental Association at its late Conferences considered the question of dental education. The following resolutions were agreed to:–
>
> That the New Zealand Dental Association begs to call the attention of the Senate to the present unsatisfactory arrangements for the training of dental students, and offers the following suggestions: 1. That all pupils or students should register on entering their pupilage, and that no pupil should be competent for registration until he had passed the Matriculation Examination of the New Zealand University, or the equivalent thereof. 2. That pupils or students should be required to pass, in addition to three years' pupilage with a qualified dentist according to the Act, one year's course in a medical school.
>
> The dental examination at present in existence in New Zealand is one of the University examinations, and is prescribed and controlled by the Senate. This examination is very meagre and insufficient, and is not recognised by any other country or colony. Even South America refuses to recognise it.
>
> In Victoria a dental school and hospital is established, and the degree of Licentiate of Dental Surgery granted. … With a fully equipped Medical School in existence here the difficulty of assimulating [sic] our regulations to those of Victoria should not be great. It is submitted that the dental examination is the only examination conducted by the University that may be passed by a candidate without doing any work whatever in connection with the University.

> Should the above suggestions meet with your approval, the Association would urge on you the desirability of immediate action.[6]

The promise of this first New Zealand Dental Association, and the hopes of Professor Scott and the Board did not come to fruition. The Trustees of the Dunedin Hospital did not at that time follow up the suggestion for a dental department, and charges that the Board was acting unfairly by not admitting some candidates to the examination increased. In 1891, in direct contrast to the proposals of the board and the Senate, the Government amended the Dentists Act by allowing additional dental examining boards to be established in the other three main centres, and took responsibility for their supervision from the Senate of the University of New Zealand. Brooking described the politicians as riding 'roughshod over the ethical dentists in 1891, defying the protests of the NZDA members with apparent glee. When the Dentists Amendment Act was passed in 1891, ethical dentistry was dealt a crushing blow which the fledgling NZDA had no hope of surviving'.[7] Brooking associated this development with the Liberal Government's desire to produce a more egalitarian society in which dentistry would not be seen as an undesirable and growing monopoly.[8] The Dunedin Board naturally deplored the Act, and promptly resigned. Responding to criticism for resigning, Scott wrote:

> I am sure I speak for all the examiners when I say that the main end towards which they directed their efforts was the establishment of a Dental School in New Zealand, so that education in dentistry might be brought up to the modern standard, and similar to what it is in Great Britain and Victoria. Until this most desirable end could be reached, they honestly did their best with the means at their disposal, to improve the standard of education in dentistry and I think a certain measure of success was achieved.
>
> The action of Parliament in establishing four examining Boards has put off indefinitely the establishment of the School and will necessarily lower the pass standard. That there should be in a small country like this four entrances to the Dental Profession is in my opinion a most harmful absurdity, and as each Board is entirely self-controlled, to practically lower the standard of entrance to what may become in time little better than a sham. We, the members of the late Board had no wish to take part in the degradation of a prestige profession.[9]

Powerful words, revealing clearly Scott's commitment to dentistry as an important health profession requiring highly educated practitioners. His support was to continue throughout his career at the Medical School.

Despite the gloom, however, 'ethical' dentists persisted in their efforts to raise the standard of the profession and the quality of training available to those seeking registration. Dentists exerting a positive influence in these times included Edwin Cox and sons Goodwin, Herbert, and Norman; H.P. Rawson, later to become the first President of the second (and present) New Zealand Dental Association; A. Hoby, LDS (Ireland); W.E. Lowe, LDS (England), DDS, who became the first Editor of the *New Zealand Dental Journal* in 1905; and its second Editor, W.H. Didsbury.

Such men, and others including Boot and T.A. (later Sir Thomas) Hunter in Dunedin; A.W. Chatfield, A.M. Carter, and J.N. Rishworth in Auckland; and F.W. Thompson in Christchurch, were prominent in agitating for a new Dentists Act that, in 1904, would set the scene for a school at the University of Otago. These men were all to become closely associated with Pickerill in major developments in dentistry.

Eventually, in the late 1890s, the Trustees of the Dunedin Hospital responded to the Board's earlier request to establish a dental department. This attracted the interest of Dunedin lawyer T.K. Sidey (later Sir Thomas), a member of the Council of the University of Otago and Member of the House of Representatives for Caversham. Sidey lobbied the Council for a dental school, and was strongly supported by Scott. Sidey's first attempt to amend the Dentists Act of 1891 was not supported by the Government but, undeterred, he introduced a private member's Bill in 1904.[10]

Enactment ensured the establishment of the Dental School, but it also gave apprentices in training until 1910 to sit their Board examinations. This long delay and subsequent extensions were to cause enormous anguish for the second New Zealand Dental Association, formed in 1905, and for Pickerill. In a paper presented to the first conference of the new Association in June 1905, A.M. Carter described the legislative history up to the time of the passing of the 1904 Act.[11] In despairing words, he foresaw the deficiencies in the Act haunting the profession for years to come:

> It is a history of the most extraordinary blundering, of steady retrogression for more than twenty years, a record of haste, carelessness and indifference to the true wants of the Dental Profession and the general public and this is a country, which according to an article by our late Governor, Lord Ranfurly is possessed of the most progressive and enlightened Government in the world.

Despite this gloom, rapid action followed the passing of the Act. Later that year, the Prime Minister approved Dunedin as the site for the Dental School and, at Sidey's urging, Dunedin dentists took the first steps in forming the second New Zealand Dental Association, the association that continues today.

The first conference of the new Association, held in Wellington in June 1905, was a momentous development in New Zealand dentistry. The discussions show that dentistry, even without a national forum, had reached a stage of advanced professional maturity.[12,13] It was vitally concerned about the state of dental health of the nation, especially of children; the education of dentists and standards of care available to the public and means to exclude from practice unqualified and incompetent operators; and how to overcome the perceived problem of 'advertising' dentists. It established a professional journal. And it was dedicated to the founding of a dental school that would fulfil aspirations to rank dentistry with medicine amongst the caring professions.

Rules related to qualifications illustrated a problem that continued for many years. Apart from the element of fraud involved by displaying bogus qualifications, certain degrees, especially some of the North American doctorates, were claimed to be not of the standard of the forthcoming New Zealand Bachelor of Dental Surgery – some could even be obtained by simply showing evidence of registration as a dentist in any country. The display of such a qualification gave the holder an unfair advantage over those who could not use the title 'Doctor'. These were to be constant problems for the Association and for Pickerill and the School.

The campaign against the continuing effort of 'unregistered men', those who were unable to gain registration under the provisions of the 1880 Act and its 1891 Amendment, was another matter that haunted the Association and Pickerill, both in his position at the School and later as Secretary of the Association, for years to come. The editorial in the second issue of the *Journal* noted with disgust that:

> these same petitioners [for registration] are *eligible* to sit the examination. But, 'wearying of good works', they now seek to throw dust in the eyes of our legislators by pleading years of experience. Experience of what? Of failure, maybe!
>
> These humble suppliants, to use their own words, 'Under the Act of 1904, *cannot rise* in their profession!' True, they cannot, by their own efforts; and now, conscious of how far they fall below the hitherto small test of ability and intelligence required of those seeking registration as dentists, with no more sense of merit than they learnt at their Sunday School treats, they pray the Government to grant a kind of consolation race in which all are to be winners![14]

The editorial in the next issue of the *Journal* reinforced this by deploring how unregistered dentists were still practising unhindered, despite the 1904 Act limiting practice only to those on the register.[15]

Before this first conference, the University had moved at great speed planning for a dental school. The Senate adopted a statute for the degree of Bachelor of Dental Surgery, and the curriculum for the degree and the Certificate of Proficiency appeared in the 1906 *Calendar* of the University of Otago.[16] The BDS curriculum was examined minutely at the conference.[17]

An important element in the debate was whether part of the course could be taken by apprenticeship with a registered dentist, or whether all training should take place at the School. There was much sympathy for the former suggestion, on the grounds that 'working men's sons must have a chance', and that spending the four years in Dunedin would impose a heavy burden. The qualification for admission as a dental student was debated, particularly whether dentistry should have the same requirements as medicine.

These matters were unresolved, and Hunter proposed that a committee should be set up to work on the syllabus – 'I do not think it would be wise for us to make up our minds hurriedly as to what is to be put before the Senate'. This was agreed, and a committee was instructed to 'formulate a syllabus' and to report to the next conference, to be held in Dunedin just six months later. The curriculum was subsequently reported back to the Council by a joint [University] Council–Association committee in January 1906,[18] and this was the curriculum in place when Pickerill arrived. A copy was sent to the British General Medical Council, which complimented the Senate on its quality, 'in some respects to be superior to the British Course'.[19] Acceptance by the General Medical Council, achieved even before the School opened, would allow registration of New Zealand graduates in Britain, a high compliment to those responsible for its design.

Meanwhile the Council of the University determined that the Dental School, including the required staff, should be ready to accept students by May 1907.[20] Building plans proceeded rapidly. An outcome of meetings of the Association and the Council was that a site had been 'recommended to be put aside' for the Dental Hospital and School,[21] and dentists promised £1,000 toward the cost of the building and equipment. Raising this amount presented some problems – the goal was reached only through a loan from Hunter – but, with the Government's grant of £1,500, building was able to start. The 1907 conference was delighted,[22] and the building was described as being:

> of seven rooms – Principal's Room, Waiting, Extraction, and Anaesthetic Rooms – a large workshop on the ground floor, lecture room and operating room upstairs. The site offers great possibility of future extension of the building. The School is built of stone, with Oamaru stone facing. The architecture is Gothic, to be in keeping with the rest of the Otago University buildings. Careful attention has been given to lighting, sanitary arrangements, etc.
>
> The Council were anxious, as it is the first building to catch the eye in the University acres, that it should be handsome and substantial.

Situated on the corner of Union and Castle streets adjacent to the Leith Stream, this dignified building, although no longer the Dental School, remains an important part of the campus, having subsequently been the home of the Registry, then the Faculty of Law, and is now the Staff Club.

In the presidential address at the 1907 conference, F.W. Thompson, stated 'the School is now in existence, and I think there is no question whatsoever that the Association is alone responsible for the fact, as we subscribed £1,000 towards it.'[23] This was going slightly too far as, although the energy, enthusiasm, and practical and financial support of the Association were all vital, the University itself had shown single-minded urgency to have this new special school up and running – at what now seems amazing speed. The University Council was no doubt driven by its desire to enhance and to confirm the reputation of the University as the nation's leading institution of higher learning, so a degree of self-interest was involved. Nevertheless, the combined forces of the profession, the University and its staff, and Sidey – the able politician and university administrator – enabled the establishment of a school highly respected internationally before it had even opened.

The search for a suitably qualified person to be its Director was a priority. A sub-committee of the Dental School Building Committee decided on 1 August 1906 that the position of Principal should now be advertised. Recommendation on the wording of the advertisement, the terms of appointment, and duties were endorsed by the full Building Committee on 19 September, and approved by the Council on 1 October.[24] The Registrar quickly arranged for advertisements to be placed in the *New Zealand Dental Journal*, the *Australian Journal of Dentistry*, and the *Commonwealth Dental Review* (Australia). Copies of the circular specifying the duties of the Director and general information also went to the Honourable W.P. Reeves, the New Zealand High Commissioner in London, and advertisements were subsequently placed in the *British Journal of Dental Science* and the *British Dental Journal*.

The advertisement that appeared in the October 1906 issue of the *New Zealand Dental Journal* was:

> SCHOOL OF DENTISTRY
>
> Applications, with testimonials, for the position of Director of the School of Dentistry will be received by the Registrar of this University not later than 31st January, 1907.
>
> Salary, £500 per annum.
>
> Duties to begin 1st May, 1907.
>
> Full particulars may be obtained from the undersigned.
>
> W.A. Mason,
>
> Registrar

The advertisement in the *British Dental Journal* of 15 December was seen by Dr H.P. Pickerill, MB, ChB, BDS, LDS who, with other aspirants for the position, quickly responded. The dream of the New Zealand Dental Association to have its own vigorous and well-led Dental School was about to be realised.

4

The call to New Zealand

By the time the University of Otago was building its Dental School and preparing to advertise for its first Director, Pickerill had completed his medical and dental studies. Although we have no clear insight into his ambitions at that point, one can imagine he was looking for an opportunity that would not only challenge his intellect, but would also be on a grand scale. His record as a scholar and his involvement in student politics suggest he would not long be content with a humble lecturer's position and part-time hospital and private dental practice. The only information found on his motivation for seeking the Otago appointment is contained in the message he prepared, shortly before his death, for the Jubilee Celebrations of the Dental School in Dunedin, which took place on 21 September 1956.

> Fifty years ago, 1906, I was a young man in England looking for a job – though I was quite unaware of the fact until I read an advertisement that a Director of a new Dental School was required at a University in New Zealand. Then I knew for certain that was what I wanted. After many enquiries and discussing the matter with our Principal, Sir Oliver Lodge, I applied, and was appointed. When saying goodbye, Lodge who was a very big man both physically and mentally, and looked like a Spanish Grandee, put his hand on my shoulder and gave me his parting advice: 'Never lumber up your mind, my boy, with a lot of facts and figures you can easily find in a book – use your brain for something better than that!'[1]

The appearance of the advertisement for the position of Director of this brand new school on the other side of the world must indeed have brought him a stunning vision. New Zealand had been promoting itself actively internationally, and especially in Britain, for many years.[2] It is likely that

Pickerill would have perceived it as an exciting, prosperous, exotic country, strongly patriotic to Britain, as shown in its enthusiastic support of the Boer War, which had ended four years earlier. Socially New Zealand was well advanced, having universal primary education, franchise for women, and a pension scheme for the destitute elderly – it was indeed the 'social laboratory of the world'.[3] The country also had an established university system and a Department of Public Health, the first of its kind anywhere. Pickerill discussed his situation with William Pember Reeves, the distinguished New Zealand Liberal politician and historian, by then New Zealand's High Commissioner in London, who would have extolled to this ambitious young man the virtues of emigrating to this 'young democratic country, still almost free from extremes of wealth and poverty, from class hatreds and fears these barriers create'.[4]

Pickerill's immediate response to the advertisement suggests this was just what he was waiting for – the opportunity to make his mark, to mould and fashion the dental profession in a young and thriving country, to pursue the research that had captured his attention as a student, and to mix in the highest circles of a university that had an established medical faculty and a growing international reputation.

According to the letter accompanying his application,[5] he saw the advertisement in the *British Dental Journal* on 18 or 19 December 1907. He would then, no doubt, have applied to the High Commission for the information about the position and for a copy of the Articles of Agreement. Allowing for the few days this would have entailed, his response was virtually instantaneous, for his application was submitted just ten days after he saw the advertisement:

Stoneleigh
Hazlewell
Birmingham
28: xii: 06

The Registrar
University of Otago
Dear Sir,

Enclosed you will find my application for the Post of Director of the School of Dentistry in the University of Otago.

I am much afraid that you will not receive this until after the prescribed time, but I sincerely trust that you will be able to accept it & place it before the Council. The Advertisement did not appear in the British Dental Journal until that number published on the 15th of this month – I received my copy on the 18th or 19th. I at once applied to the High Commissioner, but it was Sunday

22nd before I recd. my reply. It was the 28th before I'd got my Testimonials and papers in order. The delays and loss of time being due to the Christmas Season – people whom I wished to consult being out of town & and the post very late.

I had sent very few Testimonials because I think my qualifications & position here speak for themselves.

Shld. the Council honour me with the appointment, might I ask you to cable me at once (at my expense if necessary)? I shall require as long a time as possible to clear up my affairs here. Apologising for any trouble this may give you.

I am
Faithfully Yours
H. Percy Pickerill

The completed application form confirms he had the degrees of Bachelor of Medicine, Bachelor of Surgery, and Bachelor of Dental Surgery, and was a Licentiate in Dental Surgery of the Royal College of Surgeons of England; that he was aged twenty-eight, was married, and had no family at the time. He was 'engaged in Dental practice in Birmingham & on the Staff of the University & Dental Hospital'. To the section requiring information on 'Where has your knowledge and experience in Dentistry been gained?' he wrote:

1. In the workroom of Mr A.G. Levason L.D.S. (one of the best mechanical practices in the country)
2. At the Dental Hospital
3. In the University
4. In the Dental Dept. of the General Hospital
5. In Private Practice.

A 'Memorandum in Support of Application' expands on this information, and provides a background to his professional experience to this point:

I desire to bring the following facts to notice bearing on my suitability and qualifications for the post of Director of the School of Dentistry:–

I received my scientific training in the Universities of Oxford and Birmingham. Mechanical Dentistry I learnt originally with Mr. A.G. Levason of Hereford – a very old established practice – doing mostly gold tubes and spring work, and was for some time his senior mechanical assistant. I have since acquired familiarity with more modern mechanical methods, such as Bridge crown and porcelain work in the practice of Mr. Breward Neale, Birmingham, at the Dental Hospital and in my own practice. I am considered a good mechanic and in fact have a strong liking for that branch of our work.

During my student days I was awarded the following:–

1. Senior prize and certificate of Operative work.

2. Silver medal for Anaesthetic work.

3. The Ash Prize for the best Treatise on 'The care of Children's Teeth'.

4. A special Prize for a Paper read before the University Students' Society on 'The Effects of Civilization on the Teeth'.

In 1904 the Undergraduates of Birmingham University elected me as their President.

I now hold the degrees of M.B., Ch.B. and B.D.S. of Birmingham University, and the L.D.S. Eng., and was the first man to hold a British Degree in Dentistry cum curriculo.

I am on the Staff of the Dental Hospital – one of the finest and best equipped in the Kingdom.

I am Lecturer on Dental Pathology and Histology in the University of Birmingham, and a direct representative of the Students on the Court of Governors.

I am a member of the Council of the Central Counties Branch of the British Dental Association and Hon. Sec. of the Law & Ethics Committee.

It will thus be seen that my time is fully occupied, but for the work I like best – that of teaching and research – the exigencies of modern Dental Practice leave very little time, and it is in order that I may devote myself wholly to this work that I seek the honour of being appointed to the post of Director of your School of Dentistry. Should you honour me, the duties of the position will be fulfilled with the utmost of zeal, energy, and ability at my command.

H.P. Pickerill

Sir Oliver Lodge, Principal of the University of Birmingham, and Professor Gilbert Barling, Dean of the Faculty of Medicine, were his main referees, and he also named Howard Mummery, MRCS, LDS, Sir Victor Horsley, and Sir James Sawyer, MD, as persons 'to whom you would wish to refer, but whom you have not asked for Testimonials'. Sir Oliver Lodge wrote:

I have the highest opinion of Mr. H. Percy Pickerill, recently a student and now a graduate, both in Medicine and Dentistry, of this University.

While a student he achieved the position of President of the Undergraduates' Guild, always a testimony to force of character and personal influence.

In that position he came into contact with the Chancellor and other dignitories [sic] of the University, and took a leading part in important meetings, invariably conducting himself with dignity and effectiveness.

I should judge that for such a post as Director of a School of Dentistry, Mr. Pickerill is rather pre-eminently qualified.

He is now in practice in this City, and is our Lecturer on Dental Histology and Pathology, and I know that he is well thought of in the Profession.

I desire to speak highly of him as a man.

Oliver Lodge.

Professor Barling also gave high recommendation:

Dr. H.P. Pickerill tells me that he is applying for the post of Director of the School of Dentistry in the University of Otago, and I should like strongly to recommend him to the Election Committee. I have known Dr. Pickerill for some years and can testify to his marked ability as a student, to his capacity for work, his conscientious discharge of his duties and to his high personal character.

I believe Dr. Pickerill has good ability as a teacher and investigator, the qualities which should be of advantage in the post he now seeks.

Gilbert Barling

John Humphreys, MDS, FLS, LDS, Lecturer in Dental Anatomy and Honorary Secretary of the Dental Department of the University, and presumably a former teacher stated:

Mr. Pickerill's career as a student was a brilliant success, and the characteristics he then displayed mark him out as an acceptable colleague. I cannot speak too highly of his qualifications and personality.

Pickerill was not the only person to show interest. The High Commissioner's office informed the Council that twenty-seven applications had been made for the prospectus,[6] and that five candidates had told him they had sent applications. Reeves asked the Council to defer consideration of the appointment until after the arrival of the San Francisco mail, due on 7 February.[7] Later Council records indicate that eight applications were received.

The University Council met in Sidey's office on 19 February to consider the applications,[8] and resolved unanimously that H. Percy Pickerill be appointed for a term of five years at £500 per annum. The resolution was arrived at after hearing the views of the dentists present – Hunter, Swindley, Hay, Armstrong, Glendining, and Davies – and after consultation with Scott, Dean of the Medical School.

Receipt of the Pickerill application and testimonials would have caused considerable excitement amongst the dentists, fulfilling their highest hopes. They had attracted an outstanding candidate – qualified in both medicine and dentistry, and therefore very likely to be readily accepted within the Medical Faculty; a man with a strong academic record, and the first man in Britain to qualify in dentistry with a full university degree; furthermore, he had some experience in university administration through his role in student affairs and on the Council of Governors; and, importantly, he was part of the professional establishment through his roles in the Central Counties Branch of the British Dental Association. His emphasis on teaching and research as 'the work I love best' would have been a great attraction.

He was informed of the success of his application through the office of the High Commissioner,[9] subject to his providing a satisfactory certificate of health for himself and for his family. He also had to agree to the conditions given in the advertisement, which were blunt and gave no room for negotiation. The successful applicant was allowed 'the sum of Seventy-three pounds ten shillings towards the cost of his passage to Dunedin aforesaid' – no mention of family – and would need to be in Dunedin before 1 May. To fulfil this latter condition, he would have to leave for New Zealand by steamer from London on 7 March. The speed of all this was remarkable and unreasonable – the meeting of the Council took place on 19 February, the acceptance letter from the High Commissioner in England bore the same date, and the confirmation letter from the Registrar, dated 27 February, expected that Pickerill would have 'started for New Zealand long before this letter reaches England'.[10] The assumption that the newly appointed Director would be ready to sail just over three weeks from receiving word of his appointment was surely impossible, and so it proved.

The appointment was announced in the *Otago Daily Times* on 20 February[11] – the Council must have been confident its chosen one would indeed accept the offer. Brief details of Pickerill's experience and qualifications and comments on the testimonials were given – 'The successful applicant's testimonials are of an exceedingly flattering description as to his qualifications and personality …' – and included an extract from that of Sir Oliver Lodge.

Pickerill replied to the letter from Mr Walter Kennaway of the High Commissioner's office pointing out that it was impossible to leave on 7 March: he was under a three-month agreement with the man with whom he was in practice, he was in the middle of a course at the University, and had promised to finish the term that ended on 25 March. He had also ascertained from shipping agents prior to applying for the post that he could reach Dunedin in a little over thirty days by the 'A and A' route, which seems to have involved train travel across the United States. If this was not acceptable to the University, Pickerill could not take up the position.[12] The office replied that the mail service between San Francisco was then in an unsettled state and that it would be unlikely there would be a steamer which would allow him to arrive in New Zealand in early May. He was asked to provide the earliest date that he could leave England so as to get him to Dunedin as near as possible to 3 May, the date named in the agreement. Kennaway informed the Registrar that the appointee found it difficult to leave in time to reach Dunedin by 3 May, and that the High Commissioner would be asking for an extension of the date.[13]

A further delay resulted from the illness of Mabel Pickerill, who was expecting their first child. These delays obviously annoyed the University Council, to the extent of debating whether to proceed with the appointment.[14] The Registrar reported to the High Commissioner that the Council had a 'lengthy discussion' at a special meeting, but decided to accept the delay. 'The Council were more inclined to act in this way, because you said in your cable that Dr. Pickerill appeared specially qualified'. Pickerill had certainly impressed the High Commission's staff, and he emerged the victor in this first confrontation with the University authorities.

Pickerill was just twenty-eight at the time of the appointment. It was less than three years since he had qualified in dentistry, and less than two since he had received his medical qualification. He had one published paper.[15] He was thus very young and very inexperienced to be appointed to a position of such responsibility, but other senior appointments had previously gone to relatively young men.[16] For example, John Mainwaring Brown (in English Language and Literature, Political Economy and Constitutional History) and Thomas Jeffrey Parker (in Biology), were both appointed to chairs while in their late twenties, and John Malcolm was thirty-one when appointed to the Chair in Physiology in 1905. Noteworthy also is that a later Dean of the Faculty of Dentistry, Sir John Walsh, was only thirty-four when appointed in 1946.

The University and the New Zealand Dental Association had made their collective decision, and Percy and Mabel Pickerill, with their infant son, John Percival, sailed on 27 July 1907 for their new life in New Zealand.[17]

5

New country, new opportunities

The family arrived in Dunedin on Saturday 14 September 1907, and Pickerill commenced duties as Director of the Dental School on the following Monday.[1] His reaction to his new country, and some of the ideas and themes that would influence his career, appeared in the following month's *New Zealand Dental Journal*:

> First Impressions on Arrival in New Zealand.
>
> Impressions, of whatever kind, are usually damp at first, and 'first' impressions are usually unfavourable, mine certainly were – for the first few days. This, however, was solely due to the meteorological conditions. I began to think that we had come to cold, dreary, inhospitable regions, and undoubtedly should have retained that impression but for the unbounded kindness and hospitality on the part of the inhabitants, and of these, chiefly the dental section of the community.
>
> Firstly, allow me to congratulate the N.Z.D.A. on the possession of so enthusiastic an editor of their journal. Dr. Lowe evidently scented 'copy' from afar, and before the good ship Corinthic had fairly got into port was aboard seeking to entrap the unfortunate writer of these notes.
>
> Such enthusiasm was somewhat overwhelming, and I fear at first met with but a cold refusal, but like a wise editor, he made me his debtor, and I am trying to discharge it, for which, the members of the N.Z.D.A. will not thank me.
>
> One of the first things to impress me was the strong sympathy shown towards dental reform by many members of the House of Representatives. I owe it to the kindness of Mr. Allen, our Vice-Chancellor, and Mr Sidey that I was able to judge of this for myself. I was fortunate, too, in getting a talk with the Minister of Education, in whom I am sure we have a strong supporter, and who will do all in his power to help forward any matters concerning the Dental School, or

the welfare of the profession as a whole. These impressed me as the sort of friends we desire, whose friendship we should both value and endeavour to retain.

A thing which struck me – sometimes rather forcibly – was the great number of dentists at present in practice, at any rate in the larger towns, so that I feared that my office would to some extent be a 'sinecure'. But this, on the other hand, was contradicted by what I observed to be the condition of the teeth of the people one met in the street and elsewhere. Nine out of ten people appeared to have most glaring dental defects, and sometimes as glaringly remedied.

I, in my innocence, had confounded New Zealand with Utopia, and was much astonished to see so many blatant advertisements, and moreover with, what to us in the Old Country is sacred, the name of Dentist attached thereto.

I had fondly imagined that the recent dental legislation had swept away all such unsightly objects. Why it did not I have yet to learn.

As regards the Dental School, I am sure it has great possibilities. The only thing which surprised me, on hearing the numbers which had entered the profession annually of late, was that the school was not established some years ago.

The building is very satisfactory, and will be quite sufficient, when thoroughly equipped for present purposes. But I think that if the school develops as I hope it will, there will be need for extension in the future.

It appears to me a most excellent arrangement having the whole school – clinical and academical – directly under the control of the University, thus simplifying the training of students and at the same time making it more efficient. What we now require is more students. There are three classes at present for whom the school provides. Firstly, those entering the dental profession and who wish to take the B.D.S. degree; secondly, those who are taking the Board examination, and wish for a short course of surgical practice before entering; and thirdly, those who have already passed the Board examination, but who wish to make themselves more proficient in any particular branch of dental surgery before launching out into practice. And when these three classes of men realise the benefits which a Hospital and University training can confer upon them I am sure they will not be loth [sic] to take advantage of it.

In conclusion, allow me to thank, on behalf of my wife and myself, those members of the Wellington and Dunedin branches of the N.Z.D.A. who so kindly met and entertained us on our arrival in this Dominion.[2]

Pickerill's view of the political scene was no doubt coloured by his friendly reception on arrival. This perception was not maintained, for he was soon to become disillusioned by inadequately educated and trained persons continuing to be admitted to the Board examinations. He had quickly assessed the general state of oral health of the nation, and observed the unsatisfactory outcome of much of the treatment being provided. He was shocked at the extent of advertising by dentists. Indeed, he did have a 'lot to learn' about the complexities of the 'ethical' versus 'advertising' situation, and he soon became involved in the battles that occurred. The School impressed him and, although hoping for more students, he was optimistic in what it was trying to achieve through its Bachelor of Dental Surgery curriculum, its courses for those preparing for admission to the Board examinations, and its provision of refresher courses for practising dentists.

Further first impressions were conveyed in his message to the Jubilee Celebrations of the Dental School in 1956, read posthumously by his son, Paul Pickerill:

> When I took my seat for the first time at a professorial board meeting in 1907 I found myself among the great ones, and I felt very humble for they were *the founding fathers of Otago University*. Grey headed, grey bearded men, men with names still honoured and revered. Sale, classics; Shand, physics; Black, chemistry; Scott, anatomy; Gilray, English; Salmond, mental philosophy. All appointed in the 1870's and highly qualified. M.A., M.D., L.L.D., D.Sc., were usual. They had laid their foundations well and truly and had also been responsible for the drawing up of the Dental Curriculum (especially Dr. Scott). They were powerful and might easily have blocked it as I later witnessed them do with other proposed courses, but being men of good vision they fostered it. We owe them much.
>
> I still feel greatly honoured to have had the privilege of working with them. I felt then though constrained to apologise for my lack of years and experience in their deliberations but Dr. Shand interjected 'Dr Pickerill has no need to apologise for his youth, that is a matter which is only too easily remedied'![3]

The family initially lived in Cumberland Street, but no information is available on how long they stayed there, or in other homes, before they moved to a new home in Ravensbourne – described in a magazine article as a beautiful Tudor-style home overlooking the Dunedin Harbour.[4] The article states it was built in 1922 and the original owner was 'Professor Henry Pickerill, first dean of the Otago School of Dentistry. He lived there with his family for 20 years'. The latter statement is only partially correct – Pickerill left Dunedin in 1927, but Mrs Pickerill and the children stayed in the house for some years after his departure.

John Percival had been born before they left England. Their three other children were born in Dunedin – Thomas Peverel Tuakana in 1909, Kathleen Marguerite in 1910, and Ethelbert Paul (known as Paul) in 1912. Mrs Margaret Frazer, Pickerill's only daughter of his second marriage, described him to the author as 'Although of average height he was very skinny and weighed about 10 stone, but he was very vigorous. He had very blue twinkling eyes and light brown hair'.

The Council must have been happy with its choice of Director, for not long after arrival Pickerill was appointed Professor of Dentistry and Chairman of the newly created Faculty of Dentistry,[5] events greeted with enthusiasm by the anonymous writer of a report in the *Journal*. A contemporary, although in some aspects a somewhat over-optimistic review of developments since the School opened just six months earlier, conveys the pride of the Association in the School and its Director:

> A Chair of Dentistry Established
>
> Professor H. Percy Pickerill. – Progress at the Dental School and Hospital.
>
> The coping stone has been at last added to the work commenced so modestly by those who undertook the labours connected with the Dental School and Hospital scheme. The scheme began to take definitive form at the first Conference of the N.Z.D.A., held at Wellington in June 1905, and now, after a lapse of 30 months, not only has the scheme assumed the material form of stone and mortar; but the Director in charge of the School and Hospital has been raised to the dignity of Professor; New Zealand can boast a chair of Dentistry; the N.Z.D.A. representation on the Professorial Board of the Otago University, and we trust that within the near future we shall have a Dental Faculty! 'Hitch your waggon to a star' was advice given when the scheme was passing through its birth pangs, but not even the most sanguine believed that so early would the present lofty position be realised.
>
> The Dental Hospital is, we are pleased to hear, progressing satisfactorily. One of the best signs of progress being that it has been found necessary to order more operating chairs from Home. Those at present at the Hospital, together with one which has been borrowed locally, are in constant and continuous use every morning. This being so, it is unnecessary to add that the number of patients attending the Hospital is also on the increase. Just two hundred operations of various kinds have been performed during the past month, and it is satisfactory that the great majority of these have been in connection with conservative work of some kind, simple extractions being very few indeed, and anaesthetic cases only about twenty-five. The mechanical department has now made a beginning, and several cases have been supplied to patients at a charge which just covers the actual working expenses.
>
> As regards the class of patient which present themselves for treatment, they may be said to be drawn from all sorts and conditions of men, women, and children – from inmates of orphanages, benevolent institutions, and Chinese, to the somewhat elaborately dressed 'mater familias', who brings her little girl along, because the institution happens to be 'handy', and she has heard 'just as good as any other dentists,' and also (what she does not mention) considerably cheaper. Of course, this class of patient is always informed that the Hospital does not exist for people in her position (much surprise on the lady's part). She is given a form to be filled in by a clergyman, doctor, or member of the N.Z.D.A., and as she naturally fails, or does not try to obtain the necessary signature, she

> does not re-appear at the Dental Hospital. In fact, a careful watch is kept [so] that the evil known as 'Hospital abuse' should be absolutely excluded, or kept at an absolute minimum, for in a few cases it is always impossible to prevent some unscrupulous persons, who wish to get something for nothing, from persuading some benevolent clergyman or member of the medical profession that they are indeed unable to pay an ordinary dentist's fees.
>
> The majority of patients, however, at present, are children, and in many cases it is with difficulty that the low hospital fees are extracted from their unwilling parents.
>
> The students at present are all under the 'Board regulations,' but it is hoped that next session, after the results of the medical preliminary examinations are published, there will be several students for the full degree course.[6]

What Pickerill thought about the implication that he was now the 'representative' of the Association on the Professorial Board is not recorded; one suspects, however, that he saw his responsibility to the University, to the oral health of the public, and to the profession as a whole rather than specifically to the Association. He was now secure in his position – at the age of just twenty-nine possibly the first Professor of Dentistry in the Empire, and Chairman of what was almost certainly the first dental faculty.[7] He was poised to exert enormous influence on the direction of New Zealand dentistry.

6
The Dental School develops

When Pickerill arrived in Dunedin in September 1907, dental education in Australasia was advancing rapidly; the University of Otago was the third in the region to establish a degree in dentistry. The Australian College of Dentistry had been founded in Melbourne in 1897,[1] and in 1902 the Dental Board of Victoria registered thirteen candidates who had qualified with the Licentiate of Dental Surgery. The College was affiliated with the University of Melbourne in 1904, and the Bachelor of Dental Surgery (later the Bachelor of Dental Science) was first offered that year. The College opened a new building in 1907. The 1901 Dental Act, the first such legislation in New South Wales, recognised for registration any qualification in dentistry of the University of Sydney, and this stimulated the University to form a Department of Dental Studies within the Faculty of Medicine.[2] The University Dental Hospital was established in 1901, and seventeen students were admitted to study for the Licence in Dentistry. The first candidates for the Bachelor of Dental Surgery were admitted in 1906. The Faculty of Dentistry was established in 1920.

Before Pickerill arrived in Dunedin, the School and Hospital had already opened its doors to the public for treatment and to students for education, under the direction of O.V. Davies, who was a member of the first group to obtain the Licentiate of Dental Surgery at Melbourne.[3] Davies was for many years a prominent figure in New Zealand dentistry – he was in the forefront of the efforts to establish the School, was twice its Acting Director, and was a member of the staff for thirteen years, from the School's foundation in 1907 until 1920. He served the New Zealand Dental Association with great distinction in many ways, within its Otago Branch and nationally as a member of the Executive Council and as President in 1922–3.[4]

Pickerill and Davies were both strong personalities, prepared to defend their convictions vigorously. Clashes were inevitable, but there were no overt indications of these when Pickerill arrived to take over the School. But curiously, in his 'first impressions',[5] he failed to acknowledge the pioneering work of Davies and other staff in getting the School up and running. He thanked the members of the Wellington and Dunedin branches of the Association who 'kindly met and entertained us on our arrival …', but failed to mention the School's staff, and those who, with enormous effort, had brought the School and Hospital into being from a base of virtually nothing.

The formal opening ceremony, in April 1908, was a major event in Dunedin.[6] In attendance were the Prime Minister, the Right Honourable Sir Joseph Ward; the Minister of Education, the Honourable George Fowlds, who declared the School open; T.K. Sidey, MP; and a large number of civic and university dignitaries. The Vice-Chancellor, James Allen, MP, presided. Although Pickerill again failed to mention those who had worked so hard to see the School become a reality, other speakers did so lavishly. The Prime Minister 'congratulated the dentists on their co-operation with Mr Sidey, in the first instance, and with the Government in showing the way in New Zealand for the erection of a Dental School which was not only a credit to Dunedin, but would be of great value to the present generation and those who were to follow'. He described Mr Sidey as having 'almost given him toothache with the persistency and earnestness with which he hammered at his subject. Finally, he thought, in order that they might be relieved entirely from toothache the Bill was taken up by the Government and put through the House for the good of the country as a whole'.

The Prime Minister also touched upon a question that continued to vex the Association over many years – the recognition of the American qualification:

> He hoped that under Dr. Pickerill's able guidance and tuition they would be able to prevent the number of students going away to America and coming back with a three-year diploma. That was one of the things he wanted to see prevented. When he was Minister of Public Health, he heard more about the human anatomy than he had thought it possible that a Minister of the Crown could have impressed upon him, and it had been amply demonstrated by the dentists that they were desirous of having the qualifications of those practising as high as possible.

In addition to concern about the discrepancy in the length of training required to gain various qualifications that constituted the American Doctor of Dental Surgery degree, there was a perception that it conferred advantages to its holders by reason of the title it bestowed. This was the cause of much unease until the 1980s, when the Association accepted the urging of many of its members and sanctioned the adoption of the courtesy title of Doctor for all dentists, regardless of their basic qualification.

All speakers were optimistic for the future of the school under the distinguished leadership of its Director, although the Prime Minister dispelled possible doubts about having sent to the 'Old Country' for a professional expert: 'in Dr Pickerill they had discovered a most excellent man – an enthusiast, and qualified to carry on the important work for which the school was instituted'.

The Minister of Education acknowledged the dentists' contribution of £1,000 to the cost of the School, and noted that the Government subsidy had been £1,500. He believed the cost of carrying it on would be about £800 a year, and of this, £500 was assured – the rest to come from fees charged to patients.

The Vice-Chancellor also acknowledged the contributions of the dentists toward the cost of the building, stating that the University 'owed the institution and the alteration in the legislation very largely to the dentists themselves. The dentists of New Zealand put their hands in their pockets and subscribed £1,000 for the erection of the building. Not only that, but some 10 or 11 of the dentists of Dunedin were on the honorary staff and without pay or emolument gave their services ...'. He also challenged the Government by noting the research scholarships that had been created, stressing the need for the government to go further and make 'provision whereby those desiring to go in for them might have access to libraries fully equipped in all subjects necessary for research work'. It is a tribute to the University that, even at this fledgling stage in the development of its Dental School, it placed emphasis on the need for research in a fully functioning department.

Sidey covered a wide range of issues in an eloquent speech. He began by noting that whereas the number of dentists registered had increased by 40 per cent since 1904, when the new Dentists Act had come into operation, the number on the Medical Register had increased by less than 5 per cent, suggesting that gaining recognition in dentistry was far too easy, and that the University qualification was a necessity if standards were to be raised. Dentistry needed to follow the path of medicine by substituting education in properly equipped schools for education by apprenticeship, 'and as the system of free university education extended, so would the doors to the dental and other professions be opened, not to those who had the means, but to those who had the ability to qualify for them'.

Sidey went on to pay tribute to the previous Prime Minister, the Right Honourable Richard Seddon, for advocacy of the Bill that brought the School, and incidentally the Association, into existence; he acknowledged the contributions of his parliamentary colleagues, and had a special word about local dentists Hunter, Armstrong, and Hay.

Frank Armstrong, speaking on behalf of the Association in the absence of the President, compared unfavourably the Government's contribution to the foundation of the School with the £5,000 granted to establish the Mining School. 'This Dental School was not only a philanthropic work, but it was also necessary for the protection of the public. Five thousand pounds had been granted to train mining specialists, not for New Zealand, but for the world. Their locally-trained dentists would practise on the New Zealand public'. He appealed for a higher standard of facilities and equipment: 'this institution should immediately be provided with a pathological and bacteriological laboratory, electricity, a water supply to the chairs, extra chairs …', and for 'reasonable facilities' to 'encourage the 12 honorary dentists to give their services morning after morning, the two honorary anaesthetists, the honorary consulting physician and the honorary consulting surgeon …'. He then appealed for a further £2,000. 'The Government had made a good start, and the dentists hoped today the light had so shone before Ministers and members of Parliament that they had seen the good work and would grant the needed £2,000' – to this the audience responded with prolonged applause.

His appeal for better equipment echoed Pickerill's own remarks made earlier in the proceedings. Pickerill forcefully presented his concerns about the School and also gave what the report headlined as a 'grave warning' about the state of oral health of the nation:

> [Dr Pickerill] said they intended to do their utmost to make the school in every way equal to the institutions in England or America. This school might be said to have a double function, so that it would provide training for dental students, and also be a philanthropical means of charitably relieving pain and suffering.
>
> First, as to its academic progress and prospects, he would say that since it made a commencement in July they had had 10 students, the majority of whom had been qualified men. Under the old regulations a man might be regarded as 'qualified' and yet have had but little experience. These courses had already proved of obvious benefit both to the University and to the public. They now had three degree students, and anticipated three more on May 1.
>
> As to the financial aspect, there was the probability of the school, if thoroughly well equipped, being quite self-supporting; but he would point out that unless it was thoroughly equipped men would go elsewhere. There was a real danger and one to be obviated if possible, by keeping the equipment of the school

> thoroughly up-to-date in every particular … That the school had so many patients on the books at a time would seem to show that it was unable to cope with the work owing to the small number of students. This, however, was not the case. The number of patients on the books was due to the state of the people's teeth. He had been prepared for something bad, but the condition of the people's teeth here was simply appalling. It had been stated on the best authority that more physical deterioration was caused by defective teeth than by alcohol, and if the loss to the community by dental disease could be estimated the result would be alarming.
>
> It was the duty of the State to replace ignorance with knowledge. In the case of backward school children their brains were often, owing to defective teeth and the attendant ills, too ill-nourished to be able to respond to the demand made upon them, and the children, owing to the pain caused by their teeth, were often unable to pay attention to their studies. A great deal had been done in the elimination of tuberculosis, fever, and alcoholism. Dental disease was just as dangerous, and next to nothing had been done. It was treated with a deadly apathy that almost amounted to fatalism. They had a society for the preservation of the health of women and children, and its object was a worthy one indeed, and deserving the whole-hearted support of every dentist. The seed thus sown was good, but unless the conditions were altered, it stood a chance of never being allowed to mature. While children ranging from 12 months to 12 years of age were improperly fed, so would the development of their teeth and jaws be prevented. The remedy was a simple one, but it seemed hopeless to cope with it by surgical or remedial measures. Their only rational hope lay in rousing the rising generation to the danger which threatened, and by putting into its hands a weapon that would at least make the fight an equal one.

Pickerill thus laid down the dual challenge – he wanted a school fully furnished with state-of-the art equipment, and he wanted national action on the dreadful state of oral health. The former plea would subsequently be echoed by his successor Deans of Dentistry, and the latter, to be a major focus of his research, was an inspired call for the integration of oral health with other developments in health and education occurring in these early years of the twentieth century. He proclaimed that the surgical approach of fillings and extractions was not the answer. Solutions were to be found in the promotion of health on a broad scale, realising that poor oral health was associated with and contributed to poor diet and nutrition, and with inadequate child-care practices and hygiene. To this end, he commended dentists to support the Society for the Promotion of Health of Women and Children (known as the Plunket Society) recently formed in Dunedin.

The official opening was thus a grand occasion that brought Pickerill universal praise: the School was hailed as the beacon of hope for the future of dentistry, its problems were brought sharply into the focus of the decision-makers, and all who contributed to its foundation were fully acknowledged. The editorial in the next issue of the *Journal* enthusiastically took up the themes of the speeches at the Opening Ceremony. Pickerill received high praise:

> The Dental School of New Zealand is destined to grow into large proportions, and it is absolutely necessary that the man who directs its growth should possess the excellent academic qualities that Dr. Pickerill does – both academic and personal. Therefore dentists throughout the Dominion who generously subscribed to the founding of the school have nothing to fear about the future welfare of it while the present professor has it under his care.

The Editor continued by describing a circular, sent by Pickerill to all members of Parliament, which pleaded for additional funding:

> it points out the necessity of the Government making a grant to carry out, satisfactorily, many important branches of dental education. Urgent reasons are given. They are as follows:–
>
> 1. Owing to inefficient apparatus and instruments, work for patients is slow and tedious … This means that we cannot overtake the amount of work which comes in, and are hindered from doing as much good for the community as we might.
>
> 2. From a teaching point of view, *no* proper demonstration of various methods and operations is at present *possible* by the staff owing to there being *no* instruments for their use.
>
> 3. Owing to there being no laboratory attached to the school, it is impossible to make any accurate diagnosis of cases which present themselves frequently. To quote from recent cases: Is a small ulcer caused by the teeth a simple one or a *cancer?* It turned out to be the latter. Is an abscess connected with the teeth simple or *tubercular?* It turned out, on examination, to be simple, although exceedingly like the latter. Is a swelling on the jaw due to the teeth simply or to *actinomycosis?* The latter proved to be correct. Such cases at present have to be sent elsewhere for diagnosis. The student is not taught to diagnose it himself, and much valuable time is lost, which may mean life or death to the patient; it meant the latter for the patient quoted first above. Besides, students are at present passing through their course for the B.D.S. without cutting one section of a tooth and examining it under the microscope, and thus have no accurate *knowledge* of the structure even of a tooth. Such a thing reduces dental education to a farce. [*emphasis in original*]

The editorial concluded with a modest appeal to the profession for support for the School and, more forcefully, a plea to the Government to 'come forward with the necessary grant'.[7]

At the time of the opening ceremony, most of the School's ten students who had enrolled since it opened in July 1907 were already qualified to practise – that is, they had been apprenticed to dentists and had passed the Board examinations. They were classified as 'postgraduate' students and were at the School for periods of not less than six months to gain supervised experience. The School also had three BDS degree students, and three more were expected in May 1908. A year later there were eight degree and three postgraduate students.[8] This is not exactly a spectacular start, but perhaps it was all that could be expected for a pathway of training that was not only substantially different from what had been previously available, but also was of much greater intellectual challenge.

The response to the demands of Pickerill and others for additional funding was positive; the Government's 'generous grant' of £2,100 fell considerably short of the £5,000 called for, but was a substantial sum nevertheless.[9] The *Journal* item announcing this increased funding also commented on the hope that the New Zealand University Statutes 'will be so modified as to make them at least workable and understandable for all'. This call was well justified, for the situation was very confusing. The Regulations and options for students were published in an illustrated pamphlet dated 1908.[10] The honorary staff listed were Dr Colquhoun (Consulting Physician), Dr Barnett (Consulting Surgeon), and Anaesthetists Drs Fitchett and Moore. The honorary dental surgeons were the cream of Dunedin dentists, all in the forefront of the profession locally and nationally at various times – T.A. Hunter; F. Armstrong; C.W. Hay; W.A. Thomson; F. Throp, LDS(Eng); H.D. Brewer; J. Glendining; H. Ziele, DDS(Penn); O.V. Davies, LDS (Victoria); H. Dodgshun; and A.J. Chrystall.

Then follows the 'Regulations for the B.D.S. Degree' and an attempt to clarify the options for students. These pathways depended on whether the whole course was to be taken at the School or whether some of it would be based on experience as an apprentice to a dentist, how much mechanical work (making dentures) had been completed during the apprenticeship, and whether the Intermediate Examination in physics, chemistry, and dental anatomy had already been gained before the student came to Dunedin. In three options, the University was allowing for the varied educational experience of potential students and facilitating enrolment by students in distant parts of the country, but administration of such a complicated structure must have been very difficult. Confusion about training in dentistry persisted for a number of years, and may well have contributed to the enrolment of students in the early days of the School being little more than a trickle.

Adding to this chaotic situation was the course for the Certificate of

Proficiency (COP), described as being identical to the BDS course, except that the candidates did not need to 'matriculate' as students in the University. They were required to pass only the Preliminary Medical Examination, based on secondary school knowledge, and the Intermediate Examinations in physics and chemistry were set at the level required for matriculation, not at the standard expected after courses at the University Colleges. Despite the COP being in the syllabus, regulations were not introduced until 1918.[11]

The 'Post Graduade' [*sic*] courses, for 'the benefit of men who have passed the Dental Board Examination, but require further instruction and practice in Operative Dentistry', occupied mornings only, freeing the students to 'take posts as assistants with dentists in the town, if so desired'. This course was a step to competence and did not lead to a formal qualification. The requirement that 'Students are required on entry, to sign an agreement that they will in no wise use the fact of having taken a course at this School, as an advertisement when afterwards in practice' reflected the disdain felt by the 'ethical' dentists for those continuing to advertise. The brochure also noted 'The University of New Zealand is empowered to grant degrees of Master and Doctor of Dental Surgery to holders of the B.D.S. degree, but the regulations for these degrees are not yet formulated'. The estimated cost of the course leading to the BDS degree, if the full course were to be taken at the University of Otago, was £184.17s.0d.

Concurrent with his efforts in developing facilities at the School, Pickerill developed his thoughts on the whole field of education in dentistry. His important paper, 'Matters affecting dental education in New Zealand', was read on his behalf at the Wellington Conference in January 1909.[12] It began with the expectation that:

> The entrance to the Dental Profession should in a year or so be somewhat approaching the ideal. There will be a 'one portal' system, a thing very much desired in other countries … and it is to be hoped that having attained that system, the Dental profession will remain solid in the years to come, and maintain it at all costs …
>
> In Great Britain there are half a dozen different portals, all differing in character and standard. In America the means of entry are much more multiplied, and vary from the degree of a reputable University like Pennsylvania to the 'Degree' by post system. Such things not only mislead the public to a serious degree, but are exceedingly mischievous and dangerous to the Dental profession. They tend to destroy the solidarity of interest which is vital to the life and progress of the Dental Profession … the portal here will be no mean one; the standard which the N.Z. University has set is a good one. The Degree of B.D.S. will be placed perhaps somewhere between the English L.D.S and the B.D.S. of English Universities, which is exactly where it should be.

The latter statement is surprising – the suggestion that the New Zealand BDS should be something lower in standard than his own Birmingham BDS degree seems out of character for such a perfectionist. He was certainly over-optimistic in his assessment that there would soon be a 'one-portal' means of entry to the profession – through the university system and the BDS degree. This optimism was, however, widely shared – the Wellington Dental Board announced in 1909 that it would hold its 'last two Examinations on 8 September and 15 December'; the last Ordinary Examination by the Dunedin Board would be on 2 October, and it would hold a December Special Examination for those who had previously failed the examination.[13] Pickerill, now Editor of the *Journal*, applauded the demise of the Boards, noting that they had 'worked amicably with the University authorities, and did everything to facilitate the transference of their powers to the Senate…'. He contrasted this with the situation in New South Wales, where the Board seemed to work in opposition to the University.[14] R. Cape-Williamson, a prominent Christchurch dentist, expressed his delight at the Boards' demise in a letter to the Editor: 'It must be with a huge sigh of relief that the dental profession of N.Z. read that the examinations under the old Dental Boards were done with'. He deplored the incompetence of those going through that system, and condemned the

> latest doings of the Boards. It had long been a foregone conclusion that all the ragtag and bobtail of dentistry would be present at the last scene and would be pushed through. Time has proved the prophecy to be correct. From indisputable knowledge, I know that certain of the last candidates were absolutely incompetent to pass any test set for them.[15]

Pickerill added an editorial comment – 'Since every dental student now has to take the B.D.S. degree before being registered, "similar discrepancies in the future" are impossible'. Alas, another portal did remain open for many years – the 'Back Door', the term used by Pickerill in his October 1910 editorial to describe the efforts of certain dental mechanics to gain registration as dentists. Unfortunately this portal was to continue through the 1920s, causing immense frustration to Pickerill as Dean, to the New Zealand Dental Association, and to concerned Parliamentarians such as Sidey.

Pickerill continued his paper on dental education by commenting on the upgrade of equipment and the employment of a dental mechanic. He spoke highly of the 'enthusiastic and exceptionally able' honorary staff responsible for teaching in clinical dentistry. He reported that the School had seven degree students, and more would be enrolling in the near future. He then moved on to the serious issues of ethics and discipline within the profession.

> You as a profession and an Association have just emerged from a long and arduous struggle to purge your ranks, and to set your house in order, and the effort has been to a large extent attended with success. You have shepherded a great many within the fold of professional ethics, and by means of the Association brought all the members more or less into line. But is the fold sufficiently strong to hold them – the unwilling ones? Is the simple authority of the N.Z. Association sufficient to keep the line unbroken? I venture to think not. There are, and have been within my knowledge, deserters and backsliders, and the only deterrent is erasion [*sic*] from the Association membership roll. This is bad *now*. Its evils are obvious, but if such things accur [*sic*] amongst men who hold the B.D.S. Degree of the N.Z. University, if this degree is in danger, after all the travail of its birth, of being dragged through the mire of advertising and quackery, then indeed it will be *ten times worse. Our labour and time will have been nothing more than wasted.* The thing that is lacking is a controlling body, such as the General Medical Council at Home. It would be impossible, perhaps, as well as undesirable, to have such a body in this country, and the British Council is too far off to be able to exercise anything like a sufficient discipline.[*emphasis in original*]

He did not expand on why such a body would not be possible in New Zealand, or why it would be undesirable. Not until 1936 did legislation allow the establishment of the Dental Council of New Zealand. Pickerill, however, had a constructive suggestion:

> The only means of holding any real authority over the members of the profession is having the power to strike names from the Dentists' Register, and this, according to the Dentists' Act, 1904, is vested solely in the Minister of Education. If one might venture a criticism at this point, it seems strange that such authority should be vested in a member of a political party, who, theoretically at least, is subject to the influence of the party and supporters. Would it not have been wiser to have placed the control in the hands of some person or body entirely outside the influence of politics? Apart from this political aspect, it is obvious that the Minister, being a layman, would not see things in the same light as professional men, and what might seem serious to us might be trivial to him. Moreover, what one Minister thought right his successor might think wrong, and so on. There is, however, a body in this country which would seem to be eminently suited to exercising a beneficial control over the Dental Profession. I refer to the Senate of the N.Z. University. That body legally decides when a man is fit to begin practice, and it should therefore have some authority to say when he should cease. It should have the power to insist that degrees and certificates granted by it should be upheld in a worthy and honourable manner … Decisions by this body would be, I am sure, unimpeachable and just to all. It would have no desire to lessen the ranks of its own graduates or practitioners in this country, but it would have every reason to purge undesirables from its rolls. How could such authority be obtained by

> the Senate? Either, firstly, by amending the Act and substituting 'Senate' for 'Minister'. This would be far the simplest method, but perhaps undesirable from political reasons. Or, secondly, by an arrangement being made with the Government, whereby the Minister acted only upon the advice of the Senate … and should it approve of either course, to take immediate action.

Pickerill's objections – on the grounds of political expediency and potential inconsistency in rulings – to the Minister of Education having authority to remove a person from the Register are sound. But the Senate would have been unlikely to want to take on the task of judging whether a dentist was guilty of malpractice or of one of the other offences. As the body setting the standards for curriculum and examination, the Senate determined who could be admitted to the Register; discipline would have been a completely different proposition. Pickerill recognised this Senate, hence his proposed 'Penal Causes Committee', but this would also have taken the Senate outside its normal roles. From this distance in time, it seems surprising that Pickerill did not pursue the idea of a dental council analogous to the British General Medical Council, nor did he compare the dental situation with how the New Zealand medical profession dealt with these difficulties. The 1910 Medical Practitioners Act established the Medical Board of New Zealand to control registration and discipline. Although the Executive of the Dental Association explored the possibility that dentists come under the auspices of the Medical Board,[16] the medical profession was not in favour.

Although Pickerill was now thoroughly immersed in New Zealand dentistry and society generally, his diffidence about having a New Zealand registration body comparable with the British system, and his view of the New Zealand BDS course being set at a lower level than the British BDS, suggest he retained a somewhat 'colonial' or patronising view of the profession in New Zealand – a profession in which by this time he was wielding enormous influence.

In the second section of this seminal paper on dental education, Pickerill suggested that, for a limited time, a BDS degree be established for dentists already in practice. Although the proposal was still to be discussed by the Senate, Pickerill invited the Association's views if it were to occur. He was suggesting the scheme be limited to men who had been in practice at least five years, and to continue for five years from the enactment of enabling legislation. Although no formal curriculum would be involved, he considered 'it would be almost impossible to pass the examination, especially in Pathology, Bacteriology, and Oral Surgery without attending some courses'. Although an imaginative means of enhancing student numbers and raising standards, it received no support from any quarter, and was not pursued.

The third part of the paper addressed the training and standardising of dental mechanics, the workers responsible for the laboratory fabrication of dentures and crowns and bridges. In the following quotation, some marginal amendments (in square brackets) appear in the bound volume of the *Journal* held by the New Zealand Dental Association. The writing suggests the amendments were by Pickerill himself.

> The present system of training men in Mechanical Dentistry is (not referring particularly to New Zealand) at best haphazard; in fact it can scarcely be dignified by the name of a system. An apprentice pays his premium, signs his articles, and does his three or four years [2 or 3 years]; he is turned out good, bad, or indifferent; he himself has no knowledge of which he is exactly, neither has his future employer [the latter phrase deleted]. His standard is taken entirely from his ability to do the character of work which his principal is in the habit of doing. This, apart from the possibility of its being likewise good, bad, or indifferent, is often very stereotyped, and all of one sort. Everyone gets more or less into a groove, and pursues his own particular fads to the exclusion of all others. The result is that the apprentice's [pupil's] ideas of Mechanical Dentistry at the end of his time are narrowed and restricted … Even if there is a really good head mechanic in the workroom, he has no inducement to teach, no interest in seeing the apprentice make progress; in fact, often times the reverse, for sometimes a smart apprentice relieves the principal from the necessity of a highly salaried mechanic. So that an apprentice at the end of his time, although having been in an excellent workroom, has learnt one-quarter of what he ought to know and be able to do …
>
> What I would suggest briefly as a remedy is a recognised examination and certificate in Dental Mechanics, [the] holding of which would standardise the man's knowledge, and would be some guide to his abilities.
>
> I should propose that the certificate be of three grades: the third showing ability in vulcanite work; the second in plate work, gum sections, spring sets, etc.; and the first in crown, bridge, and porcelain work. The examination for each to be separate and distinct, but capable of being taken at one or several times.

This was a revolutionary proposal, as he concluded the article by pointing out 'It is a reform badly needed at Home, but which has not yet been attempted. Can not New Zealand in this, as in other things, show the way?' He did not suggest who would examine the apprentices, but presumably he would have seen a role for the School, there being no other body able to ensure a consistent standard in examination. The suggestion was undoubtedly an attempt to raise the standards of laboratory work throughout the country and thus ensure a well-trained workforce.

Unfortunately, the *Journal* contains no feedback on any of these proposals. The three propositions presented were novel and thought provoking, but there is no indication of how they were received, or whether they were pursued.

Pickerill acknowledged the confusion over the pathways to the BDS degree described in the 1908 syllabus by publishing an explanatory notice in the *Journal*. He prefaced this with 'In spite of the fact that some time ago a syllabus of the Dental School explaining the necessary curriculum in detail was sent out to every dentist on the register … very hazy notions seem still to obtain …'.[17] The explanation was somewhat helpful, but the complexity of bringing in the new system continued. Qualification solely by apprenticeship was now impossible but, despite this stricture, 'back-door entry' was to remain for some years yet. A minimum of four years had to be spent studying dentistry after passing the medical preliminary examination – any mechanical or other work done before passing this examination would not count toward the degree. Three years of mechanical work subsequent to the medical preliminary could be taken with a private practitioner or at the Dental School. If the latter, lectures and other practical classes could be taken concurrently – spending just the two final years of the course at the School was discouraged. Spending all four years at the School in a structured timetable was the recommended and least expensive pathway. The three examinations after the medical preliminary were 'Intermediate', which could be taken at any of the affiliated colleges of Auckland, Wellington, or Christchurch, or at the University of Otago. The first part of the First Professional Examination consisted of anatomy and dental metallurgy; the second comprised physiology and *materia medica*, and was taken at the end of the third year. The Second Professional, comprising dental surgery, dental mechanics, and pathology, occurred at the end of the fourth year.

The promised additional facilities at the School were described, with photographs, in the March 1910 issue of the *Journal*. The writer, presumably Pickerill, enthusiastically announced: 'The equipment of the Dental School is now practically complete. And, speaking of British Schools, we may say we think with truth that it is *Nulli Secundus*'.[18] Electricity was provided for each dental chair, the lecture room had a 'modern electric lantern for use in illustrating lectures, and the museum cases are gradually getting filled with interesting specimens'. The pathological laboratory had 'all requirements for cutting sections in every method, with a number of very fine "Leitz" microscopes, and with all the bacteriological apparatus necessary for the conduct of such work, and for opsonic and vaccine methods of treatment'. Electric lathes were installed in the 'mechanical room', and the students' room had been added. A full complement of students for operative work was expected, and it seemed probable that some would have to be refused.

The effort that had gone into establishing, staffing, and equipping the

Dental School at last bore fruit when three students completed their final examinations for the BDS degree at the end of 1910: A.J. Hansen, C.E. Hercus, and W.S. Seed. Hercus, later Sir Charles, did not practise dentistry; graduation was followed by a distinguished career in medicine – he was appointed Professor of Bacteriology and Public Health in 1922, and was Dean of the Medical School from 1937 to 1958. It is likely that Pickerill encouraged Hercus into medicine – a paper by Hercus, describing treatment of a patient with fractures of the upper and lower jaws, listed him as 'Dresser to the Case' under Dr Pickerill.[19] Hercus was not lost completely to dentistry, however, as the bacteriology of the mouth remained an interest and, as Dean of Medicine, he was closely associated with the Faculty of Dentistry over a long period. Seed was to work with Pickerill at The Queen's Hospital, Sidcup, during the First World War, and later assisted in the continuing care of returned soldiers back in Dunedin, before he practised in Christchurch.

Throughout these early years of the Dental School the administrative, teaching, research, and clinical load of the Dean, the only full-time academic staff member, must have been enormous, even with the able support of the eleven honorary staff. The 1908 *Syllabus* shows he was responsible for the subjects of pathology and bacteriology; orthodontics; dental mechanics, which included dentures, crowns, splints, obturators used in the treatment of cleft palates; and dental surgery, which was described as covering:

> the diagnosis and treatment of caries (remedial and prophylactic), dental arthritis, alveolar abscess, erosion, necrosis, fractures of the teeth and jaws, tumours and cysts in connection with the teeth, neuralgias: and a consideration of those reflex and other lesions liable to be caused or aggravated by diseased conditions of the teeth.[20]

Pickerill would not have given all the lectures in these subjects, but he bore responsibility for teaching standards. Adding to this was the remarkable extent and quality of his research and publications, on which his teaching was based. His long-held interest in tooth decay would have been reinforced by his observations on the appalling state of oral health in the colony, especially in children, when he arrived. His research is covered in more detail later, but an outline of his major publications reveals the incredible energy of the man.

The Cartwright Prize, awarded quinquennially by the Royal College of Surgeons of England to the author of the best essay upon a subject relating to dental surgery, was a major honour received by Pickerill in 1911. Two publications arose from his 'essay'. His major textbook, *Prevention of Dental Caries and Oral Sepsis*,[21] was internationally acclaimed, and proved so popular that a second edition appeared just two years later; the third edition was published in 1923. *Physiological Secretion of the Salivary Glands in the Human Subject* recorded his investigations on saliva and its role in the aetiology and prevention of dental caries [22] – in this field he was a world leader. It had formed part of his thesis for the Doctor of Medicine degree from the University of Birmingham in 1912, the title being *Lactic Acid Fermentation in the Mouth and the Normal Function of Salivary Glands in the Prevention of Oral Sepsis*. That year he also achieved his Master of Dental Surgery degree from the University of Birmingham, his thesis being *The Enamel Surface. Its Normal and Abnormal Conditions and Powers of Resistance to Acids*.[23]

Adding to these achievements was another major textbook – *Stomatology in General Practice*, subtitled *A Textbook of Injuries and Diseases of the Mouth and Teeth for Students and Practitioners*.[24] In this book, also published in 1912, he attempted to bridge the gap between medicine and dentistry, the subtitle referring to members of both disciplines. Pickerill was at this time also providing a series of lectures for medical students,[25] and, as a member of the British Medical Association, stressed to medical colleagues the link between oral and general health at every opportunity. The preface to the first edition of *Stomatology* included:

> There is a somewhat ill-defined territory lying between medicine and dentistry, which to many practitioners is to a certain extent a *terra incognita*.
>
> There is also practically the whole field of dental disease and its treatment which is certainly the same to the general practitioner of medicine … An attempt has been made to throw a beam of light *across* this territory, so that its main features and important points will stand out in bold relief …
>
> … no one can doubt at the present time that it is *absolutely essential* that practitioners of medicine should be familiar with the pathology and means of treatment of the more common diseases arising in connexion with the oral mucous membrane, teeth, and jaws.

The contents of the book reveal the wide range of his interests and expertise. After a review of the history of medicine and dentistry, the topics covered developmental anatomy, deformities of the teeth and jaws, inflammatory conditions in the mouth, the nature and prevention of dental caries, alimentary secretions, surgical treatment of oral conditions, fractures of the jaws, tumours, the manifestations of systemic diseases in the mouth and the systemic effects of oral sepsis, the relationship of oral disease to various conditions of the nervous system, and local and general anaesthesia.

Pickerill's teaching in *materia medica* was based on the text *Otago Medical and Dental Schools' Pharmacopoeia*, which he co-authored with Dr Falconer, the Resident Medical Officer, Dunedin Hospital, in 1909.[26] The review by Davies correctly suggested that the title was misleading, as the formulae are for oral conditions, not of medicines for general medical purposes.[27]

To gain two major additional degrees and to publish three books over a space of two years were remarkable achievements, notably so when it is realised that he was also fulfilling all his teaching and administrative tasks, and at this time was Secretary of the Association and Editor of the *Journal*.

The Dunedin Hospital recognised Pickerill's surgical expertise by appointing him Honorary Dental Surgeon in March 1909. When requesting the Council's approval of him accepting the appointment, he sought the result of the Council's consideration of an earlier letter,[28] presumably a request for a salary increase – this rose to £600 from 1 April. He thought the prosperity of the School through its fees would justify the increment, and estimated that the total receipts of the School over the previous five months had been £326.[29]

Just a year later, the matter of salary was raised again, this time in the context of an invitation from the University of Sydney for him to take up the position of Dean of its Faculty of Dentistry. He wanted the advice of the Council to help him make the decision – he was reluctant to move, especially now that the School was well equipped and running smoothly. If he did accept the position he wanted to know whether the Council would insist on the 'payment of £70 as per agreement'.[30] His employment contract included a clause calling for repayment of £73.10s, the cost of his passage out to New Zealand, should it agree to any application for him to resign within five years of appointment.[31] He also asked whether there was any probability of his present salary being increased should he remain. He pointed out that in the last two summer sessions he had held classes in dental surgery for senior medical students – previously optional, these classes were now compulsory, yet no fee had been charged. Although he said he did not expect one to be paid, he would like to hear the Council's views on this before the next class commenced.

His natural desire for a quick response from the Council caused him to write to the Registrar just five days later asking if the 'most important letter of the 3rd' had been received and considered. If not, could the Registrar ensure the Chancellor or the Finance Committee see it.[32] Pickerill stayed in Dunedin, but the matter of teaching medical students arose again toward the end of 1911. He pointed out to the Council that a Mr Malcolm gave five lectures to mining students and ten shillings and sixpence were charged; the same amount was charged for Dr Fitchett's (presumably still the Dental School's consulting anaesthetist) three lectures. In contrast, in Pickerill's ten lectures in stomatology, he went to 'a good deal of trouble in arranging demonstrations and no fee is charged'.[33] He later suggested that a portion of his salary be a charge on the Faculty of Medicine.[34] The outcome of this request is not known.

Pickerill's initial five-year appointment expired in September 1912. Presuming the Council still wanted his services, he was 'very happy to continue' in the position. 'Considering the adverse circumstances under which we have laboured, the Dental School has I think during the past five years made satisfactory progress'. He admitted, however, that the number of students still 'leaves something to be desired', but he believed the numbers would rapidly increase in the near future. He took the opportunity to mention his salary once again, noting that he was the only member of the University staff who 'has classes running continuously from 9 to 5, every day, Summer and Winter sessions'. He had lectures twice every day, sometimes three times, plus practical classes. Yet, he pointed out, his salary was less than that of other professors who had winter sessions only and less than that of other professors who had less arduous summer sessions. He asked whether the Council 'in the near future', could increase his remuneration consistent with his responsibilities and duties.[33] The Registrar replied saying this request would be considered when 'finances allow it'.[34]

Pickerill undeniably had an enormous workload of teaching, research and writing, and administration – he was still the only full-time member of the professional staff of the School. By this time, too, the family had grown – an increase in salary would no doubt have been very welcome and well deserved. His University activities were, however, not his only commitments – the New Zealand Dental Association quickly recognised his outstanding organisational and administrative abilities, and in 1909 had elected him its Secretary and appointed him Editor of the *Journal*. The load further increased when the Association, largely led by Pickerill as Secretary and Hunter as Chairman of the Council, lobbied hard for dental services for Army recruits after the declaration of war in August 1914.

Although responsibilities to the Association entitled him to no additional compensation, it is understandable that he felt he should be appropriately rewarded for all he was doing for the University. He applied yet again for a salary increase in May 1915, on the grounds that his work was more onerous than that of any other member of staff and that it included normal professorial duties plus the supervision of patients attending the dental hospital; furthermore, there were few men able to fulfil the teaching in the various subjects, including stomatology for the medical students. He also repeated his belief that he was the only member of staff who worked during the winter and summer sessions; his methods of teaching were being adopted in Great

Britain, and his research work was widely recognised, adding that although a professor was always prepared to make sacrifices for love of his work, in this case the disparity between his income and a private practitioner was too high. He further added that the finances of the School were good; the cost of living over the past eight years had increased and, unlike a private practitioner, he could not raise his fees. He suggested his services were equal to that of the Professors of Anatomy and Clinical Pathology, and his pay should equal theirs.[37] At this time his salary was £600 per annum. His convincing case was at last recognised by the Council, which approved an increase to £700 at its July meeting.[38]

Pickerill was granted six months' sabbatical leave in 1914. He took the family with him to England, and they had a happy family reunion in Hereford. He also visited his *alma mater*, and he proposed the toast to the University of Birmingham at a meeting of the Central Counties Branch of the British Dental Association. In his speech he reviewed reasons for the shortage of dental students, a topic of vital interest to his own faculty.[39] He reported that he visited 'nearly all schools and clinics in England and Australia', and was convinced that 'ours compared favourably in equipment, organisation and teaching'.[40] He was in London at a meeting of the International Dental Federation when war was declared. The School was soon involved in the war – Pickerill himself in establishing dental services for recruits, and students and recent graduates amongst those immediately enlisting.

Despite his satisfaction with the state of the School, the chronic lack of students was a major problem. His solution in 1916 was to invoke the provisions in the Dentists Act for the Certificate of Proficiency. He wanted it to be 'workable and suitable for such dental students as find it difficult or impossible to attend University for the whole four or even three years …'. His proposed course was initially strongly opposed by other members of the Faculty,[41] and was held over until the Dental Association could consider it at its next annual meeting. Faculty approved the regulations at its next meeting nearly a year later,[42] but the need to introduce the lesser qualification confirmed the seriousness of the situation – there had been just six students in 1914–15 and five in 1915–16,[43] and only three in 1917.[44] Even though the country was at war, something had to be done, both to maintain an adequate number of dentists to meet public needs, and to show the University and the Council that the School continued to be viable. This major problem, however, was to be solved not by Pickerill, but by O.V. Davies.

The faculty meeting of December 1916 covered important matters.[45] Until this point, the honorary staff had all been unpaid, but now there was 'need for inducement for Honorary Staff'. The meeting suggested five be appointed at £50 per year plus a guinea a visit to cover two hours' teaching in clinical dentistry and one hour per week in vacations. At the same meeting Pickerill protested strongly at the move of the Auckland University Council to establish a dental school in Auckland, not the last time that such a suggestion would be made. He had already brought this to the attention of the Council, which echoed his alarm and resolved to protest strongly to the Senate.[46]

Pickerill then 'mentioned there was probability of his going Home on Military Service', though he had 'received no communication from the Defence Department personally about the matter'. He reported he had made suggestions to the Council about the management of the School during his absence, and replied to a complaint over lack of prior consultation by pointing out that, due to the uncertainty of the matter, he had been unable to do anything more. By that time, however, matters were pretty certain – the first hints had come from the Ministry of Defence as long ago as October, when Pickerill requested leave of absence if asked to go overseas by the Defence authorities. The Council agreed to this if his services were formally requested, provided financial arrangements could be made in consultation with Pickerill and Davies.[47] A letter from the Minister of Defence[48] was received at a special meeting of the Council on 8 December:[49]

> It is considered necessary that Major Pickerill of the New Zealand Dental Corps should proceed to England as Jaw Specialist. It is quite possible that arrangements could be made for Major Pickerill to start and organise the work in England, the Director of Medical Services in England then finding someone to take his place to enable him to return at an early date to the position and duties he now holds under you at the Dental School of the Otago University.
>
> I would be glad to know at your earliest convenience what date Major Pickerill could proceed to England. It is possible that he will travel on one of the Transports as an Officer of the New Zealand Dental Corps.

Pickerill's proposals, dated 7 December, for the conduct of the School during his absence were accepted, subject to Davies and Frank Throp accepting the positions offered and to Pickerill arranging for payments to them. Davies would attend every morning, and in the afternoon would deliver lectures; he would be responsible for the proper conduct of the school, with the suggestion that he be appointed Acting Dean of the faculty. Pickerill proposed that he would personally pay a remuneration of £500 to Davies, 'approximately the salary I should receive for my Military duties'. He would therefore be employing Davies as a *locum tenens* during his absence.

Pickerill's forthcoming departure was not well received at the Faculty meeting, for he had kept the Faculty in ignorance of this major change in the conduct of the School. Nevertheless Davies unhesitatingly accepted the position offered,[50] and events moved rapidly – on 20 December, Pickerill confirmed to the Chancellor that General Henderson wanted him to 'go to the front to undertake the treatment of gunshot wounds to the jaw'.[51] The Council formally granted him leave of absence at its meeting the next day.[52] The Chancellor and Vice-Chancellor were to attend to the financial arrangements between the Registrar and the War Expenses Office of the Ministry of Defence, in consultation with Pickerill and Davies. The complicated nature of these arrangements[53] added to later dissension between the two men – while Pickerill was on active service, the Council paid Davies' a salary of £200 and paid Pickerill a salary of £700. Pickerill paid Davies £500 out of this salary. To allow Davies to pay for the rent of his rooms while he was fulltime at the Dental School, the Council increased his salary to £250.

When Pickerill departed for England in December 1916, the School was in its tenth year of existence. It had developed into an internationally respected institution, and was regarded with enormous pride by the Dental Association which, with considerable justification, felt responsible for its founding. The selection of Pickerill had proved an outstanding success. His achievements in research, teaching, and writing show he was a man of enormous energy and vision. His roles in the Dental Association as Secretary and Editor cemented the close relationship between the School and the profession in a way that has never been equalled. The disappointment of these first years of the School was, however, the small number of students it had attracted – Pickerill had neglected this problem in the midst of all his other activities. But he had on his staff a person who had carefully analysed the situation and, fortunately for the School, this man had been appointed Acting Director while Pickerill was overseas. Pickerill was to inherit, as he did on his arrival in 1907, the outcome of the foresight, energy, and administrative abilities of a great servant of New Zealand dentistry, Owen Vivian Davies.

7

Research: focus on caries

Pickerill had a gift for recognising and defining problems, plus the energy and intellect to seek and find solutions. These qualities were displayed immediately he arrived in New Zealand when he noted the public's appalling state of oral health. The two serious problems were dental caries (tooth decay) and periodontal disease (diseases of the gums and tissues supporting the teeth in the bone). Caries was undoubtedly a major scourge, the cause of much pain, especially in children, and disfigurement through the destruction of the crowns of the teeth and, eventually, extractions and the fitting of dentures, often in early adulthood. Abscessed teeth were extremely common and often associated with chronic general ill health. The severest forms of periodontal disease, known at that time as 'pyorrhoea' (literally 'flow of pus'), also had devastating effects on the teeth. Modern understanding of periodontal diseases has resulted in improved methods of management – the term 'pyorrhoea' is now outmoded and, fortunately, the fatalistic view that periodontal disease inevitably leads to loss of the teeth no longer pertains.

Pickerill focused his attention on caries rather than periodontal disease, a logical development in view of his research as a student at the University of Birmingham.[1] When he arrived in New Zealand, the alleviation of the ravages of tooth decay and the provision of care for children and the indigent were dominant topics at meetings of the Dental Association and its constituent societies and branches. Repeated calls were being made for the systematic examination of children in schools and for the establishment of dental hospitals in the main centres. The whole situation presented a tremendous research challenge, and one can imagine Pickerill bursting to become involved. The outcome of his caries research was to bring him international recognition and acclaim. He came to stand in the foremost ranks of the researchers of the period, and his contributions are still acknowledged today.

He withheld publication of the results of his Dunedin research until he could bring together all his findings in *Prevention of Dental Caries and Oral Sepsis*, published in 1912. Of particular interest to modern researchers is his emphasis on the role of saliva in resistance to caries.[2] The review in the *Journal* included the following:

> The passive resistance of the teeth themselves, has been the subject of considerable experimental work; and the enamel is shown … to vary considerably in hardness and resistance to acids. The active part played by the saliva and oral fluids in producing a physiological immunity to caries, is very exhaustively treated; and we gather that the author is of the opinion that the chief means of natural prevention of dental and oral disease, and of building up the resistance of the enamel surface, resides in the saliva. A considerable amount of this work on salivary glands is of physiological interest, since it is the first record of complete analysis of saliva obtained from the human subject, during the mastication of ordinary articles of diet. The extraordinary variations in the composition of saliva, from various dietetic stimuli is extremely interesting: in fact, it is concluded that the saliva, both as regards amount and composition, is completely under control, and may be varied at will.
>
> A curious paradox is evident from the author's work, namely that although acids cause caries, acids also are the chief excitants of the protective forces of the mouth. Experimental evidence is quoted to show that a sequence of ordinary caries-producing food and salivary stimulants will entirely negative any acid production in the mouth.[3]

This was a completely revolutionary view of the mechanism of caries and how it might be prevented. The reviewer also commented on an aspect of Pickerill's research that has very modern connotations – the introduction into the oral cavity of bacteria that might have protective functions. This was not a new concept, even in those days, as antagonistic interactions among bacterial species were proposed by Pasteur in 1877;[4] the modern equivalent is the BLIS technology – Bacteriocin-Like Inhibitory Substances produced by bacteria that have antibiotic activity against other, closely related bacteria. This is a major research emphasis in the Department of Microbiology in the University of Otago. As the *Journal*'s reviewer stated: 'The proposal to inoculate the mouth with organisms which will rapidly disperse the carbohydrate food adhering to the teeth, is quite a fresh departure, and one which apparently, has very great possibilities.'

His research on the structure and development of the teeth gave rise to the term 'Imbrication Lines of Pickerill', minute horizontal corrugations on the tooth surface indicating the end points in the formation of the layers of enamel. He believed these imbrications indicated that the teeth had erupted before enamel formation was complete, and that they contributed to the teeth's susceptibility to decay.

The book was received in New Zealand with enormous pride and enthusiasm, its author viewed almost with awe. Herbert Cox, for example, in his presidential address to the Auckland Branch claimed:

> As the result of these [studies by Pickerill and others] and similar researches, we may confidently predict that at last there is a gleam of hope that the ravages of dental disease may not only be checked as hitherto, but absolutely prevented. Professor Pickerill … has written a work, which I claim will rank among the classics of dental literature, and which was awarded the distinguished honour of the Cartwright Prize for original research (1906–1910) by the Royal College of Surgeons of England, and will do much to revolutionise some of our ideas as to how to prevent teeth decaying. New Zealand is to be greatly congratulated in having secured the services of such an able, scientific, and practical teacher as Dr. Pickerill …[5]

Later that year, Pickerill lectured the Auckland Branch over two evenings, the report suggesting it could have been a rehearsal for his presentation to the International Dental Congress in London the following year. He attracted 'a record attendance of members, and the lecture was without doubt the most interesting ever given before the branch'.[6] As a result he was elected honorary life member of the branch, and was presented with a silver soup tureen and a case of pipes.

The renowned caries researcher C.F. Bödecker of Berlin was more restrained but nevertheless complimentary in a letter written in November 1913:

> Today I have finished reading your excellent work on the 'Prevention of Dental Caries and Oral Sepsis' and I wish to express my great esteem for the man who has gone through the many years of work in order to place the above book before the profession. I can readily understand the painstaking labor you have gone through, in making all those experiments …
>
> It is a wonderful theory you have evolved, one which is entirely new to me and I am sure to most of our profession. To discard the alkaline tooth paste and powder as useless, even harmful, is a matter which will not be understood by the public, even the dentists will be sceptical for some time …
>
> It gave me great pleasure that you have finally and absolutely defined the different classes of teeth, the malacotic and sclerotic. As you say, during the last ten years one did not dare mention hard and soft teeth, even though the clinical experience endorses this view daily …

I intend reading a paper before the American Dental Society of Europe … next July at their meeting in Paris upon the subject of caries. Your work will find the most prominent place in the article …

One clinical feature of immune patients you have not mentioned, but probably thought of, is the effect of smoking. Here in Germany it is claimed that smoking causes an excess of potassium sulphocyanate to be secreted in saliva. I think your theory explains this heightened resistance to caries more surely and simply, namely to a greater flow of saliva. The chewing of gum or tobacco probably has a similar effect.

Considering that a greater flow of saliva is beneficial, would not the chewing of licorice wood, especially by children be useful? Besides stimulating the salivary glands, it would also develop the muscular and bone tissue. By previously saturating this licorice wood in lemon or orange juice and then drying, the effect would be a sour sweet taste. What is your opinion of this means to induce children to masticate thoroughly.[7]

We do not know Pickerill's reaction to this latter suggestion, but he certainly endorsed the value of chewing fibrous food. Bödecker's remark about chewing gum foreshadows the modern advocacy by the Wrigley Company that increased salivary flow, produced by use of its products, neutralises the acid produced by fermentation of carbohydrate. Pickerill's theory of the importance of stimulating salivary flow, developed over ninety years ago, has been soundly endorsed by modern dental research. Bödecker seems not to have fulfilled his promise to incorporate Pickerill's research into papers he presented in Paris,[8] and no further correspondence between the two men has been found.

Although he confessed to not yet having read the book, Charles Tomes, another giant of the dental world, wrote in 1912 'a glance at different subjects has impressed me with the care and thoroughness with which you have treated the subjects …'.[9]

The book was translated into German,[10] and attracted much interest and some criticism in that country. An anonymous reviewer in the *Journal* praised it as being 'for the most part' faithfully done, but then deplored some liberties in translation and the omission of certain highly important material. 'The edition is not free from some serious errors, due to faulty proof reading, and several of the illustrations are reversed'.[11]

The German researcher Theo von Beust sharply criticised yet another German reviewer:

The tone adopted by the critic, Prof. Williger of Berlin seems little becoming to a man of science when criticizing the works of a colleague. You can be assured that it is only an expression of the attitude assumed by the German dentists

> toward all foreigners. Soon you will find your original ideas going the rounds of the German literature and no credit given to the author.[12]

Editions were also published in Japan and America, and although the German translation was not a complete success, Pickerill was now firmly established on the international stage. His research was not, however, confined to clinical and pathological aspects – he also had great insight into the epidemiology of the condition. He opened his paper to the 1912 Annual Meeting of the Association with an optimistic statement:

> In proposing to bring before the Association a simple method of charting teeth, my object was to provide for the time when we should be able to induce the Government to arrange for the inspection of the teeth of school children. That hope has now been realised, for the Minister for Public Health has today given us an assurance that the dental inspection of school children will be arranged for; that it will be carried out by the medical officers who are to inspect the schools in other respects. It is necessary that these officers shall have some instruction in the diagnosis of the various dental diseases and the various stages of dental caries, and in methods of charting which shall be simple, rapid, and effective.[13]

He then asked practitioners to put aside their own personal charting preferences in favour of a method that, with minimum training of the examiners and recorders, would produce reliable and comparable results quickly and simply. Such data would, he claimed, allow the caries problem to be examined objectively, for treatment and preventive services to be planned for each child, and for the overall problem in the population to be assessed. Overlooking the facts that recording the extent and severity of caries still exercises the minds of epidemiologists to this day, and that examinations for epidemiological purposes are not necessarily suitable for planning treatment for the individual, the paper displays a remarkable clarity of vision. He continued:

> With an assistant to take down the items, the time occupied in each case would not be more than two or three minutes … while the result will … give a reliable basis for statistics … a dentist examining the chart afterwards will be able to tell quite easily and rapidly, what line of treatment should be adopted. From the information so collected, it will be possible to ascertain the number of carious teeth, the percentage of carious teeth in each child, the percentage of sound to carious teeth, the amount of sepsis present … the total available masticating area, and the probable amount of pain. These calculations could be made by the clerks in the Public Health Department from the figures ... My whole anxiety is to save the professional man as much as possible, and throw as much as possible upon the clerical staff of the Department, because therein lies, I believe, true economy of time, energy, and brain power.

This approach is echoed by epidemiologists today.

The *Journal*'s review of the second edition of *Prevention of Dental Caries and Oral Sepsis*, published in 1914, was the work of 'AMC', presumably A.M. Carter, a prominent member of the Association and committed advocate for the education of teachers and school children on the prevention of caries. Carter ponderously but lavishly praised the style of the book and the quality of its language:

> To the average dental reader who is merely desirous of keeping himself in touch with the latest developments of dental science as reflected in the literature of the profession, Dr Pickerill's works prove attractive because of his pureness of diction and lucidity of style alike, under his meaning at all times readily intelligible, a marked contrast to many scientific writers; whilst from those who are themselves more seriously engaged in trying to solve the urgent problems presented, our author commands both attention and respect, his arguments being difficult to controvert, based as they are for the most part on exact observation and experimentation.

Pickerill, as Editor, refrained from simplifying this tortuous sentence, but he must have been tempted. Carter criticised aspects of a chapter on mastication and sections dealing with jaw position in chronic mouth-breathers, which today certainly seem extraneous topics in a book on dental caries. But the possibility of the use of 'good' bacteria in caries prevention intrigued Carter:

> In order to justify conclusions arrived at, as recorded in the first edition, on the possible utilization of the antibietic [*sic*] properties of certain mouth organisms [*sic*]. A chapter, partly bibliographical and partly detailing further experiments, is added, on the alimentary secretions considered as a whole.
>
> The question of thus cultivating one organism with a view to inhibiting the proliferation of another more noxious form is one of the most fascinating problems of modern bacteriological science. We are but on the threshold of our knowledge, and it is along this line as applied to the oral secretions we would like to see our author devote his further energies.

Although a great deal is now known about antagonism between bacterial species, many would argue that we are still 'on the threshold of our knowledge' in this field. Carter concluded:

> On these distinctive arguments which made the first edition of his work epoch-making in dental science Dr Pickerill is Dr Pickerill still. His views on the acid-diet-dentifrice question receive remarkable confirmation from investigations into the nature and action of sugar cane, observations which should be read to be appreciated. No one who is a real lover of his profession or who is desirous

> of keeping abreast of modern dental thought can afford to be without this book.[14]

Carter noted that this edition of the book included a 'brief resume of the research carried on by Prof. Champtaloup, among the natives of the Uriwera [*sic*] country as to the cause of their immunity from dental caries ...'. Pickerill had raised this project at a meeting with the Minister for Public Health in July 1912:

> [Dental researchers] did not know at the present time the bacteriological difference between the mouths of people who were susceptible to caries ... and the mouths of those who were immune ... It would be an extremely important matter to know in the case of a race like the ancient Maoris – who were afflicted with caries to a very minute degree – whether their mouths were free from the conditions giving rise to dental caries ... Professor Pickerill mentioned that the Royal Society of Medicine in London had instructed him to carry out this enquiry, and had made a grant of £50 to forward it, with a promise of further support, if necessary ... The New Zealand Dental Association had also voted a similar sum for the purpose of the inquiry. The available funds might or might not be sufficient to cover the cost of the enquiry, but ... they would like to have the moral support of the Health Department ... It might not be possible to find in this country a tribe of Maoris sufficiently uncivilized for the purposes of this inquiry. In that case they proposed to take an expedition down to one of the islands. Should this be necessary they might ask for a small grant from the Government.[15]

Presumably 'uncivilized' Maori meant those having limited or no contact with pakeha, who had diets containing few refined carbohydrates. The Minister was cautiously supportive of the bacteriological research – perhaps he realised that the project was anything but a 'little point' that Pickerill had mentioned in his introductory comment. In the subsequent 'brief conversation' it was revealed that 'at this stage it appeared that Professor Pickerill proposed in the first place to go into the Urewera Country, taking a full equipment of bacteriological instruments and appliances'.

The report of the findings of the two expeditions he made to the Urewera was a landmark of Pickerill's research. The numerous photographs display the bacteriological findings and something of the life of the people he studied. The journey itself and the people of the region of the Urewera, which lies inland from Gisborne on the East Coast of the North Island, obviously fascinated him. His observations are also of great interest today:

> Information from various sources as to the conditions of life of the natives in the Urewera country were so varied that it was determined that the only

satisfactory method of ascertaining the truth was to go through the country. Professor Champtaloup, at the time, was unable to leave his laboratory so, perforce, one of us (H.P.P.) had to make the journey alone. The Government could not spare an interpreter, since all the Native Land Courts were then in session; an introduction was, however, given to the Chief Judge of the Native Land Court sitting at Taneatua, to whom also was explained the object of the proposed visit. The Government Survey Department had previously advised that we should probably find more Natives of the type required at Maungapohatu, the headquarters of the prophet Rua, than anywhere else. The latter place it was therefore determined to make the objective *via* Taneatua.

I (H.P.P.) took with me a certain amount of bacteriological apparatus, sufficient to enable me to make 200 smears from the saliva and materia alba [bacteria and food debris scraped from the teeth], in order to gain a general idea as to the character of the bacteria present. I also took a small number of swabs (as used for diphtheria) to take material from the gums. The idea being to get these out of the country as quickly as possible, and posted down to Dr Champtaloup at Dunedin, in order to ascertain whether the organisms would survive for that length of time – more particularly with a view to testing their actions on carbohydrates. I proceeded to Taneatua by train, steamer, coach, and buggy, a distance of about 900 miles; there, by the courtesy of the Judge, and by the aid of his interpreter, I addressed the assembled Maori. They showed every sign of considerable interest and appointed a guide, who would also act as interpreter, to accompany me round their country. It then rained heavily for several days, and it was a week before the rivers were sufficiently low again for me to be able to induce my Maori to start, he also seemed to require that time to collect three horses and a pack saddle. I spent the next eight days in the saddle riding from pah [village] to pah through the dense primeval forest, along and across river beds (one river alone, the Waimana, we crossed over 200 times), over wooded spurs and hills, two of which were over 2,000 feet in height. The narrow and almost prehistoric Maori tracks were so rough and precipitous that it was clear that it would be absolutely impossible to take a full bacteriological equipment in by that route at least. Arrived at Maungapohatu on the third day, I found it veritably a 'deserted village'. On enquiry I elicited the information that 'Rua, he humbug, no good to Maori: Maori he go home'. [Rua was subsequently arrested during a raid by police in 1916, during which two of his followers were killed.[16]] So that my Government information had been very misleading. I subsequently visited the pahs at Tatahauta, Omakoi, Matatua, Waikirikiri, and Ruatoki, and here I found more than a sufficient number of children and adolescents immune to caries, from whom to take swabs and smears.

I found more caries present than I had hoped to find, but still only to a very slight extent in any one mouth, and I saw more perfect sets of teeth than I had ever seen before.

The 'Bacteriology' had to be done under very adverse circumstances, such as in the corner of a plantation, in a whare (hut) by the riverside, or just wherever

> the Maori children could be caught. I limited my investigation to young Maori, since I found that a considerable number of adults had been out of the country on visits to civilised parts on one or several occasions.
>
> As regards food, I found that in great part, the Maori have forgotten the food of their ancestors. At present their principle [*sic*] diet seems to be riwai, kumara, maize (rotten), pig, and occasionally mutton. Fruit grows wild in the country and they are very fond of it, but I did not ascertain that they stored it at all. European flour, tea, and sugar, they are all very anxious to obtain, and when it is obtained consume in considerable quantities until the stock is exhausted. The old stores of kumrra [*sic*], etc., were nearly exhausted at the time of my visit, the new supply was not yet to hand, and the partition between the Natives and starvation in some places seemed very thin indeed. Yet, withal, they were quite happy, always smiling, ever ready for a joke, and to share with the pakeha … their last riwai [potato]. They feed squatting on the ground, without either knife or fork, and these characteristics I shared with them during my visit.[17]

Pickerill had a great love of the outdoors, and was an enthusiastic mountaineer and fisherman; his sociological comments suggest he thoroughly enjoyed the whole experience. His photographs are of high quality. The swabs and smears he stained himself, and presumably took them back to Dunedin for examination by Professor Champtaloup. Not surprisingly, the results are primitive by modern standards but, given the circumstances, this was quality research. Several days' journey by horseback into a very remote area, packing in all his equipment, and working under what were undoubtedly trying and difficult conditions, were major achievements.

The second part of the article reports a second visit to the region. This is stated to have occurred in November–December 1914, but as the article appeared in the March 1914 issue of the *Journal*, it must have taken place in 1913.

> On this occasion it was decided to take as full a laboratory equipment as possible, and to make Ruatoki the centre for investigations. There are about five or six pahs in the surrounding district, and the children were selected from these. The Government Health department fitted up a shed as a laboratory for the work, and though the space was somewhat limited it served the purpose well. An oil incubator was taken, together with tubes and dishes of culture media, and all the apparatus and re-agents necessary for salivary analysis. Despite the fact that the last hundred miles was across country everything arrived intact.

The tests on fifty 'perfectly immune children' included 'as complete an analysis as possible of each child's saliva', its viscosity, the amount of acid production from biscuit detritus from the mouth after incubation for twenty-four hours, and bacteriological cultures.

Pickerill's access to the *Journal* was undoubtedly enhanced by his being its editor – the March 1914 issue contained the results of the Urewera investigation, and the editorial, presumably written by him, justified the novelty of comparison of susceptible and what he called 'immune' groups.[18] Editorial comment on articles published in the same issue is a common practice of modern editors, but comment in this way on one's own work certainly opens up implications of lack of objectivity.

After acknowledging the financial support of the Dental Association, the writer of the editorial continued:

> It has been well said that *science is measurement*, and the problem of the causation and prevention of dental caries can only be solved by the most rigid scientific enquiries … It is necessary to have a standard measurement with which others may be compared in order that the deviation from the normal may be more or less accurately estimated. It is precisely in this respect in which scientific investigations of dental caries in the past have been lacking. Many have worked at the subject … but their enquiries have, of necessity almost, been limited to susceptible individuals. We knew what the organisms were which were found in susceptible mouths, we had a fair knowledge of the histology and morbid anatomy of the tissues affected, we knew the role played by fermentable carbohydrates, we knew something of salivary secretion – but in what way these differed from conditions found in immune mouths we did not know.

If the writer was indeed Pickerill, he then ventured an opinion that should have been left to others. 'The investigations published in this issue supply to some extent at least standards of measurement, and therefore cannot fail to be important.'

The editorial went on to state that the bacteriology of the mouths of immune Maori children 'does not materially differ from that of susceptible European children'. Pickerill did not promote the theory that race *per se* was a determinant of disease, even though he did not distinguish clearly whether he thought the children were truly immune to caries, or whether they had no or very low rates of caries simply because they had not been exposed to the conditions conducive to the disease, for example, of diet. But this is a statement commonly made even today – that because a condition is not present in a person, that person is immune. Nevertheless he acknowledged the role that the encroaching 'civilised' diet was likely to have, and enlarged on this when he described in the article some general health issues:

> On the outskirts of the country the tubercle bacillus is reaping a rich harvest, and unless something more is done by the Government to educate the Maori as to the nature of phthisis [tuberculosis], and proper hygienic methods of its prevention, I fear that the genial Tuhoi people of the Urewera are doomed to a

> process of slow decimation. In particular should Government inspectors refrain from inducing the Maori to give up his pine slab whares in favour of sawn wood huts, with iron roofs and tightly sealed windows and doors. In fact, the very best thing for the Maori would be for the Government to close the country to the pakeha entirely and let the Natives develop slowly along their own lines.[19]

A provocative comment, but one that seems to be made with genuine concern about the future of a population he seemed to respect and admire.

Pickerill took his conclusions on caries to the Sixth International Dental Congress held in London, 3–8 August 1914. The first part of his paper introduced the history and geographical distribution of caries, recognising:

> the increase in wealth and luxury, in refinement of thought, habits, and food occurring in any nation. Where these latter attributes have evolved slowly the progress of caries has been slow, but where they have come rapidly or been thrust suddenly upon a nation or community, the destruction of the teeth has occurred with an equal speed and certainty. The Maori in some parts of New Zealand, in a single generation passed from a state of immunity to one of susceptibility equal to that which took European nations some 2000 years to reach.[20]

Although he still used 'immunity' carelessly, he recognised the overwhelming effect of the changes in diet on what were, in reality, highly susceptible teeth. He broadened the discussion to include geographical variables; dietary customs; and the nature of the diet of various ethnic groups, including the diets of Maori, African, and Asiatic people. An indication of the magnitude of his research is given in his comparison of these diets with results of a 'detailed examination of the dietaries of 1500 primary school children'. He quoted from the work of others in his discussion of the associations of occupation and social class on caries, and on the influence of heredity. He also reviewed work on caries in adolescents who were, 'either by disease or by operation, suffering section or destruction of the nerves supplying trophic function to the teeth'. This section of the paper is not Pickerill at his best, but he presumably included this discussion because of the current speculation on the relationship between mental health and degenerative conditions. He concluded the first part of the presentation with a discussion on the theories of causation and the nature and pathology of the carious lesion.

In the second section he discussed the nature of the organisms causing caries, quoting his Urewera bacteriological findings, repeating his conclusion that 'we are unable to find any distinctive difference between the organisms present in these [the Urewera children's] mouths and those found ordinarily in the mouths of civilised communities'.

The third section opened with a carefully reasoned argument opposing the commonly held belief that saliva in some caries-susceptible people contains carbohydrates capable of being fermented into acid. He continued with evidence supporting his view that saliva was essential for the enamel to reach maturity after the tooth erupts into the mouth. This section had a modern ring to it – dental enamel is indeed not fully mature when the tooth erupts, and minerals from saliva contribute to the ongoing development of the hydroxyapatite crystals that form the enamel, the outer covering of the tooth.

After discussing other factors influencing the quality of enamel, he turned to 'The Fourth Factor – Deficient Salivary Secretion', arguably his most significant contribution to caries research. When the production of saliva is low, such as can occur when the salivary glands are affected by disease, by irradiation during cancer treatment, or by many modern medications, the risk of caries increases greatly. The flow of saliva is enhanced, as Pickerill suggested, by vigorous chewing and by the acids in fruit. This increased flow has a protective function, as proclaimed by the chewing gum companies.

This long discussion led into the possible influences of the secretions of the thymus, thyroid, and pituitary glands on saliva and thus on caries, and the intriguing speculation that 'cerebral stimulation leads to salivary depression, and this, if continuous, certainly means caries'. He unfortunately did no further investigation of these theories – salivary flow can indeed be affected by emotional states. He concluded with a summary of his own research and that of others, expounding eloquently on the multi-factorial aetiology of caries:

> It is obvious from what has been said that to the etiology of dental caries a large number of factors may or do contribute. There are two chief attacking – carbohydrates and organisms – and two defensive – the resistance of the enamel surface and the protective action of the salivary secretion. Each of these may vary more or less, and so the possible permutations and combinations favouring caries are approximately twenty-four. But each of these factors is composed of a large number of contributing factors: the variations in the fermentability of the carbohydrates consumed, the number and type of organisms present, the different possible weaknesses of the enamel surface, and the varying amounts of the chemical constituents of saliva …
>
> There is no golden key to be discovered to unlock the riddle of dental caries. Although we may safely generalise to a certain extent, each case must be studied as a distinct clinical entity ... No one would be bold enough to assert that the etiologies of all cases of heart disease or of diabetes were identical, though the obvious symptoms might be quite similar. Just as it is necessary for the physician to study each case of any particular disease, to analyse the excretions

> and examine the blood before a correct idea of cause can be formed, so it is necessary in our speciality to examine each case minutely (visually, chemically, and bacteriologically), and to submit it to critical judgment before an opinion as to the *exact* cause of the lesions present.

He ended his mammoth presentation with a plea for further research on the causes and pathology of caries, so that the condition 'may be placed on the solid foundation that is demanded by its superstructure – national preventive measures'.

This had been his first public presentation of his research to an international audience, and he did it in a grand manner – he was a major speaker at a major conference, and the extent of the reporting suggests he made the most of the occasion. The Congress was cut short by the declaration of war, and no discussion of his paper, if it did occur, was published. This is unfortunate, as he had presented new and, probably to many in the audience, startling material.

Pickerill's energies at this time were being diverted away from caries research by his military duties, and his subsequent work in plastic surgery was a further interruption. But others seem to have taken advantage of his absence from the research scene. His military files include an attachment describing the recognition he had received internationally for his research. This was indeed substantial – in 1912 the prize from Vienna for a monograph on the anatomy and physiology of the palate and the repair of clefts; in 1913 the offer of a Chair in the Royal University at Budapest; in 1914, presumably an outcome of his presentations at the London Congress, an invitation to lecture at American universities; and publication of his research in American, German, and Japanese editions. Then appears the following:

> Volunteered for active service August 5th, 1914 … Since then wholly occupied with Military duties in various capacities.
>
> As a consequence Research work wholly neglected, and position which I had attained almost entirely lost through:–
>
> (1). Attacks by others in America and Sweden which I have been unable on account of Military duties to answer.
>
> (2). Other investigators who had not been engaged in War work taking up my researches where I left off and going on in the same direction.[21]

These bitter comments could have marked the end of his caries research, but there was still work to do. In 1923 the third edition of *Prevention of Dental Caries and Oral Sepsis* was published. In the foreword, Pickerill noted the cessation of his research during the war, but that his interest in caries had been 're-awakened'. New diagrams were included that 'render the wonderful adaptability of the salivary secretion to be better and more quickly grasped'.[22] There was also more on the 'immunity' of Maori children.

The nature of the attacks on his work became clearer in a paper he published in 1924.[23] The criticisms of his work included his opposition to the use of alkaline toothpastes and powders, and among his critics were the powerful tooth-product manufacturers. He therefore reviewed the evidence on the importance of saliva in neutralising the effects of acid arising from the fermentation of carbohydrate, and re-emphasised the importance of a copious flow of saliva to ensure the teeth are bathed in the fluid, especially after eating acidic foods. The most effective way of ensuring this flow is not by alkali, but by acidic stimuli, his hypothesis still being quite revolutionary at the time. He also rebutted criticisms of his research methodology and pointed out examples where he had been misquoted.

This is a very well reasoned article, but it must have been very hard to write. Not only was he facing the indignity of having to defend his work, he would also, no doubt, have suspected his rebuttals would not carry much weight, published as they were in the rather remote *New Zealand Dental Journal* – probably not noted at that time as being in the forefront of international research publications. From the adulation heaped upon him in earlier years, the ill-informed criticisms must have been a bitter pill.

At this time, however, an earlier interest in the diet of native peoples was rekindled, for his correspondence reveals extensive enquiries to many countries.[24] Some of his contacts were supplied by church mission societies, and his papers contain letters, for example, from the London Mission Hospital in India, the Methodist Missionary Society of New Zealand, Knox College (Presbyterian) in Dunedin, the New Zealand Anglican Board of Missions, and Holy Cross College (Mosgiel, Dunedin). He accumulated information on the nature of the diet and its preparation from India, various countries in Africa, Papua New Guinea, the New Hebrides, and Madagascar. The collection of this information does not seem to have resulted in any formal publications, and it probably represents pursuit of a personal interest rather than formal research. His research on caries ended at this point, its place to be taken by his commitment to plastic surgery.

A detailed critical review of Pickerill's caries research is not appropriate in a biography. In the light of current knowledge obtained through the advanced research techniques and equipment enjoyed by today's researchers, criticisms can indeed be made. But this could only denigrate the work of a true scientist, a man with the enviable combination of incredible energy and an enquiring mind. His research was of the highest quality. Where it would have led if he had continued with it is impossible to predict, but undoubtedly he would have further cemented his place as a world leader in the field. Pickerill today is remembered largely for his plastic surgery, but this should not overshadow his contributions to research on dental caries.

8

Involvement in the New Zealand Dental Association

Pickerill became involved in the affairs of the New Zealand Dental Association within days of his arrival in Dunedin. Initially this was with the Otago Odontological Society, soon to become the Otago Branch of the Association, but the national Association quickly sought his services – in 1909 he was elected Secretary and also appointed Editor of the *New Zealand Dental Journal*.[1]

Pickerill as Secretary

Pickerill made two substantial contributions to the Association's 1909 annual meeting, the first being of a controversial nature that could have had profound implications for the future directions of the Association. He could not attend, but Hunter read on his behalf the paper 'New Zealand or British Dental Association', in which he argued, perhaps not surprisingly given the short time he had been away from the 'Old Country', that the Association should become a branch of the British Dental Association, analogous to New Zealand's medical practitioners being members of the New Zealand Branch of the British Medical Association. This was also a proposal made by another speaker, Frank Armstrong.[2] Pickerill's paper was never published, but the discussion of the two papers was vigorous. Dr Norman Cox, the first speaker opened with scathing words:

> I think this is a very serious subject, and the short time we have to take it in is not enough, but I should like to point out a few things worth considering. It is very easy to see that Dr. Pickerill is quite English. Well, I, from a dental point of view, am quite American; both my degrees were obtained in America, and I suppose I look at things from an American point of view. Professor Pickerill

has not a true grasp of affairs here. He doesn't know that for the last twenty years we have been struggling to advance ethical dentistry in New Zealand. Those who have helped to form the Association look upon it as their own child. The N.Z. Dental Association had an independent birth; if we had started as a branch of the British Dental Association it would have been all right, now it is slightly different. We have got a sturdy child, and all we have to do is to see that it develops into strong manhood …

… we shall get just as much value … out of the British Dental Association if we go Home as visitors … I think it would upset the whole arrangements; we should have to change our name and our bylaws … Professor Pickerill doesn't understand the position. When we started five years ago, a good many men had to be coaxed in. We would not have had an Association at all then if we had been under the B.D.A.[3]

Armstrong sprang to Pickerill's defence by pointing out that 'all sorts of local prejudices' would be got rid of if the Association joined the BDA. He felt that '… we have progressed to the position that even if we get rid of half our members we will still be a strong Association; and we had better be a strong Association, with fewer members, than a big Association of which a number are more or less breaking the laws'.

This latter view, as might be expected, brought immediate reaction, including discussion on whether dentists without degrees were even eligible to be members of the BDA. Pickerill's absence from the meeting was regretted, and criticism of the lack of information came from Davies:

A man who writes a paper like that should provide for discussion, so that the one who reads the paper may be fully prepared to answer. If two-thirds of our funds are going Home, how are we to do our business? A scheme should be laid before the Association before we can consider it at all.

At that point discussion was sensibly adjourned, but the matter was raised again in the Auckland branch. W.F. Goulstone, addressing the questions 'How can we raise the standard and professional tone of dentistry in New Zealand? How can we help in the real education of the public?', said he had written to Pickerill on the matter and received this revealing reply:

I regret to say that I cannot send you my paper which was read in Wellington, as I have not seen it since I gave it to Mr. Hunter … I have recently taken over the editorship of the *Journal*, and all papers etc, have been sent to me from Wellington, but my paper is not among them. The advantage of joining the B.D.A. would be a far more complete and homogeneous organisation, more especially in the relationship of the branches to the General Association – it would tend, I think, perhaps, to help in raising the whole professional tone of Dentistry. I am sure that as a Branch of the British Dental Association we

> should carry more weight and prestige in any official dealings with the public, Government, or University Senate, in any litigation we may take up, and in our associations with the medical profession. This I regard as most important, especially from a *'Preventive Dentistry'* point of view. If we are to save the teeth of the people we shall have to work in close association with the 'Medical Men', and our professional standing in the eyes of the public must be of the highest standing, and, if it is seen that we are recognised by the Home authorities, I think this would be more readily attained. We should, in fact, have the advantage of the moral support, advice, and experience of the Home Association.
>
> As regards the vital point of the qualifications for membership, I think all members of the N.Z.D.A. both should and would be accepted *en bloc*, but I am unable to state anything definitely. I wrote Home about the matter, hoping for an answer before the Conference, but so far have heard nothing.[4]

Perhaps it was just as well that Pickerill had not read the paper himself at the Wellington conference and that it had been lost. His arguments would have been shredded, as would his vague opinions, such as that prefaced by 'it would tend, I think, perhaps, to help …'. This unusually defensive stance would have been scorned by the many members who were passionate about their organisation and proud of what it had achieved.

The matter was not, however, quite laid to rest, for it surfaced again at the 1912 annual meeting, which embroiled Pickerill in further controversy. Moving rather tortuously from a motion about what dentists may publish in newspapers as 'a card' before it transgressed to become an 'advertisement', he:

> looked forward to the time when we shall have one great British Dental Association throughout the Empire – all the dentists of the British Empire welded into one great whole. Then we shall have the prestige of the Old Country behind us, and shall have large accumulated funds, and a vast amount of power that we have not at present … we should, as far as possible, be bound to our fellow-men across the seas in one great association, just as the British Medical Association is throughout the world.[5]

Opposition to his utopian dream was once again instantaneous. Goodwin Cox was scathing – he took a 'different view from our esteemed professor. I emphatically protest against his attitude'. Part of the advertising argument was focused on the suggestion that any announcement in newspapers should not include the word 'Dentist', and this, it was claimed, would be to the great disadvantage of those whose title was 'Mr' rather than 'Dr', although the latter, as Dr J.Y. Warren pointed out, 'would be more likely to come to me for attention to broken arms and legs and disordered stomachs than for treatment of their teeth'. Pickerill's desire to remove the word 'Dentist' from any announcement was clearly viewed as ridiculous, and he also received no support in his further attempt to include the Association within the British Dental Association.

Meanwhile, at the 1909 meeting, Davies had proposed Pickerill for the position of Secretary despite his criticism of the inadequacy of the BDA–NZDA information at the meeting, and despite not knowing whether Pickerill would accept. Referring to the Association's legal actions against unregistered practitioners, he added 'He is a man who is an organiser, and if there were any prosecutions wanted you could not have a keener man for prosecuting'. The meeting was very likely influenced in its decision to appoint Pickerill by his major paper on dental education,[6] also read at the conference by Hunter. Davies was elected Treasurer, and Armstrong was elected President. Armstrong accepted the position at the time, but he did not serve the full term and was replaced by Hunter.

Pickerill was to prove a hard-working and effective Secretary until he resigned to go overseas early in 1917. Then, as now, the Executive of the Association had a busy schedule, and no doubt the main workload was borne by the Secretary. Matters handled by the Executive over a short period included a deputation to the Registrar of the University of New Zealand regarding the recognition of the American DDS degree; the suggested incorporation of the Association; a review of the ethics of lists of dentists appearing in the telephone directory; the question of the formation of a Defence Union, a topic vigorously pursued by Davies; attempts to organise the Association throughout the country by persuading local societies to become properly constituted branches of the Association; and the care of children's teeth. The prosecution of illegal practitioners was a recurring and no doubt very time-consuming theme.[7]

The 1910 conference in Dunedin certainly proved a busy one for Pickerill, not only in his role as Secretary, but also because the conference was centred on the Dental School. The annual meeting had no sooner opened than he was in the midst of a debate on the interpretation of the Rules and how they could be changed, followed by a debate on the decision of the Senate on the recognition of overseas qualifications; he reported on the status of the application for incorporation of the Association, and took part in the debate on the listing of dentists in telephone directories,[8] a contentious ethical matter until the 1980s when relaxation of guidelines allowed advertising in the *Yellow Pages*.

Pickerill also led the discussion on the possibility of including dentists in the proposed Medical Practitioners Bill, which, as it stood, would result in the medical profession being controlled by a board with the same functions as the Medical Council in Great Britain. Pickerill argued that:

> The present position was most autocratic and most unsatisfactory. The Dental profession was at present under the thumb of the Minister of Internal Affairs, a man who was avowedly antagonistic to their interests, and who stated that they had formed themselves into a close corporation simply for the purpose of raising the fees. To be under the thumb of such a man, who could strike any of them off the register without appeal, was most unsatisfactory.

The chances of including dentists in the Bill were remote, not least because the Medical Association itself was doubtful about the proposition, but Pickerill pressed on. The subsequent debate was one-sided – a strong argument against the motion was that doctors were indifferent to dentists in many places in the country and, to the despair of Dental Association members, commonly referred patients to unregistered practitioners. Despite his lonely but vigorous defence, Pickerill conceded that the motion would be lost, reiterating the need for a mechanism to suppress 'quackery'. The situation in one form or another would continue for many years, for the Dental Council of New Zealand was not established until the passing of the Dentists Act, 1936.

The members must have been satisfied with the work of their Secretary, for he was re-elected and his work was praised by retiring President and colleague Thomas Hunter, who had been elected to the newly created position of Chairman of the Executive. Frank Throp completed the strong Dunedin executive team when he was elected Treasurer in place of Davies.

Another item to rumble on for many years was raised at the 1910 conference – the acceptance of the Toronto degree of Doctor of Dental Surgery. The Executive had declined to admit to membership Dr J.F. Yule of Invercargill, on the grounds that his was the DDS from Trinity, a Toronto college that admitted without examination dentists registered anywhere in the Empire to the DDS of the University of Toronto. Although there was uncertainty at the meeting whether Dr Yule's degree was indeed from Trinity and whether he had undertaken course work at the University of Toronto, the Executive decided he could not be a member of the Association while he displayed the degree and used the title. The Southland Dental Association had staunchly supported its highly respected member to the extent that it would remain a 'local association' and not a branch, even though all its other members were also members of the New Zealand Dental Association. The Association's stand on the matter was based on the perceived unfairness of a dentist calling himself 'Doctor' without having undertaken any advanced training whatsoever. Some members had American doctorates from reputable schools such as the University of Pennsylvania, although even with these the impression was that the training, mostly over three years, was not as rigorous as New Zealand's own Bachelor of Dental Surgery. The real concern, though, was the Toronto DDS degree which, it was claimed, could be obtained *ad eundem gradum* – without any course work, just the payment of a fee and the submission of evidence of registration in the applicant's own country. Such a situation was anathema to Pickerill, who believed it undermined the standing of his own school and mocked efforts to raise admission and examination standards. In this he was strongly supported by Hunter and others associated with the School.

The Toronto doctorate affair continued to haunt the Executive over the succeeding year, for at the next annual meeting, Hunter moved that 'the use of the degree of D.D.S. Toronto *ad eundem gradum* ... is sufficient to constitute a breach of Rule 10'. The motion was passionately seconded by Pickerill who described the degree as '... very poor, weak, and almost valueless ... from my point of view I think we should take strong action and show our unqualified dissatisfaction with the granting of such degrees by refusing to receive the holders of them in an Association of this sort'. He quoted from the Regulations for the degree – 'all legally qualified practitioners of dental surgery of Great Britain, or of any portion of the British Empire, will be admitted to the final examination without passing their matriculation and without further attendance at lectures'.[9]

The opposition was led immediately by Warren (the father of a future dean, J. Le B. Warren), speaking for the Auckland branch, which had previously voted to support continuing membership for the holders of the degree. He called for charity and forgiveness for men who had made mistakes in their professional conduct. He also recognised the distinction between the Toronto degree and that obtained from 'reputable American colleges' (Warren's own doctorate was from Pennsylvania). Davies suggested the problem would be solved if the holders agreed to drop the use of the title, albeit over a period of time so that their patients would not be alarmed at a sudden apparent loss of prestige. The debate ebbed and flowed, always in an objective manner, with great concern for the members affected, who apparently numbered just three at the time. In his reply, however, Hunter was more personal and outspoken:

> We ask these men not to be so terribly selfish as to say 'You the whole of the members of this Association must alter your rules, your ideas, and your ethics for three men'. I consider it gigantic selfishness on the part of these men to ask such a thing. I say it is moral cowardice on our part if we do not take a stand and say you shall not do this thing. We cannot regard it simply from the point of view that these men are jolly good fellows and say 'We do not think they ought to do this sort of thing, but it is here we plead for charity.' It is a question of principle versus expediency. It is an easy matter to slide down and hope that

> perhaps nothing of the kind will happen again; but it may happen again and that is what I am looking to. I want nothing of this sort to ever occur again.

This long debate at the 1911 annual meeting ranks as one of the most eloquent and thoughtful in the history of the Association, conducted with restraint and without rancour, although it did not achieve the result Hunter and Pickerill wanted – it was lost by twenty votes. Now that the holders of this particular degree had been endorsed as members of the Association, Dr Yule was eligible for admission, and not long afterwards, in 1912, the Southland Dental Association became the Southland Branch of the national Association. But the matter of the American doctorate was not yet over, for it was to surface again in 1913.

Petitions of unregistered 'dentists' to gain registration caused the Association and its Executive great anguish over a long period. Pickerill was a leader in the skirmishes to defeat once and for all the entry into the profession by the 'back door.'[10] The Act of 1904 had allowed those who had been in practice 'as a dentist' for three years prior to November 1904 to be registered without examination. By 1911, over six years later, applicants were still coming forward expecting to be registered under this provision, submitting affidavits that they were engaged in the practice of dentistry between 1901 and 1904. The Executive strenuously opposed almost all these applications, claiming that, during the specified time, one applicant was a housepainter, one a cycle expert, and another a monumental mason.[11] Other latecomers were required to sit an examination set by an examining board in Wellington, and the Executive demanded of the Board of Examiners that it set an examination at the same standard as the final examination of the BDS degree. In a curious lapse in his otherwise unwavering commitment to the Dental School and the need for high standards of training, Sidey supported the Dentists Amendment Act (1911) in Parliament.[12]

Even these legislative concessions were insufficient for those still fighting to gain registration, as a further Dentists Amending Act was passed just a year later.[13] Pickerill commented in his January 1912 *Journal* editorial that 'forsooth, a few incompetents are unable to pass the Board examination in the already extended time, and heigh presto, the wires are pulled, and the Ministerial hand again opens the back door to our profession for whose elevation we have been striving these many years!' The Act extended the time for candidates to sit the examination (without course study) until September 1912; if they fail at that attempt, Pickerill asked, what happens then? 'If the Minister for Internal Affairs [the Honourable D. Buddo] is still in possession of that portfolio, we have to look forward to still another amendment, for the Government have so frequently promised finality in this matter, that we have ceased to expect it from them; it would seem that the only finality we can hope for is a change of Government.' He went on to further criticise the Minister:

> We [presumably speaking for the Executive] believe, too, that the Minister for Internal Affairs treated the Board of Examiners with scant courtesy after the last examination, and we very much doubt whether, after having broken faith with the dental profession in the manner in which he has done, he or anyone else will find it possible to secure the services of any self-respecting medical or dental practitioners to act on an Examining Board which is told, almost as plainly as possible, that the candidates have to be passed.[14]

This was plain speaking indeed, but at that time, toward the end of Sir Joseph Ward's Liberal Government, when industrial discontent was growing, the Government may have felt that the elite profession of dentistry should not continue as a perceived 'closed shop'. Subsequently, at the 1912 annual meeting, Maurice Denniston, one of the Wellington members of the Council and a future president of the Association, reported that he and Arthur Hoby, a past president, had lobbied the Minister and other Government members to vote against the Bill. At that time, Denniston noted, 'members lacked the moral courage to do anything. They were at the end of the session and they could not see their way clear to block any business. They wanted to get away to the elections. That is the real reason why the Dental Amendment Bill went through.'[15] The Government lost the forthcoming election, and William Massey, leader of the Reform Party, became Prime Minister. Speaking to the annual report at the 1912 annual meeting, Hunter was optimistic that the new Government, 'composed of educated men who will listen to reason, and will not have their minds made up before you lay a matter before them', would not allow further amendments and back-door entry. Unfortunately this did not end the matter, and registration problems were to persist for some years yet.

The 1912 report confirmed Pickerill's contribution to the business of the Association. During the previous twelve months the Council of the Association had met eighteen times. The Secretary had attended all meetings. Membership stood at 269, less than half of all registered dentists, a distinct disadvantage to the Association in negotiations with Government and in its image with the public – dentistry was hardly a united voice. The Council was pleased to report that all local societies were now legally constituted branches of the Association, this important result having been gained, after 'prolonged negotiations', much of which, it might be expected, had fallen to the Secretary. The 'satisfactory' financial report would show that the balance in hand was £290 15s 6d, but outstanding subscriptions totalled £385 12s 6d – a ratio that would appal any present-day treasurer. Davies would have been pleased the Association now had an indemnity scheme, although not in the form he had advocated. The Executive had authorised three prosecutions against unregistered practitioners during the year, and had 'taken steps' regarding the examination and treatment of the teeth of the Territorial Forces, the latter a topic to be pursued vigorously by both Hunter and Pickerill.

A great deal of discussion occurred at the 1912 conference about the state of children's oral health, and Pickerill, in his roles as Dean, Secretary of the Association, Editor and, by now, an international authority on dental caries, was deeply involved, politically and publicly. At this time, the Association was united in its agitation for recognition of the problem, but later became embroiled in controversy over the means by which the treatment needs of children could be managed. The events leading up to that point and the outcome for Pickerill are described later, but it should be noted here that the Association's Secretary and Editor made important contributions in raising the awareness of the profession, the public, and the politicians to the appalling state of the oral health of the nation's children.

The recognition of foreign degrees again became a topic of importance for the Executive in 1912, when Warren, noting that 'Last year there was rather an unpleasant time for all of us over the question', pointed out that the matter had not closed – he had learnt of a college in America that was issuing a DDS degree after just one year of study. In ten or twelve years, he believed, New Zealand could have great numbers of such graduates 'with degrees that we cannot respect, and the public cannot respect'. Hunter, as Chairman of the Executive, brought to the next (1913) annual meeting an addition to the Rules whereby the Association would only recognise foreign degrees issued by a reputable college that had a curriculum of three years. In proposing the motion, he must have come close to offending Warren, for he concluded:

> Now, it might seem that there was always the old sort of feeling that he was up against the Americans, but what he wanted to point out was that some of the American training was not of a character that they should countenance. They had men going to America simply for advertising purposes. We were British, and ought to go on British lines. The degree given in America was not worth the name of doctor. They had no curriculum there worth the degree of doctorship.[16]

Pickerill drew applause for his defence of New Zealand's own four-year course. He felt it was 'unfair and unjust' that they should impose certain conditions on the product of their own country, and not at the same time impose the same conditions on students from other countries:

> any practitioner coming from elsewhere, should, at least, have gone through a similar curriculum to our college ... Here we had a bachelorship, and a mastership before a doctorate, because the doctorate should be for work done after graduation and show ability in research work.
>
> He thought a man would spend his time more profitably and they would honour him far more, if he took a four years' course and then went to America and took a special course of training, and devoted his time to advancing his real knowledge, but it was not logical, and not fair to our students that a man could go to America and get a degree inferior to our own, and then compete with our home-trained practitioners on terms of equality.

The next speaker churned up the meeting by stating he had never heard of an American degree which did not have solid teaching behind it. He failed to see 'why this Association, which consisted largely of men of no degrees at all ... should spread its tail in the air, and say "We won't recognise you, because you came a little later than we did"'. He did not see the Association as others did – the 'be-all and end-all of everything'. The Immediate Past President, J.N. Rishworth, calmed things down, but the debate ebbed and flowed on various grounds, including whether Canada, being 'British', counted as foreign, and what happened when successive years of training were taken at different colleges, as was apparently common. Pickerill reminded the meeting of the need to conserve the interests of their own students, but seemed reasonably content with the final motion, 'That this Association recognise only outside degrees issued by a reputable dental college after three consecutive years, from and after this date'.

This was an extremely busy period in Pickerill's career. Not only was he heavily committed to the Association as its Secretary and Editor, and to the University as Dean of the Faculty of Dentistry, but his caries research was coming to fruition, and he was becoming increasingly interested in international dentistry – he chaired a New Zealand committee planning for the Panama–Pacific Dental Congress to be held in 1915 in San Francisco. The oral health of children gathered momentum as a major initiative of the Association, and he was a member of a deputation to the Ministers of Education and Public Health in July 1913. At this time, leading up to the First World War, the Association was also advocating a dental service for the Territorial Force that was soon to involve Pickerill and Hunter as prime movers of what became the New Zealand Dental Corps after the outbreak of war. As if in anticipation of his future role in the repair of wartime facial injuries, he had a growing number of publications in the fields of fractures of the jaws and in cleft lip ('hare lip') and palate. All this, as well as his routine teaching and administration of the School and Dental Hospital, represented an enormous load, which he seemed able to bear efficiently and effectively.

Some of this load was temporarily relieved for several months by D.V. Donaldson, who became Acting Secretary, and R.B. Cape-Williamson, as Acting Editor, when, in March 1914, Pickerill had sabbatical leave, and he and Hunter attended the Sixth International Dental Congress in London. On behalf of the New Zealand Dental Association, Pickerill applied for recognition of the Association and the appointment of one representative on the Executive Council of the International Dental Federation, in which the Association has had distinguished commitment ever since. The outbreak of war no doubt shortened this trip, for he was back in New Zealand by September 1914.

Conferences were not held in 1914 and 1915, but the 1916 meeting was a busy one for the Secretary. The Association was determined to tidy up once and for all the ongoing problem of practice by unregistered practitioners. To achieve this goal, the Association adopted the motion that 'No person, unless registered under the Dental Act of New Zealand, shall carry on the practice of dentistry; and the N.Z.D.A. be urged to have the Act amended to safeguard the interests of the public'.[17] In effect this was a despairing move, as only dentists already on the Register were legally entitled to practise as dentists – the problem was enforcement of the law rather than the law itself.

This was Pickerill's last conference as Secretary, a position he had held with distinction.

Pickerill as Editor

The *New Zealand Dental Journal* was founded at the inaugural meeting and conference of the New Zealand Dental Association, and the first issue, July 1905, appeared just a month later. The first Editor was Wellington dentist William Ernest Lowe, LDSRCS(Eng), DDS(University of Pennsylvania). In addition to his own practice, Lowe was the co-principal, with W.H. Didsbury, of the Wellington School of Dental Therapy, which provided formal courses for candidates preparing for the examinations of the Wellington Board of Examiners.

Lowe set the style for future issues of the *Journal* for many years – editorials on topical issues, papers presented at conferences, news from branches of the Association, personal items, brief notices of general and clinical interest, letters to the editor, and professional advertisements. Early records of the Association were destroyed by fire, so the custom of publishing very full, almost verbatim, reports of discussions at annual general meetings, minutes of meetings of the Executive Council, and reports of other important meetings and delegations to the Government meant that the *Journal* became the archives of the Association. Original articles were encouraged, but their frequency proved to be erratic, and reprints of papers published in other journals were common. Reports of court proceedings, generally related to practice of unqualified persons or involving recovery of unpaid accounts, were no doubt of great interest to readers at that time, as they are now to readers of those early issues.

Dr Lowe edited the *Journal* until the January 1908 issue, when he left New Zealand. He was succeeded by Didsbury, who maintained the same high standard. The event that cut short Didsbury's term was probably the debate following the proposal at the conference in January 1909 that the Editor should be a member of the Association's Executive. The tone of the discussion suggested that the Executive wanted to rein in the Editor to ensure that items in the *Journal* were always in accordance with Association policies. The issue of March 1909 still shows Didsbury as Editor, but it had no editorial; it is likely that Pickerill, just appointed Secretary, had stepped in and was responsible for it. The May 1909 issue bears his name as Editor. Keeping the *Journal* under control, if that had been the problem, had been solved by the Secretary being appointed Editor.

Pickerill was the first of three deans of the Dental School – the others being Professors Sir John Walsh and John Le B. Warren – to hold the position. He brought some changes in style: the editorial was no longer placed at the front of each issue, and the month and year were removed from the running head on each page, the latter a frustration to those searching bound volumes for particular articles. He later changed the numbering system so that the issues were numbered cumulatively rather than 'No. 1' being the first issue of each volume. This system continued until 2003, when the newly appointed Editor, Alan Roddick, commented: 'With the current issue, Volume 99, No. 1, March 2003, we are returning to the system which was lost 92 years ago'. Roddick thus broke the link back to Pickerill, but reintroduced the original style.

A notable new feature of Pickerill's first issue was the appearance of book reviews. O.V. Davies reviewed *Otago Medical and Dental Schools' Pharmacopoeia* by Pickerill and Dr Falconer, Resident Medical Officer at Dunedin Hospital. The reviews of *Diet and Dietetics* by a Dr Sutherland, and *Notes on Practical Physiology* by John Malcolm, Otago's own Professor of Physiology, were both unsigned, but were probably written by the Editor himself. Another new section, 'Miscellanea', contained comments on 'Oral sepsis and its dangers', which reported the death of a dentist after being bitten by a patient, and an item of dental interest from the Annual General Meeting of the British Medical Association. These features reflected the more academic and international approach of the new university-based Editor, who would have had greater access to developments overseas than did his predecessors in private practice. Who, if anyone, assisted him with the *Journal* is not known, although it would be surprising if he did not seek assistance in various aspects of its preparation – Davies, who nominated Pickerill for Secretary of the Association, could very likely have helped, despite the testiness between the two men.

The work involved in some issues was enormous. For example, the July 1910 issue contained the first part of the report of the Sixth Annual Meeting of the Association, which ran to over twenty pages of closely set, small print. Presumably the huge responsibility for preparation of this report (and a further four pages, albeit in larger type, in the following issue) was borne by the Secretary, who, as Editor, then had to ready it for publishing.

The printer during Pickerill's time as Editor was John McIndoe of Dunedin, a family firm that served the Association well over many years, including printing T.W.H. Brooking's *A History of Dentistry in New Zealand* in 1980. McIndoes would no doubt have provided proof-reading services, although the standard slipped in Pickerill's third issue, October 1909, which contained many typographical errors.

Pickerill did not hesitate to use the pages of the *Journal* to push his own agenda. Generally, because he was also the Association's Secretary, this was in accordance with the Association's policies. On some matters, however, he used editorial and secretarial privilege to attempt to move the Association faster and further than it was prepared to go. Nevertheless, during his time as Editor he enjoyed the complete confidence of the Association. His editorials were always respected and frequently applauded. Some of them deserve particular mention. His first was an impassioned plea for action over the dreadful state of oral health of children,[19] a topic he returned to on other occasions, it being a matter of intense concern of the Association as it fought to involve the Government in providing a public health service.

His belief in the need for a strong association came through in 'Organisation' (October 1909).[20] He called for unity in the profession, urged all registered dentists to join the Association, and encouraged all local dental societies to become branches. The theme of unity also came through in 'The parting of the ways' (March 1910), in which he commented on the move to biennial rather than annual conferences. This change did not occur, but he used this opportunity to appeal once again for strength in the Association – 'we must at all costs have unanimity on our ideals and in our actions'.[21] Unfortunately, he himself was to ignore this ideal when attacking plans for the School Dental Service after the First World War.

Education was another major theme in his editorials. In the January 1910 issue he praised the dissolution of the Wellington and Dunedin Boards of

Examiners, and applauded dental education being now entrusted entirely to the University of New Zealand. He contrasted the New Zealand scene with that in New South Wales, where the equivalent board seemed to work in opposition to the University of Sydney – here in New Zealand the bodies 'worked amicably with the University authorities, and did everything to facilitate the transference of their powers to the Senate …'.[22] Unfortunately his applause was premature, for 'back-door' entry into the profession was to continue for many years. He vented his frustration, and that of the Association, when, in the issue of October the same year,[23] he deplored the continuing efforts of unqualified persons to force themselves onto the Register. He returned to it in the next issue with eloquent passion:

> With supreme contempt for the advice of this Association, utterly regardless of the representations made by deputations, by circulars, by letters and telegrams from all Dental Societies in the Dominion, and ignoring the *real facts*, the Government have amended the 'Dentists' Act' of 1904, and we are practically back again to where we were at the beginning of 1905. Five years gone by the board, and all in the name of 'justice' forsooth! Where, may we ask is the justice to the public in allowing untrained men to practice upon them? Where is the justice to those students who complied with the law and took the full degree course at the Dental School? Where is the justice to the dental profession which subscribed £1,000 in order that students might be trained in full assurance that the Government would make such training compulsory?[24]

This was Pickerill at his very best – righteous indignation, broad targets to attack, flowing language, even a classical reference to 'Scylla and Charybdis' to reinforce the argument. He published the Parliamentary debate on the Dentists Amendment Bill in full in the same issue.

The 1910 annual meeting of the Association had resolved that 'all persons holding the Board of Examiners' certificate, and who are on the New Zealand Dental Register, be permitted to sit for the final B.D.S. examination (*sine curriculo*)'. The purpose was to give those who had qualified for registration prior to the Dental School being established the opportunity to gain the BDS. The situation was contrasted with those who gained a three-year degree overseas and then were permitted to sit the examination for the degree without further study. The matter was raised again at the 1911 annual meeting by a member who sought the outcome of the previous meeting's request that the Secretary apply to the University Senate to allow registered dentists '… to get the B.D.S. (*sine curriculo*) of the University of New Zealand'.[26] Pickerill, no doubt wearing his dean's hat at this point, corrected the speaker for not mentioning that passing the final BDS examination was a requirement in the original motion – applicants had to prove they were worthy of the degree.

Hunter announced that the Executive had considered the matter but, being sure there was no chance of success, had not pursued it further. In '*Sine Curriculo* Degrees', a well-reasoned and positive editorial in the same issue in which this discussion was published, Pickerill very carefully explained the situation in other countries, and stated 'Should such a degree be instituted, we may take it as a *sine qua non* that an examination of sufficient standard would be insisted upon to safeguard the interests of the graduates *cum curriculo*'.[27] Pickerill himself would have nothing to do with a move that would undermine the status and quality of the BDS programme.

In the July 1911 issue he took his impatience over several issues to a new dimension, not entered by preceding or subsequent editors. He urged members to take advantage of the forthcoming general election by seeking from candidates their views on three major topics of the day – the dental inspection of schoolchildren, the training of primary school teachers in 'dental prophylaxis', that is, education on oral health, and the appointment of dental surgeons to the Territorial Forces. After calling for dentists to '… sink personal feeling, opinions, and dislikes, and unite for the welfare of the race – let this spark of patriotism unite the dental profession throughout the Dominion, and we shall become an *irresistible force*', he implored dentists to:

> assert our rights and privileges; hitherto it would seem to have been anybody's privilege to trample with impunity on the dental profession. Is this to continue? Or are we now to make it quite clear and apparent that the Dental Association is a power of good in the land, and one neither to be despised nor neglected?
>
> … let it be clearly understood that unless the candidate is prepared to support such measures for the welfare of the community, no vote will be forthcoming on their behalf.[28]

But the profession continued to be trampled upon, for yet another Amending Act was passed in 1911 to extend the allowable period for 'back-door' entry. This brought forth another stinging editorial in January 1912, as mentioned previously.

Overall, the *Journal* prospered during Pickerill's tenure, but criticism surfaced at the 1911 annual meeting. R.B. Cape-Williamson (Christchurch) wanted to 'pass a few remarks' about the *Journal*, and he hoped they would be taken in the spirit in which they were intended, namely as a friendly criticism. He thought the *Journal* was not giving 'full accounts of their Association all over the Dominion'.

> His chief objection to the Journal was the re-production of papers from other magazines. Were they so unoriginal that they could not scrape up a paper from their own men from the North Cape to the Bluff. In one Journal they had a

> reprint of Dr Stuart Moore's paper delivered in Dunedin 13 months ago. Did the Editor not get any papers from local Societies? He had sent down papers read at his Branch, and they had not been published, including the presidential address. He wanted to hear through the Journal what the Auckland men were doing, and he supposed they wanted to know what the Christchurch fellows were doing. He had a suggestion from Wellington for personal notes, and he had gone to infinite pains to get personal tit-bits of interest to other members, but they had been ignored. He thought it would be a good idea to have a social page, and he was sure members would appreciate it. He thought the Editor should consider local papers. They might not be up in the very first rank of dental science so far as work was concerned, but they had some original ideas, and they must come out in papers. He would also point out that there was no statement of assets and liabilities to show how they stood.[29]

In his patient but deliberate response, the Editor described for the meeting some of the same difficulties that were to trouble his successors down the years. Although he was delighted the members were taking sufficient interest in the *Journal* to criticise it, he had previously expressed disappointment at the lack of any opinion either for or against the *Journal*. 'One could not please everybody, but if one knew the general feeling one could aim at that'. He went on:

> Mr Cape-Williamson apparently did not realise the difficulty and trouble he [Pickerill] had in getting reports from the various branches. He had to write and write for them. Notices also appeared in the *Journal* asking for reports on the first of the month, but he never remembered a single case since he had been Editor, of a report having been sent in without being asked for; and usually when it did come in response to his requests, usually it was a scrappy little report. Well, that was their fault and not his. If they knew the Editor's work, they would know it only made his heart rejoice to see copy come in.

Pickerill apologised if he had published articles that readers had already seen, but his idea in publishing abstracts from other journals was to bring to readers information that he did not think would be read in this country. Because of the volume of material presented at conferences, he could not publish everything in only four issues per year. Referring to the suggestion of a 'personal column', he made his objections clear to the meeting:

> he thought it would be degrading to a professional magazine, and no magazine which had an official standing like theirs should descend to that sort of thing: as long as he was Editor, nothing of that sort would go in. He should be only too pleased to put in original articles from anybody and everybody, but he did ask members of branches to write good papers for the local Associations, and send them down to him. The Auckland people were the only people who were keeping up-to-date with their papers, and he got them in as soon as he could.

Claude Moses, Secretary of the Auckland Dental Association and a future president of the national Association, then congratulated the Editor on the improvements that had been made since he had taken the *Journal* in hand. He certainly thought it was conducted on good lines and well worthy of perusal – not exactly a ringing endorsement, but it brought the spat to an end.

Cape-Williamson had a further attempt at changing the style of the *Journal* at the 1912 annual meeting. He wanted the Association 'to do something with the huge balance', that is, £290, and he would like to see the *Journal* brought out every two months rather than quarterly.[30] He constructively suggested that each branch should set up a small committee to get material for submission to the Editor. He repeated his earlier suggestion of including small personal items about dentists, and a practical hints column. He asked what had happened to items sent from a Christchurch study club, but nothing had been published.

The Editor rose to this latest challenge. He was scathing about what could become 'paragraphs to the effect that Mr. So and So is the proud father of twins, or that Mr. So and So is enjoying some fishing at Rotorua'. He rightly refused to be drawn into public discussion about why a particular article was not accepted for publication, and was critical of the study club mentioned by Cape-Williamson; he believed that if he published its material, he would be doing a disservice to the local branch. His duty was to publish, firstly, papers and work done by the Association, and secondly, to publish independent articles which would be of interest to the Association. 'If I were short of Association material, and had not any brilliant abstract matter, I should be quite willing to insert material from the Weddelstadt Searle Study Club, or any other club …'. He strongly supported the suggestion of a two-monthly journal, 'But that is only practicable if the local Branches will yield more papers and send them for publication. Unless the Branches do that the Journal will become the Journal of the Auckland Branch pure and simple', the latter comment referring back to the strong support received from that branch. After another member spoke in support of the Christchurch study club, the meeting quickly moved on to other business.

Under Pickerill's guidance the *Journal* was generally error-free, but with one notable exception – the July 1910 issue bore the heading that it was the July 1909 issue, this unfortunately coming immediately above the black-bordered tribute to the passing of King Edward VII – 'The Passing of Edward, *Rex et Imperator*'. After August 1914, the war and the dental profession were dominant subjects of Pickerill's editorials through to his last issue, which was either September or November 1916. These strongly patriotic editorials reflect, no doubt, the views of the Association, but they would certainly have positioned him for the significant role he was soon to play in the Dental Corps.

Davies edited the January 1917 issue, and A.M. Carter then took up the appointment with the March 1917 issue. Thus ended Pickerill's seven years as Editor of the *Journal*. In this role he further displayed his characteristic qualities of intense commitment, superb organisational skills that enabled him to manage multiple tasks, and facility of language that allowed him to identify and evaluate major issues in forceful and elegant prose.

His services as Editor and Secretary were greatly appreciated by the Association, but looming on the horizon, beyond the more immediate development of his surgical expertise in the care of facial injuries, was the post-war furore over what was to become the School Dental Service. This was eventually to result in his censure by, and resignation from, the New Zealand Dental Association. In 1917, however, he left New Zealand for war service, highly respected by a grateful Association.

9

War service in New Zealand, 1914–1917

New Zealand's dental profession is proud, and rightly so, of the dental care of those in the armed forces. The Dental Association, even before the outbreak of the First World War, persistently and forcefully advocated for soldiers to have good dental care – one cannot be effective in battle while suffering toothache. The New Zealand Dental Corps, subsequently the Royal New Zealand Dental Corps, has a long and distinguished history, and has set world standards for the provision of oral health services for the forces. Pickerill was in the vanguard of the campaign leading to the formation of the Corps.

Support for the concept of Empire and national patriotism was running high when the Liberal Government brought in the 1909 Defence Act, which established a territorial force to be recruited by means of compulsory military training. Although not universally popular, the outcome was that New Zealand had almost 60,000 trained soldiers by 1914.[1]

The Dental Association was involved from the outset – it wanted to act patriotically, but it was also upset that doctors, not dentists, were providing dental examinations for recruits. The 1911 annual meeting learned that 'medical men were already examining the teeth of cadets and were getting paid two shillings and sixpence per cadet …'. A large number of cadets were being rejected owing to the shocking state of their teeth. Davies moved, strongly supported by Hunter, who was eventually to command what became the Dental Corps, 'That, in the opinion of this Association, it is eminently desirable that dental surgeons should be appointed to the Territorial Forces on the same basis as surgeons; and further, that such dental surgeons should necessarily be commissioned officers'. Before the motion was carried and left in the hands of the Executive to bring before the Government, Denniston warned 'if there was going to be any expense in this respect, he was afraid the Government would shut down on it. He had reason to believe that when the Bill came in it would prove a regular staggerer.'[2]

Although most notably honoured for his care of New Zealand troops with facial injuries during the second half of the First World War, Pickerill, as Secretary of the Association, was involved from the start in establishing general dental services for men in training. War was declared on 4 August 1914 when he was in London for the International Dental Congress. He volunteered for active service the following day and was immediately appointed Honorary Civil Surgeon to the Bristol Engineers.[3] This appointment was brief, for by September he would have been back in New Zealand – the hard-hitting style of the editorial in that issue of the *Journal* suggests it was written by Pickerill rather than his acting editor. The editorial stated that the profession had good reason to congratulate itself on what had already been achieved in the few weeks since war had been declared.

> To our knowledge, and we speak under correction, this is the first time, in a British dependency at least, that the mouths of the troops have been regarded with so much official care, and have actually had officers appointed for the sole purpose of attending to any trouble that might eventuate in connection with those organs.[4]

Already dentists had been appointed to the military, with a commissioned officer posted to each troopship. The editorial went on to comment on the appalling state of the mouths of recruits, and pointed out that if the regulations concerning teeth were strictly adhered to, the number of men going overseas would be very small. The writer linked this with a cry that perhaps now the Government and the public would realise the seriousness of the oral health problem in the country. He deplored the 'scandal' of inadequate equipment and materials available to dental officers, who were forced to 'pay for indispensable items out of his own exchequer'. The result was an inefficient service, but his novel yet practical solution – that dental officers have their own accounts at supply houses – was soon implemented by the authorities.

The speed of mobilisation seems remarkable, even though preparation for war had been underway in Britain and in the Empire for some time. Just weeks after war was declared, New Zealand soldiers, accompanied by dental officers, were already heading overseas. But dental services at this early stage remained primitive, and urgent action was required.

Such urgency was apparent when the Auckland Branch, at a special meeting on 12 August, decided to offer treatment at no cost to the Auckland contingent in New Zealand's Expeditionary Force. Every member present agreed to devote a whole week to providing this care. The branch also noted that B.S. Finn, had been commissioned – thus began the distinguished career of a future Director of Dental Services in the armed forces.[5]

The following issues of the *Journal*, still edited by Pickerill, traced his and the Association's role in the foundation of the Dental Corps. One decision of the Executive seems now to be a quaint reminder that motorised army transport was very much in the early development phase:

> The Chairman of the Executive [Hunter], after consultation over the telephone with the other Executive members, wired Branch representatives, suggesting that funds for the purchase of two horses be donated. Favourable replies were received, and it was resolved that the sum of sixty pounds be donated for the purchase of two horses, at thirty pounds a-piece. One horse to be sent from each Island. A telegram was received later from Lieutenant Colonel Reakes, Director of Remounts, advising that the Minister of Defence highly appreciated the generous offer.[6]

The Executive also reported progress in upgrading dental services.

> The President of the Association and the Executive have been in touch with the Minister of Defence and the Comptroller General of Medical Supplies, and as a result of representation definite promises have been given, as follows:–
>
> 1. Dentists to be appointed to every contingent.
>
> 2. The honorary rank of Lieutenant conferred, with attached pay.
>
> 3. The sum of £50 allotted to each man for dental outfit.
>
> 4. For the future, appointments not to be made without the Executive being consulted as to the qualifications of applicants.
>
> The President, Mr. Carter, has been especially energetic, and a great deal of praise is due to him for the expeditious manner in which he arranged matters for the welfare of the troops as regards dental treatment. The following telegram was sent by the Chairman of the Executive through Mr. Denniston, to the dental surgeons attached to the Expeditionary force:–
>
> 'The Executive Council, on behalf of the Association, wishes God speed and safe return to members going to the front. Hopes each man will prove value of dentists with Forces.'[7]

The reason for the Association to be consulted by the Government before dental officers were appointed was to ensure only suitably qualified dentists would be selected, but it also excluded non-members. The Association was thus in a position of great strength and influence in the direction and personnel of the fledgling Dental Corps. Advantages to the Government, however, would have been confidence that only capable men would be appointed, and no risk of rivalry or animosity between members and non-members in service at home or overseas. The obvious body to which the Government could turn was the Association, there being no other with the expertise and organisational skills to advise and lead. The Association made the most of the opportunity, and to its great credit, the outcome was eventually a largely efficient and well-organised unit.

Pickerill maintained intense pressure on the Government to improve dental care for servicemen. In January 1915 he reiterated the serious situation of oral ill health as the main cause of rejection from the services, and the unsatisfactory method of examination, and he deplored the continuing dental examination of recruits by doctors.

> The point is this – Can a medical man say just exactly from the necessarily hurried examination he must give of the mouth, and without a special dental knowledge, what constitutes a good dentition? … A dentist could almost tell at a glance whether the mouth was all right. Can a medical man?[8]

He argued that only the trained dentist could adequately assess the mouth for sepsis, and appealed for dentists to be appointed to each recruitment centre. He also sensibly suggested that, because so many recruits were rejected on dental grounds, the dental examination should come first – only when they had passed the dental examination would they move on to the medical examination.

Through Pickerill's writings, the Association continued to express frustration with the slow developments, although viewed ninety years later, remarkable progress was made from a zero base. By May 1915, fifteen dentists were serving in their professional capacities with the Expeditionary Force. Ten had left with the main body for Egypt; three dentists had accompanied various reinforcements, and two were in camp at Trentham.

But lack of consultation was a sore point – Pickerill complained that, although branches of the Association had been consulted over appointments, consultation should have been with the Executive. In this he seemed to be expressing a personal grievance that he, as Secretary of the Association, was not being consulted on its behalf. He acknowledged, however, that in the 'majority of cases' the branches were being consulted, so the Government was certainly trying.[9]

He continued to stress the unsatisfactory arrangements for dealing with recruits, and he appealed again for the Government to 'appoint dentists with commissions in each recruiting centre to treat those recruits who would otherwise be rejected, or it should ask the New Zealand Dental Association to organise a suitable scheme for such treatment.' He went on emotionally:

> We believe that each member of our Association would be only too glad to 'do his little bit' to enable some man who was willing and able to go to the front, that he might help in the humanitarian task of ridding the world of those traitors and renegades of civilisation who have dragged the respected name of 'German' into the mire of everlasting shame and infamy. We think that a simple scheme might easily be evolved whereby the cost of materials for dental treatment might be met partly by the funds of the Dental Association, and partly by individual members. A man who is prepared to offer his body as a defence and shield for our hearths and homes is not the man we want to take fees from for anything we may be able to do for him.[10]

Treatment of recruits was becoming a major task of the Dental School. A deputation from Dunedin's Recruiting Committee sought help from the Hospital Board, which then asked the University Council if the School would provide free treatment for these men under the current arrangement between the Board and the School.[11] Pickerill pointed out to the Council that the School had been treating rejected recruits for the previous month, all except one being treated free of charge. This resulted in 'considerable disorganisation of work and a loss to the School of at least £50'. Although he agreed that recruits should not have to pay for their treatment, he did not think the University should pay £50 per month. He was also frustrated that, after recruits had been made 'dentally fit', some recruits were not subsequently required.[12] He noted that students had given up holidays and worked late at night for the recruits, but apparent wasted energy resulted in enthusiasm waning. He followed this up by reporting that in Auckland and Christchurch the majority of recruits were being treated at the expense of the Hospital and Charitable Aid Boards; in Wellington, nothing seemed to be done; and in South Canterbury, members of the Dental Association were doing the work at no charge.[13]

The Registrar referred these matters to the Minister of Defence, resulting in the Director of Military Hospitals replying that the matter was receiving attention, and that 'Dr Pickerill and Mr Hunter, representing the New Zealand Dental Association, waited upon the Minister yesterday.' As a result the Ministry hoped that all matters relating to the dental treatment of recruits would be 'placed on a proper footing'.[14]

In addition to the students assisting with treatment of recruits, others were quick to enlist and to serve either as dental officers or in the front line. Pickerill reported to the Faculty that the School was being deeply affected by the war – 'for a comparatively small University Department I think the Dental School has contributed its quota to the defence of the Empire'.[15] Two students were admitted to special final-year examinations in September 1914, enabling their early graduation and commission as lieutenants in the Expeditionary Force.

One student was a non-commissioned officer in the infantry; one a lieutenant in the infantry; and one was serving as a private.

The trials of dentists on active service on Gallipoli were described by Captain J.H. Don, who was constantly involved in the repair of dentures – 'The hard biscuits are playing havoc with the men's dentures, and most broken ones are not worth repairing.' He noted that 'Finn, of Auckland is also here doing all the extractions, but he has a fairly easy time'; Finn may not have agreed with that statement. The pioneering nature of the service being provided was suggested by Don's concluding sentences:

> General Godley [Major–General Sir A.J. Godley, the General Officer commanding the combined New Zealand and Australian Division] comes round and has a look at my work once or twice a week. He expressed himself the last time as very pleased with the excellent work I was doing, and said that it was making history to be doing dental work within a few hundred yards of the enemy. The other day I was visited by five generals altogether, so I am getting quite swelled-headed.[15]

In September 1915, Pickerill optimistically announced in his *Journal* editorial that the Government had accepted the Association's proposals. The Ministers of Public Health and Defence agreed to recognise the members of the Association as part of an 'Official Dental Service for the Troops', and asked the Association to nominate two of its members as supervising officers. Pickerill also appealed to members to accept nominal payment to treat recruits, pending the formation of a fully-fledged dental corps. At present, it was not logistically possible for treatment to be left to the dental officers in the camps – involvement of local dentists was essential, and he called for dentists' support as their patriotic duty. Treatment in the camps was to be re-organised, and the Association offered £100 toward such improvement. The Government doubted this would be required, but it nevertheless was remarkably generous. The cynical view might be, however, that it was part of a public relations campaign to ingratiate further the Association with the Government – other matters were still being pursued, including the care of children, unregistered practitioners, and 'back-door entry'.[17]

The Government's request for the Executive to nominate two persons to the key supervisory positions in the armed forces dental services was a most unusual way of appointing commanding officers, but was certainly practical and effective in this instance. Dentists already serving as commissioned officers were apparently not considered for elevation. Instead, the Government approved the two most senior men in the profession, the Chairman and the Secretary of the Dental Association, on the assumption that they had the necessary stature and administrative experience. The duties of the officers were to

> supply reports upon a very large number of questions affecting the official dental service for the troops. The function of the supervising officers will be to advise the director of military hospitals on all matters relating to the dental service, whether in camps or out of them, to organise details, and to a certain extent to be responsible for their execution.[18]

Pickerill had been commissioned as a territorial captain in the New Zealand Medical Corps (Territorial Force) from 1 June 1915,[19] and was transferred from the New Zealand Medical Corps to the New Zealand Dental Corps from 7 November 1915.[20] Under the section of the *Gazette* relating to the New Zealand Dental Corps, Thomas Anderson Hunter was appointed Director, with the rank of Lieutenant Colonel, and 'Captain Henry Percy Pickerill, from the New Zealand Medical Corps to be Assistant Director, with the rank of Major'. The appointment of J.N. Rishworth, later to be an associate of Pickerill's at Sidcup in England, was announced as Executive Officer with the rank of Major.

Pickerill now had another large responsibility added to those of Dean of the Faculty of Dentistry, Secretary of the Dental Association, and Editor of its *Journal*. His editorials at this time described the significance of further developments, although at times he may have presented a rosier picture than was actually the case. He optimistically viewed the formation of the Dental Corps as an indication of better things to come in the advancement of the public health:

> It is a matter of congratulation for the Association that its long-continued efforts to get the Government to recognise the necessity for State dental treatment on properly organised lines for certain sections of the community have at last begun to come to fruition. …
>
> Given hearty and loyal co-operation between all three sections [administrative, executive, and civilian] of the corps, it should be a complete success; the whole field is covered, no recruit can now say that 'he cannot go, because he can't get his teeth fixed,' and no soldier should leave this country handicapped by septic or deficient teeth. In doing this, the New Zealand Dental Association will have contributed its 'war quota' in full measure. It will be its proud boast that no section of the community has done more, and we doubt whether any other has done or offered so much.[21]

By January 1916 he reported that organisation was well advanced, all recruits were being properly dentally examined by dentists, and many previously rejected men were now being enlisted after treatment. Dental officers had been appointed to practically all recruiting stations, albeit with some difficulty in smaller places. Progress had indeed been substantial:

> Work in the camps is now in full swing. Dental hospitals have been erected at Trentham Camp and Featherston Camp. These are both 'permanent' buildings, and comprise in each case a surgery, a work-room, and a waiting room; water is laid on, and each hospital is quite well equipped. At Trentham and Featherston there is a staff of three officers, a sergeant-mechanic, and two orderlies in each place; and there is accommodation for addition to these staffs should this be necessary. At Maymorn Camp there is one dental officer and a mechanic, and a similar staff at Rangiotu Camp. Awapuni and Narrow Neck Camps, being smaller, have only one dental officer each. …
>
> The motto of the Corps is *'Ex malo bonum'* – Out of evil, good. This we regard as particularly appropriate to the time and occasion, and it might be applied in quite a variety of ways – to make something good out of something bad should be the motto of every member of the corps.[22]

The glowing tone aside, his editorials recorded a truly remarkable achievement, unmatched by any other country, with the possible exception of Canada, which also quickly developed a dental corps. The foundation of the scheme was developed within the Executive Council of the Dental Association, in which Hunter and Pickerill were the prime movers. The inclusion of civilian dentists to provide care for the recruits at the recruiting centres was an imaginative response to the enormous problem of so many being unfit for service because of dental problems.

Up to this point, Pickerill had managed his involvement with the Dental Corps from his Dunedin base. The time came, however, when a more 'hands-on' commitment was necessary. He informed the Chancellor in December 1915 that General Henderson, the Surgeon General, wanted him at Defence Headquarters in Wellington to assist in the organisation and control of the Corps, and trusted 'the Council will have no objection'.[23] Whether he had previously sought approval to accept the role of Assistant Director of the Corps is not recorded, but this may never have occurred to him: a job needed to be done, he was the best person to do it – worry about the implications later. He anticipated the necessary work could be done before the beginning of the next university session in March 1916. The Council granted the leave at its meeting the following day.

As soldiers were being treated in preparation for overseas service, others with disabilities were returning to re-enter civilian life. Their dental care was another aspect of the scheme organised by Hunter and Pickerill, and consultant dental surgeons were appointed to the discharge boards. Each soldier appearing before a board received a dental examination, and prescribed treatment was provided by either a civilian dentist already treating recruits, or by the soldier's own dentist. An itemised price schedule was designated, and the consultants were to be paid 'at the rate of one guinea per Board at which he attends, irrespective of the number of soldiers examined by him'.[24] Davies was involved in this work in Dunedin as an officer in the Dental Corps and described his duties as 'solely of examining, with Major Pickerill, soldiers returning in transports to Dunedin'.[25]

Despite all that had been achieved, and the appeals made to support the scheme as a patriotic duty, complaints about treatment of recruits surfaced at the annual meeting of the Association in May 1916. The criticisms included the level of fees payable to the dentists treating recruits, the scheme being thrust upon members by the Executive, and whether all treatment should be provided in the camps rather than initial treatment being provided in the recruitment centres. Hunter was far from impressed with the emphasis on fees: 'The whole thing was evolved originally from a patriotic point of view ... There were lots of difficulties to overcome, and mistakes made which everybody admitted, but nothing better had yet been suggested. They were forgetting that the effort made was a patriotic one. They were all talking fees, fees, fees.'[26]

Rather surprisingly, this challenge was not resented – rather the opposite, as Hunter's concluding statement: 'I do hope that at this period of our history we will not make the mistake of rejecting this proposal – it would destroy all that we have gained at one swoop' was greeted with applause. The outcome was adoption of a scale of fees to present to the Minister of Defence. The scheme was safe.

An ironic feature of the long, wide-ranging discussion on the subject was that Pickerill, as Secretary of the Association and one of the scheme's founders, had to support the interests of its members, yet as Assistant Director of the Dental Corps had to defend it. Hunter was in a similar situation, as he was still the Chairman of the Executive Council; Rishworth, by now designated an Assistant Director of the Corps, also criticised the scheme. It was a remarkable balancing act, yet the report of the meeting shows that personalities did not intrude and the discussion was constructive and restrained. The election of officers at the conference resulted in Captain Denniston becoming President and Major J.N. Rishworth Chairman of Council – the military continued to have an influential voice in the affairs of the Association. C.H. Moses was elected Secretary, relieving Pickerill of that responsibility.

The Defence authorities perceived the University of Otago as an important source of officer material, and the Medical Unit of the University Officers Training Corps was established. Pickerill became the representative of the

Faculty of Dentistry on the Military Committee which, at its meeting of 10 August 1916, gave power to a subcommittee of members of the Medical and Dental Faculties to arrange parades. In December that year, the Military Committee took up Major Pickerill's suggestion 'that a General Army Order be obtained stating that students who obtained A and B Certificates in the Officer Training Corps should gain preference in the matter of commissions'.[27] Pickerill thus had a guiding hand in the establishment of the Otago University Medical Corps, an organisation that until recently was an important contributor to New Zealand's military service.

During this period Pickerill was preparing the ground for his subsequent role in the war; his release from the Dental School was announced on 21 December 1916.[28] The *Journal* recorded in March that:

> For the first time for many years our *Journal* fails to bear the imprint of Dunedin on its cover, that of Auckland being substituted. Under the able conductorship of Dr. H.P. Pickerill, it has appeared for so many years that one had come to regard it as inseparably connected with his name, and with that of the Queen City of the South.
>
> The departure of Dr. Pickerill has been due entirely to the exigencies of war, his services, as expert in injuries of the face and jaws, having been requisitioned by the authorities. We regret to lose him from our midst for a while, but congratulate him and ourselves in that his special gifts have been recognised.[29]

The temporary departure of Hunter 'to play his part in the Empire's struggle' was also noted:

> To him will fall the onerous task of organisation of and construction in connection with the New Zealand dental service at the front. We wish both him and Dr. Pickerill, when their tasks are completed, a speedy return to our midst, as we can ill spare them.

Lieutenant Colonel J.N. Rishworth was appointed Director of Dental Services in Hunter's absence.[30]

An aside from the Pickerill story, but highly relevant to the New Zealand Dental Corps, was Captain B.S. Finn's paper read to the Annual General Meeting of the Metropolitan Branch [London] of the British Dental Association in December 1916. He castigated the British War Office for allowing so many dentists to enlist in the ranks rather than using them in the urgently needed dental care in the forces. He noted that the state of oral health of British Forces in the Mediterranean was so bad that seven New Zealand dentists in England were requested to provide additional care, and Australian dentists also provided assistance. He praised the dental health of German soldiers, and deplored treatment by means of 'wholesale extractions'. Among other criticisms of the British system he made was the 'immense waste of money in equipping your dental officers. The equipments I have seen have not been chosen with a view to general utility and economy, nor is there any uniformity as to supplies; the dental dealers seem to have the responsibility of providing, irrespective of conditions.' He pointed out the need for a director of dental services, and contrasted the British situation with the New Zealand Dental Corps, established by such hard and persistent efforts. Not surprisingly this outspoken address provoked a vigorous discussion at the meeting, but most speakers endorsed the criticism of the British system.[31]

The contrast Finn portrayed between the British and New Zealand approaches was, to a very large measure, due to the work of Pickerill and Hunter, with generous and patriotic support from the majority of members of the New Zealand Dental Association. This was indeed a united response to the appalling state of oral health of the recruits. Pickerill and Hunter were the men for the moment. They enjoyed great respect within the profession, they were vastly experienced, Pickerill in particular being able to exert great influence in his roles as Secretary, Editor, and Dean. Pickerill's war service is usually recognised in relation to his skills in plastic surgery. His role in the establishment of what became the Royal New Zealand Dental Corps must also be acknowledged.

10

Preparation for Sidcup

The *Journal* continued the tribute to its former Editor with comment on the humanitarian nature of Pickerill's future role in the war:

> We rejoice the more because his departure means a reduction of suffering for those who are bearing our burdens at the front. Shell and gunshot injuries of the jaws and face have proved one of the most appalling features of the war. The suffering involved, the protracted and difficult nature of the treatment required, the imperfect results so often obtained, the hideous deformity which, in many cases persisted, all combined to make up a picture of hopelessness only too frequently seen in the early stages of the war. But, happily, scientific plastic surgery has risen to the occasion …[1]

In what seems at first sight a remarkable transition, Pickerill, the renowned researcher of dental caries and university teacher and administrator, went overseas as a 'jaw specialist' to take command of the unit treating New Zealand servicemen with facial injuries. He seems not to have taken any special courses, and at that time had no postgraduate qualifications in surgery. He did not follow the usual pathway to specialisation by obtaining the Fellowship of the Royal College of Surgeons – his Australasian Fellowship was to come much later. He would have gained experience in the principles of general and maxillofacial surgery during his undergraduate years in medicine and dentistry at Birmingham. In the nine years from arrival in New Zealand, and amongst all his other roles, Pickerill built on those foundations to earn recognition as a specialist in a challenging field – further testament to his remarkable energy and commitment.

Confirmation within the University of Otago of his growing surgical expertise came at the April 1911 meeting of the Dental Faculty, which approved a recommendation from the Medical Faculty that he be allowed to see 'Special Cases of Medical and Surgical Disease having a possible causal connection with the teeth', and to operate when requested by medical or dental practitioners – 'it being recognised that the operation shall be such as would not be performed by a dentist'.[2] It is presumed these 'cases' were beyond the expertise of the general dental practitioner, yet not within the recognised domain of general surgeons, many of whom would, just as today, find the presence of teeth and the complex musculature of the jaws and face to be daunting and best avoided. Pickerill was, in effect, New Zealand's first maxillofacial surgeon, to use the specialist title now generally adopted. His patients would have included those with tumours and cysts of the mouth and jaws, and it might be expected that, just as today, he would have worked in consultation with surgeons specialising in the ear, nose, and throat areas.

The treatment of fractures of the jaws and facial lacerations, common injuries resulting from falls and blows, would have been a routine part of his clinical responsibilities, but he also moved into much more complex surgery, such as the removal of sections of the mandible to correct protrusion of the lower jaw.[3] His review of the sparse literature on this topic implied that the operation he performed was rare, and his may well have been the first authoritative article on what is now included in the definition of orthognathic surgery. In two separate operations, he removed a section of bone on each side of the lower jaw, thus allowing the front portion to be repositioned backward and wired to the remaining part of the jaw. Now a relatively common operation in facial surgery, in 1912 it was a heroic approach to the correction of an aesthetic disability. It would have required very careful planning and meticulous technique to avoid penetration into the mouth and hence infection of the surgical site by oral bacteria. Infection that did occur after the first operation had to be controlled before he could operate on the second side. The successful outcome for the patient was an improved profile and the ability to enjoy a better diet – the patient quickly gained thirty pounds. Pickerill here displayed the expertise of a highly skilled surgeon working in an area where nerves and blood vessels had to be avoided, infection prevented as far as possible, and the mobile bone ends wired together accurately and retained against the complex forces of the muscles controlling the lower jaw.

Also in 1912 he described the treatment of a patient with a very nasty fracture of the mandible, complicated by infection that was possibly life-threatening.[4] Two treatment principles illustrated in this patient were later of great importance in surgery associated with war wounds – the management of gross infection in an era long before antibiotics, and the retention of teeth, even though septic, so that they could be wired or splinted together to aid fixation of the bone ends.

He was also at this time displaying his expertise in the treatment of cleft palate, a field of plastic surgery in which he was subsequently to excel. The illustrated lecture and demonstration he presented to the Southland Branch of the Association was a notable event, for he not only illustrated the lecture with 'various slides thrown on the screen', but also used a 'phonograph record' to show improvement in an adult patient's speech after surgery. After reviewing common techniques, he described the 'latest method' involving the surgical construction of a soft-tissue bar across the palate to act as a support for an artificial palate.[5] On the following day he demonstrated the technique on an adult patient, with apparently good results. To do such an operation, in strange surroundings, and no doubt with a critical audience pressing in to observe what the surgeon was doing in a very constricted field of operation, confirms Pickerill's very high degrees of skill and of confidence. His expertise in cleft-palate surgery was acknowledged by the award of 500 kronen from Vienna specifically for his research into the treatment of cleft palate[6] – the name of Pickerill the surgeon was becoming widely recognised.

In addition to his major paper on dental caries at the Sixth International Dental Congress in London in 1914, he presented a paper on cleft palate. Here his expertise was on international display, but unfortunately the full paper was not published. A résumé, however, shows it was an authoritative presentation in which he reviewed the aetiology, anatomy, and physiology of normal and cleft palates, described original investigations, and reviewed current methods of treatment. He also described a 'new method' based on his investigations.[7] No discussion of the paper was reported, so it is not known how it was received. It would, however, have added to his growing reputation, as surgery at that time almost invariably resulted in poor appearance and speech.

In the period leading up to his departure overseas, he showed he was right up to date with the management of the severe trauma arising from gunshot wounds to the face. In an extensive review, he compared the principles of treatment of simple fractures of the mandible with the challenges of repair when there was loss and fragmentation of bone, associated loss of muscle and skin, and serious infection. He also described some 'new methods' in the wiring together of the jaws, an important technique to allow the jaws to be held immobile while union of the bone occurred.[8] He did not state who these patients were, but presumably they were returned servicemen – the specialised units for this type of treatment had not yet been formed in England. This was an authoritative paper reviewing deficiencies in current techniques for repairing serious jaw injuries; he proposed original methods, including a description of the 'Pickerill splint'. This is the work of a knowledgable and skilled surgeon, who appreciated the difficulties associated with realigning bone fragments in a highly infected operative field.

In addition to developing his practical skills, he also had access to developments overseas – for example, the extensive supplement on war injuries published in 1916 in the *British Dental Journal*.[9] This contained reprints and summaries of articles by British, French, American, Italian, and German authors, and presumably represented the most up-to-date review of the topic. It would have given surgeons such as Pickerill a broad overview of contemporary knowledge and management methods.

The combination of his advanced surgical expertise, his understanding of the principles involved in the management of disfiguring war wounds, and his thorough knowledge of the musculo-skeletal system of the face and jaws, fully justified Pickerill's designation as 'jaw specialist'. The Ministry of Defence sent him overseas safe in the knowledge that he was the best man for the job – indeed, one of the few in the world ready to cope with the challenges presented by the horrifying outcomes of trench warfare.

11

Rebuilding faces, 1917–1919

On 30 December 1916, Major H.P. Pickerill, NZDC, left Wellington with the 20th Reinforcements on the troopship *Athenic*. He disembarked at Devonport, England, on 3 March 1917. After transfer back to the New Zealand Medical Corps, he was appointed on 30 March to establish a jaw department at the Second New Zealand General Hospital at Walton-on-Thames, a few miles south-west of London.

The hospital was based on two old mansions set in very attractive surroundings. It became a large hospital, able to accommodate nearly 1,900 patients. In 'normal' times there were usually 1,000 patients under treatment or convalescing, but after a 'push' it could be full to overflowing. This large New Zealand presence in Walton-on-Thames is still remembered in the village, especially at St Mary's Church of England where the New Zealand flag is displayed beside a plaque bearing the names of New Zealand servicemen who died while at the hospital. Prominent in the church's graveyard are two white stone monuments to the deceased New Zealand servicemen. The annual Anzac Day service is an important event attended by diplomats, military personnel, and members of the public.

Pickerill was initially in charge of a general ward of fifty beds, but none of the patients had facial or jaw injuries. He reported to his dental colleagues back in New Zealand that the patients were 'all medical and surgical cases of every conceivable type, so that of necessity I had to furbish up my surgery and medicine'. For a maxillofacial surgeon, this period must have been a challenging learning curve, but he soon gathered more patients with facial wounds:

> There were, however, two jaw cases in Hospital, and these I collected and started work – with no work-room and only a visiting mechanic, who knew nothing of any kind of metal or splint work. It has taken two months hard work to get all this changed. I now, by a process of elimination, have my ward nearly full of jaw cases (40); a work-room built and equipped, and a competent mechanic for the making of splints etc.

He described those first patients as '... old cases which have been treated elsewhere, and, from various points of view, these are not so satisfactory as the cases one gets fresh from the front'.

In this same report to colleagues, he reviewed the various situations encountered, mentioning that the 'kind of projectile that does the most damage ... is the glancing or tangential projectile; this always produces much comminution [pulverisation of the bone].' The difficulties with the 'old' cases were adhesions, un-united fractures, and fractures with loss of bone. He described management of the latter condition:

> These are the most difficult of all cases to deal with if disability and deformity of the patient is to be remedied. At present there is only one method of treatment, and that is by 'bone grafting.' For this operation of course the wound must have healed perfectly, and it must be possible to open up the wound and get at the ends of the bone without in any way communicating with the mouth.
>
> This having been done, a piece of bone is taken from the tibia (or a rib), and, having been cut with a special circular saw to the right dimensions, is fitted into slots in the two ends of the fractured jaw. It is an operation requiring, of course, the most rigorous asepsis, and opinions are at present, I find, doubtful as to what is going to be the future of the method. All cases are not successful – the graft does not 'take', just as the graft on an apple tree may not take. But when it is successful, there is no doubt about it – the result is excellent in every way, and a loose wobbling jaw, swung over to the affected side is converted into a rigid functional jaw, with but a slight 'bump' where the new bone is inserted. Up to the present I have only done one such case, and although I cannot yet say what the functional result is going to be, it appears to be quite successful. In this case I took the bone from the tibia. I have several other cases waiting to be 'done', and hope to be able to report on them later.[1]

Pickerill was not the first to attempt bone grafting, but he was certainly amongst its pioneers. In the forefront was the New Zealand-born surgeon, Major Harold Gillies. Gillies had volunteered in 1915 for service with the Red Cross and worked with and assisted Major Charles Auguste Valadier, a French-American dentist who used bone grafts in the treatment of serious facial wounds at a surgical unit in Wimereux, France.[2] The use of bone grafts was an enormous development. Without the insertion of a graft to replace shattered or lost bone, attempts to secure union between the bone ends resulted in gross distortion of the lower third of the face. The outcome was not only a grotesque appearance, but also compromised speech and mastication.

Although Pickerill had used the bone-grafting technique at this point on just one patient, his typical confidence was shown in this authoritative description of the technique. He found being within twenty miles of London allowed him contact with other surgical units, and he may well have observed the technique performed by Gillies who, after returning from France, was stationed at the Cambridge Military Hospital, Aldershot.

From his observations, Pickerill described two distinct approaches to the management of facial fractures:

> one of which believes chiefly in maintaining asepsis, or, should I say, cleanliness, by the extraction of any teeth in the neighbourhood of the fracture and the extraction of the upper teeth also, on the fracture side, to allow the posterior fragment to swing inward and so shorten the lower arch, splints being used to a minimum degree. The other school relies on splints and elaborate and ingenious appliances almost entirely.

Pickerill refrained from final judgement on the two techniques – 'As always, I think we shall find that the right line lies intermediate between these'. But he no doubt would have been appalled by outcomes of the former technique, and would have enthusiastically embraced new methods to prevent shortening of the lower jaw and the resulting serious effects of asymmetry on appearance and function.

A feature remarkable to modern readers is that advanced trauma surgery was being successfully practised without the benefit of antibiotics. Wounds were grossly contaminated – the dirt and mud of Belgium and France made this inevitable – but infection could be brought under control to allow repair and reconstruction of shattered faces and jaws. This is revealed in his description of the management of infection in the 'fresh cases'; these men would have received at the Front just enough attention to control bleeding and to stabilise the airway.

> These always arrive in a very septic condition, and have, first of all, to be cleaned up and X-rayed. This being done, one decides on the line of treatment … Usually there is a piece of shrapnel somewhere embedded in the tissues which has to be removed, and it is wonderful how easily one can miss these. Although the X-ray shows them quite plainly, they have, I find, a habit of moving about, and may be quite an inch from where they were when the skiagram [radiograph] was taken.
>
> At the time of removing the 'F.B.' [foreign body] the bone may be wired, a splint inserted, or intermaxillary lacing [wiring the upper and lower jaws together to

immobilise fragments of bone] adopted ... I like to immobilise completely for at least a fortnight, and then to allow a certain amount of movement of the jaw – not at the fracture line …

Septic mouths are atomised with a pressure atomiser, using peroxide or weak iodine lotion, from two to six times a day, depending on the case. Every mouth must be kept clean.

Patients are weighed once a week, and I expect them all to put on weight, if not, there is an enquiry. No special method of feeding is required, even if the two jaws are firmly laced together; the patient will feed himself and put on weight, if he is given the right kind of food, and in sufficient quantity. One cannot expect a patient to overcome sepsis and to regenerate bone if he is at the same time losing weight.

These patients, when they come in, are of all the most miserable, and most sorry for themselves, but under the above treatment they rapidly pick up, and, I think, I may safely say, that my ward is the most difficult in which to maintain discipline in the whole Hospital.[3]

The control of infection is described here almost nonchalantly – remove foreign bodies, keep the wounds and mouth clean by the trusty means of irrigation with peroxide and iodine solutions, and keep the patient well fed. Later, at The Queen's Hospital, eusol, a chlorine solution, replaced iodine for irrigation of wounds, and the liquid diet was egg-based. He did not dwell on any complications, although they must have existed. Basic surgical principles produced good results – to the extent of converting his patients, miserable and sorry for themselves on admission, into the undisciplined and 'cheery' group he described in the caption to a photograph he sent home. This shows him as the sole officer, surrounded by wounded servicemen, nurses, and a corporal and a private, presumably his only auxiliary staff. The caption includes:

Herewith … some of my 'jaw' cases, those able to be up and about. They look cheery enough, don't they? Yet all have had face wounds with compound comminuted fractures of the jaws. Many of them have had portions of jaw missing, but of course you see them with the splints in situ. Several of them I have bone grafted from the tibia or rib, or both. What I am liking best at present, and is new as far as I know, is a combination of tibia and rib cartilage. It is giving excellent results. I have at present 66 cases in my ward.[4]

He had quickly developed his bone-grafting skills, possibly pioneering new methods. Here, apparently, was a successful, innovative unit, with a confident and expert solo surgeon as its commanding officer. But one suspects that in such reports for home consumption he made light of the appalling wounds he had to deal with, and the effects these had on the men themselves. Dealing with such injuries, including the constant efforts to control infection and ensure adequate nutrition, would have caused emotional stress to the nursing staff, and no doubt to himself.

A major event at Walton-on-Thames was the visit of King George and Queen Mary, a visit that Pickerill recalled sentimentally when the Queen died in 1953. He wrote at that time:

> I feel I have lost a friend, for many years ago it was she who changed the whole course of my life by persuading me to become a plastic surgeon …
>
> The procession trailed around the ward, the King stopping every now and then to speak to a patient and airing his knowledge … by telling me that he had been told of some doctor who had 'invented' a very simple way of treating fractured jaws by wiring the top and bottom jaws together. He said to me, 'Have you heard of that?' … I said 'I use it frequently' but might have added that I happened to be the 'some doctor' who had described this simple method in the British Medical Journal for the previous year'.
>
> The techniques of skin grafting and rebuilding faces were then in their infancy; tin masks, painted as best as possible to blend with natural colouring and sometimes to replace missing eyes, were still in use in severe cases to replace lost parts of the face, and were much hated by the men and the surgeons alike. The alternative entailed grafts the like of which no plastic surgeon had then envisaged … the Queen said she hoped I was going to the new Empire Hospital at Sidcup … for such cases. My reply was I thought I would rather stay at my own hospital where I believed I could serve New Zealand soldiers better. Then the Queen did a wonderful thing. By her friendliness, graciousness and tone of voice she made me forget that she was a Queen and we talked on the subject without reserve … When I had to leave her, in shaking hands she said, 'Well Major, to please *me* I would like you to go to Sidcup' … my opposition evaporated … I have been a plastic surgeon ever since …[5]

On 9 January 1918, Pickerill, his dental mechanic, and twenty-nine patients were transferred from Walton-on-Thames to The Queen's Hospital at Sidcup, Kent, a new establishment, founded specifically for the treatment of facial and jaw injuries. Major J.N. Rishworth, NZDC, arrived on the same day from headquarters for duty with the New Zealand Section. They were assigned three wards, and many of the British patients already in those wards were taken over. Before the work of the section could be properly started, however, Pickerill contracted acute tonsillitis and he spent three weeks at the convalescent home for New Zealand officers at Brighton.[6]

Sidcup became synonymous with the name of Gillies, who was Dunedin-born but qualified in medicine at Cambridge University and St Bartholomew's Hospital, London.[7] Working as an ear, nose, and throat surgeon in London when war was declared,[8] Gillies convinced the authorities that the best treatment results were to be achieved in specialised units. After returning from France, he was allocated 200 beds at Aldershot, but the number of casualties soon proved overwhelming. The establishment of a convalescent home to overcome the problem was initially proposed, but Sir Charles Kenderdine, one of the founders and organisers of Queen Mary's Hospital at Roehampton, where the treatment of amputees was centred, wanted a more ambitious scheme – a specialised hospital with facilities for surgery and for long-term convalescence of large numbers of wounded soldiers.[9]

A strong supporter of this proposal was Sir William Arbuthnot Lane, the Senior Surgeon in the British Army, to whom Pickerill was to give primary credit some years later:

> It might not be out of place at this distance in time to remind readers that Lane was really the founder of modern plastic surgery. Not that he did any himself, but his was the conception in 1916 to have an Empire Plastic Surgery Hospital at Sidcup in Kent, to which all British Empire casualties with facial losses, from all fields of war should be sent. His greatest difficulty was in getting us together. All of us, British, Australians, Canadians and New Zealanders wanted to stay with our own hospitals. But Lane's persuasiveness eventually prevailed and a large and well run hospital resulted … Lane's interest did not cease with this for he stayed with us as a very active consulting surgeon to the last. His advice was much valued, for if we were stumped as to the best way (or indeed any way) of dealing with some terrible mutilation, Lane could always draw upon his vast experience and tell us how he had seen a somewhat similar case in America or Italy, or Germany, or Vienna … and the surgeon did so and so. For it must be remembered that then we had no textbooks or published papers on plastic surgery to guide us, and most of our instruments were improvised. If we wanted more operating theatres and more wards, Lane was the man who pulled the strings and got them quickly …[10]

Rivalry and even jealousy between the surgeons existed at Sidcup, and here it seems that Pickerill, through his praise of Lane's contribution to the success of Sidcup, may have been subtly attempting to undermine the eventual acknowledgement of Gillies as 'the father of plastic surgery'. Lane was later to write the glowing Introduction to Pickerill's *Facial Surgery*, so the two men apparently had great mutual respect. Lane certainly made an enormous contribution to the success of Sidcup as an enabler who got things done.

The hospital was on the Frognal Estate, the former residence of the late Earl of Sidney. The existing mansion was used as administration offices, mess room for convalescent officers, and living accommodation for nursing staff. Kenderdine organised the scheme along the same lines as at Roehampton; Queen Mary took a great interest in the development, and commanded that it be named after her. It was supported financially by the Queen's Special Fund, by individuals, by government and private organisations, and by the Red Cross in New Zealand, Canada, and Australia.[11]

The estate was obtained in 1916, construction began in February 1917, and the hospital was opened in July that year.[12] It consisted of wards, operating theatres, and departments for physiotherapy, dentistry, and radiography, facilities for photography, an artist's studio, and areas for convalescence and recreation. Later in 1917 the hospital was designated as the central face and jaw hospital for all the Empire's forces, and enlarged to 560 beds. With the inclusion of local auxiliary hospitals, over 1,000 beds were available. By January 1918, the Army Council instructed that all soldiers with 'serious injury to the face requiring plastic surgery when evacuated to England will be specially labelled "Facial Injury" for the Queen's Hospital, Sidcup'.[13] All soldiers with these injuries in hospitals elsewhere were to travel to Sidcup as soon as they were fit to do so.

Arbuthnot Lane is recorded as telling Gillies in September 1916 that 'I want to make Sidcup the *biggest* and *most important* hospital for jaws and plastic work in the world and you consequently a leader in this form of surgery', and in a further letter: 'The larger the hospital, the bigger the men associated with it the stronger will your position be. We must work together to this end'.[14] Lane clearly singled out Gillies to be the driving force in this new venture. Lieutenant Colonel J.R. Colvin, a former Army Service Corps officer in the Indian Army, was appointed to administer the hospital, which was in five sections – the British had the equivalent of two sections, and the Australian, Canadian, and New Zealand forces one each. An American contingent of surgeons joined the team toward the end of the war, but their role was largely observational. In his reminiscence of the Queen's visit to Walton-on-Thames, Pickerill noted: 'I was looking at a photograph of a group of American plastic surgeons recently and they had nearly all been initially instructed by us at Sidcup in 1918'.[15]

The pioneering nature of the plastic surgery undertaken at The Queen's Hospital became increasingly appreciated when Professor A.D. (Sandy) Macalister presented the 1987 Menzies Campbell lecture to the Royal College of Surgeons of England.[16] Professor Macalister held the Chair of Oral Surgery and Oral Medicine at the University of Otago from 1972 to 1984. Pickerill brought back to New Zealand a large number of Sidcup records. These eventually came to be in two locations. One group was saved from destruction by Professor Macalister and, through his son, Dr Donald Macalister, was donated back to the hospital, arriving some seventy years after they had left. The other group, now in the Hocken Collections of the

University of Otago, was donated to the University of Otago Medical School by Dame Cecily Pickerill in 1981, some twenty-six years after the death of her husband. The Pickerill records, together with the Australian records held at the Royal Australian College of Surgeons in Melbourne and the British records held at Aldershot, are thought to be the only surviving medical records of the First World War.[17]

Maintenance of meticulous records was seen as a crucial goal for Gillies and his colleagues, who relied on them not only in planning the details of surgery, but also in assessing outcomes and techniques. Records are in the form of files of individual patients, and include brief surgical notes, superb photographs, and radiographs and watercolour paintings of some patients. Together they are a unique record.[18] Those returned to Sidcup form the basis of what has been named the Macalister Archive. The records illustrate very clearly the shocking nature of the wounds caused by high velocity bullets and shrapnel, and the heroic nature of the repair. Some of the records are incomplete and many do not reveal long-term outcomes. They do, however, show the outstanding results that were achieved in many instances. Those with the most disfiguring injuries were by no means returned to an unblemished appearance, but final results showed restoration of lost tissue – noses, ears, lips, cheeks, and jaws – and function and appearance that would undoubtedly allow an acceptable return to civilian life for many severely wounded men. The accompanying illustrations are examples of the nature and quality of the records.

Pickerill was the Officer in Command of the New Zealand Section at Sidcup. The British Section was commanded by Gillies, the Canadian Section by Major C.W. Waldron, CAMC, and the Australian by Lieutenant Colonel H.S. (later Sir Henry) Newland, AAMC. These officers formed a medical committee to advise the Commandant on all purely medical matters affecting the administration of the hospital. Newland was elected chairman, Pickerill vice-chairman, and Waldron the secretary.[19]

The surgical staff included many who were to become famous in plastic and maxillofacial surgery – Gillies, Waldron, Newland, Kelsey Fry, Kilner, Blair, Ivy, McGee and, of course, Pickerill. Macalister recorded that these men 'made their contribution and established their reputations at Sidcup. Concept and organisation was unique and a large credit for support and for the enthusiasm must go to Sir Arbuthnot Lane, who was at that time Consulting Surgeon to the Aldershot Command …'.[20]

Pickerill was now part of a large team of specialist surgeons and dental surgeons dedicated to rehabilitating the many soldiers who had the dreadful face and jaw injuries resulting from trench warfare. Pickerill's own staff included Captain W.S. Seed, NZDC, one of Pickerill's first three Otago BDS graduates, and Major J.N. Rishworth, NZDC. Rishworth returned to duty at headquarters, possibly temporarily, in May 1918, and Captain J.M. Turner, NZDC, joined the team. Captain S.D. (Tommy) Rhind, MC, NZMC, twice wounded in France, came to Sidcup from the New Zealand hospital at Brockenhurst, where he had been a patient after being gassed. He became Pickerill's surgical associate. The *War Diary*, dated 14 July 1918, shows that the British Unit was providing the anaesthetists, but later, Captain A.McP. Marshall, who had been severely wounded just before the Battle of Messines,[21] became Pickerill's anaesthetist. Major McGee and Captain Stone of the American Army were appointed to the New Zealand Section for training in plastic and jaw surgery.

Despite the Queen's urging, Pickerill initially was not pleased at moving to Sidcup. Two days after he arrived there he reminded the University of Otago Chancellor that he left New Zealand to set up a jaw department for New Zealand casualties in England and that he was then to hand over the work to others.[22] With the unit now established, he believed he would be of more service in New Zealand. As some of the reparative operations could not be undertaken for many months after healing of the original wound, he was sending these people back to New Zealand. If granted approval by the University Council, he would operate on them at the Dental Hospital. The move from his sole position at Walton-on-Thames to the large team at Sidcup was a major change for him – he would no longer be in complete control, and perhaps he wished to return to New Zealand to run his unit in his own way. His rather curious request – a military surgeon asking permission from a university to operate on returned servicemen in university facilities – was denied,[23] on the grounds that his services had been specifically requested by the military, that the Council had made arrangements to carry on his university work during his absence, and that the military situation was critical.

His attitude changed rapidly, however, for on 7 April 1918, just the day after the Registrar replied, Pickerill wrote again, stating that he could not then return to New Zealand.[24] His perspective of the situation in England had altered – he listed an acute shortage of medical officers, British and New Zealand; the massive German offensive on the Somme to open the road to Amiens had flooded all hospitals with wounded soldiers;[25] in addition, the British Red Cross had voted £5000 for a new ward and operating theatre to accommodate his section at the hospital. Under these circumstances he thought it not surprising that the Director of Medical Services did not want him to return yet. He also felt it would not be right for him to leave 'at the present critical juncture when the Empire requires the utmost of every man'. He said he was in good health, but very busy, and that they were only taking the worst face and jaw injuries, 'but they are pouring in every day and night from France. This war is truly a ghastly business'. Pickerill was now part of the team.

Correspondence beginning in June 1918 between Pickerill, the Minister of Defence, and Brigadier General G.S. Richardson, the Administration Officer of the New Zealand Forces in France, suggested that New Zealanders had been sent home against Pickerill's wishes, but whether this was the group he referred to earlier is not known. Pickerill claimed he could not have prevented it without having the rank and the status of consultant, but his application for promotion was not approved.[26] The Minister did not reply until September, when he apologised for the 'difficulty' over Pickerill's appointment as consultant, and acknowledged '… there is no doubt that some jaw cases were returned to New Zealand improperly treated, with the result that little or nothing could be done for them here. I am very anxious that every soldier should receive every benefit that we can bestow upon him in the way of treatment'.[27]

Pickerill performed the first operation by the New Zealand Unit on 11 February 1918 – 'a rib-graft to make good a portion of the malar & zygomatic arch on the right side'. At that point he had no assistant, 'Major Gillies kindly lent Lieut. Birt RAMC to assist, & this officer was, a few days later, temporarily attached to the N.Z. Section, until a permanent N.Z. officer could be obtained'. The section was divided into three wards:

> Ward 10 – Fresh septic cases from France. Ward 8 – clean cases requiring daily dressing. Ward 9 – plastic operation cases. This has turned out to be an excellent plan, & if small wards could be set apart in all hospitals for 'clean' cases i.e. plastic or orthopaedic, it would be of great advantage.[28]

Whether this segregation of patients was adopted throughout the hospital is not known, but it ensured a logical progression from admission and initial cleansing and removal of dead tissue from wounds, to reducing and controlling infection, stabilising mobile sections of bone by means of splints and wiring, and then on to the stage when the series of plastic surgery operations could begin. This would have reduced the risk of cross-infection, a subject that was later to contribute greatly to Pickerill's success in plastic surgery for infants.

In the following five months, the section performed 113 plastic operations, which included operations on the face, nose, lips, eyelids, and palate. Ten grafts using rib cartilage and two grafts of bone from the tibia were performed. The *War Diary* indicates some of the logistical problems encountered:

> The number of plastic operations has been somewhat limited for want of theatre accommodation, it being possible to allot only three half days per week to each Dominion section.
>
> In addition, 56 operations have been performed in the septic theatre, comprising currettings [removal of superficial dead tissue], sequestrotomies [removal of dead bone], openıng abscesses, & removal of Foreign Bodies, Cysts, Glands & Tumours of the jaws, ligation of arteries for secondary haemorrhages & saline and blood transfusions. During this same period, there have been in the dental department, a large number of splints of considerable ingenuity, & have attracted attention outside this hospital, & similar devices to those originating in this section are now in use in France & in London hospitals. Such credit is due to the dental mechanics for the careful, thoughtful, and thorough way in which instructions have been carried out by them.

Splints and fixation devices were indeed essential to ensure immobilisation of healing fractures and provide stability where bone grafting had been performed. Gillies acknowledged this aspect of the New Zealand Section's expertise in *Plastic Surgery of the Face*,[29] attributing the invention of a particular splint to Rishworth.

The rivalry between the sections at Sidcup has been the subject of much speculation. Generally it is spoken of as being 'friendly', as in the comment of Sir Arbuthnot Lane in his Preface to Gillies's book: 'Major Waldron and Captain Risdon … Colonel Newland … and Major Pickerill, and the officers serving with them joined in heartily in friendly rivalry and healthy competition to the great benefit of their poor *mutilés'*. Gillies's biographer noted that

> their differing surgical hallmarks were obvious to the expert eye. The Gillies nose was apt to have a patrician curve. The flap transferences of Risdon, the Canadian team leader [jointly with Waldron] were as distinctive as the pedicles of Pickerill … and the excisions of Ferris Smith, the American. Gillies was the doyen …
>
> He was jealous of his leadership in the new surgery and showed it strongly when an Australian surgeon seemed to be gaining favour with Arbuthnot Lane. He had a certain thrustfulness of manner disliked by some of his English colleagues.[30]

Gillies and Pickerill had strong personalities and it could be expected that they would indeed have had their differences from time to time. An insight into this, and even some long-held bitterness, is shown in a note attached by Pickerill to the cover of a reprint he sent to Gillies in 1955: 'Reprint extracted and sent to Gillies 29.3.55. So that there should be no doubt as to who first skin grafted a buccal sulcus [the depression or channel between the cheeks or lips and the bone of the jaw] with open free graft under pressure'.[31] The sulcus is an important and necessary feature for successful construction and retention of dentures. Before this development, a complicated, two-stage operation to insert an inlay of epithelium had been used. Gillies acknowledged Waldron as the first to perform this modification, and added, 'He was closely followed by … Pickerill'.[32] The new method was a big advance, and Pickerill was clearly annoyed that he was not given primary credit.

Pickerill also wanted to justify his own reputation in other areas. He claimed, for example, ownership of a pressure method for skin grafting, and a graft used in the replacement of lost tissue in the forehead: 'so far as I know, I was the first to originate the method … Naturally it was rapidly adopted by others, especially at Sidcup'.[33] He also described and claimed to be the originator of a method to repair perforating wounds of the maxillary antrum. The American author H.L. Hunt, who had possibly been at Sidcup, acknowledged him to be the originator of a technique of using a particular form of pedicled fat graft (that is, the graft remained attached to its base at one end to maintain vitality while it 'takes'), to fill depressions or restore mobility to adherent scars.[34]

Controversy existed on who first devised the tube graft, a technique for replacing lost skin with healthy tissue from adjacent areas such as the forehead, neck, or chest. In order to keep a blood supply while the graft or flap 'took', one end of the flap stayed attached in its original position. Between the attached base of the graft and the area where the free end of the flap was sutured into position, the bridge of tissue rolled itself into the form of a tube. Gillies claimed credit for the tube graft, but was dealt a 'bitter blow' when he learned in 1919 that Filitov, a Russian surgeon, had been the first.[35]

Pickerill acknowledged: 'The tube flap probably was first extensively used as a means of maintaining the nourishment of large flaps at the Queen's Hospital, Sidcup, during the war, when it was used by Lieut. Col. Newlands, Major Gillies, Major Waldron, and myself'. He then went on to describe a modification he used '… for the first time on 26th June 1918', the date apparently being crucial to substantiate his claim to indeed be the first.[36] He also implied that he was the first to use what became known as the double tube flap, used for restoring simultaneously the inside and the outside of the mouth, and that he originated the living-bone screw – that is, made from the patient's own bone – for fixing bone grafts into position.

The nursing staff was well aware of the rivalry existing between the sections – 'They all vied with each other – at the same time sharing information', wrote a senior theatre sister, who worked with all the sections, to Pickerill's daughter, Margaret Frazer, many years later. 'They were very happy days at Sidcup – everyone so keen and the work so exciting … We all had our favourite teams – and I am not making it up just to please you – but the New Zealand "Team" were my favourite – they were quicker and more gentle than the Australians or Americans'.[37] So although the rivalry was 'healthy', and many of the important developments at Sidcup arose from the teamwork of highly skilled surgeons, they were, not surprisingly, also jealous of their own reputations and felt the need to claim ownership of new developments and techniques.

But respect for one another's skills was also displayed. Gillies' respect for Pickerill's work, even if many years had elapsed, is shown in the reference in the Gillies biography to the 'Pickerill pedicle'. In 1955, Gillies sought Pickerill's permission to publish details of a patient Pickerill had treated using the technique:

> Dear Pickerill
>
> I am trying to get a little book[38] out on Plastic Surgery and in the historical part of it, in regard to Sidcup, we talk about how each surgeon develops his own characteristic style. There are, for instance, pictures illustrating 'A Risdon Transformation', 'A Gillies Hook' [of the nose], and we also have two photographs of the famous case you did for a British boy with immense loss of the upper cheek and nose which you repaired most beautifully and we call it 'A Pickerill Pedicle'.
>
> I should hate not to use your name because I would like to pay such a tribute to the work you did. I am enclosing a little drawing which may possibly help you to remember the case. Unfortunately, I do not remember his name and his notes are way back somewhere. As the book is on the verge of being handed over to the printers, it would be charming of you if you could let me know your views.[39]

Pickerill, however, was not so generous in return in *Facial Surgery*. In the Preface, he mentioned the 'healthy rivalry existing between the various sections', but did not name Gillies or the other team leaders. He did, however, attribute much of the success of the hospital to the tact and sagacity of the commanding officer, Lieutenant Colonel Colvin. He does not even acknowledge any of his own staff – Rhind, Rishworth, or Seed, or his technical staff – although he does praise his anaesthetist: 'Both during and after the war practically all my patients, military and civil, have been anaesthetised by Dr A.McP. Marshall, to whose skill and devotion to the work I am very much indebted'. He continued by pointing out 'All the cases to be described are those which have been entirely under my own care, and many of the methods utilised in treating them are original'. Pickerill did not operate alone – he was the leader of a team – and it is curious and even churlish that he did not acknowledge the highly skilled support of his surgical and technical assistants in this his major work on plastic surgery.

Pickerill continued to keep the profession in New Zealand informed of the activities in his section. A photograph in the July 1918 issue of the *Journal* shows staff and patients on the occasion of the visit of General Richardson and Colonel Heaton Rhodes to the Section. Major B.S. Finn, DSO, the Deputy Director of Dental Services, was also present. The note accompanying the photograph outlined the work and the problems encountered:

> The patients … are just half of the total under my charge … they are not all New Zealanders; in fact I have at present more British than New Zealand patients, and the majority of the British are extremely bad cases, since this Hospital is the British centre for all severe face and jaw injuries, fractures and simple face injuries are sent to other purely 'Jaw' Hospitals.

He described the work as being very heavy at the time because of the current German offensive, and that the wounds were more severe than had been seen before – scarcely a day passed without a death from secondary haemorrhage, presumably as a result of infection, or from pneumonia. In such a period, the team was engaged in saving lives, and plastic surgery was almost at a standstill.[41] The casualty rates were astounding. New Zealand, with its population of less than one million people in 1914, contributed nearly 20 per cent of its eligible manpower, a higher proportion than any other allied country except Britain itself.[41] Over 90,000 were sent overseas, and of these, nearly 17,000 were killed and 41,000 injured. At the battle of Passchendale alone, in October 1917, the New Zealand Division lost 640 men killed and 2,100 wounded. Pickerill would no doubt have treated some of the casualties of this and earlier great battles – the Somme in September 1916 and Messines in June 1917, for example – at Walton-on-Thames, but it is likely that many of these early casualties with facial injuries received inadequate treatment, and could have been among those referred to by the Minister of Defence as having returned to New Zealand prematurely.

Pickerill found the plastic repair work 'exceedingly interesting, making new noses, new lips, ears or eyelids, and bone grafting, all from the patients own tissues. It is the more fascinating, because it is all pioneer work, and one has to think out and devise each case for oneself.' Here he did acknowledge his staff, for he noted that Major Rishworth's roles included the design, supervision of manufacture, and placement of splints. 'We are getting some quite good results, which according to some authorities we certainly should not be getting by our conservative methods.' These methods included preserving as many teeth and fragments of bone as possible, to be used as points for fixation by wiring or by splints, and for ensuring a final repair as close as possible to the original contour of the face and jaws.[42]

Details of the nature of the surgery undertaken by Pickerill and his team can be found in the Sidcup records in the Hocken Collections, Dunedin, and in the Macalister Archive at Sidcup, in Pickerill's own articles, and in his last major text *Facial Surgery*. A detailed description is not appropriate in his biography, but an outline provides insight into the complexity of the surgery and what could be achieved.

A crucial principle in treatment was control of the sections of shattered bone. Pickerill described these in a major article reviewing the nature of the injuries, which were dependent on the site and the angle at which the missile struck the bone; the effect of contraction of the tissues due to scarring; how the various muscles of the jaws and face displaced bone fragments; and the techniques used to join and immobilise the fragments by wires, screws, and splints. He made an interesting comparison of the criteria for removing comminuted bone fragments in military and civilian practice. He had formerly believed that such fragments should be removed in the

> unhealthy, cantankerous, and alcoholic individuals whose resistance and reparative powers are not very high. The majority of our present patients are, however, extremely 'fit', respond wonderfully to treatment, and one can retain fragments and adopt a much more conservative line of treatment than one could for civilians.
>
> … there is no reason why small fragments of bone or a tooth should not survive partial detachment provided they are relatively immobilised within reasonable time and not allowed to be more or less permanently bathed in pus.[43]

Flexibility and innovation were features of the pioneering methods at Sidcup. A dramatic example was the Pickerill team's management of a soldier with a perforating injury of both cheeks. He had fractures of the upper jaw and the nasal and cheek-bones. The injury had occurred nine months before admission to Sidcup and, although the wounds had healed, no attempt had been made to restore function and appearance. The deformity was severe – 'the whole of the upper face had fallen backwards, the nose was sunken and depressed, the maxilla [upper jaw] was too far back by three-quarters of an inch, zygomas [cheek bones] had united but were in mal-position and bulging outwards; there was also a long scar, and an unsightly swelling on the right cheek'.[44] This was 'an old case', that would have been managed quite differently if admitted 'fresh'. Because of his debilitated state due to long-standing chronic infection, this patient was not fit for surgery. Instead Pickerill devised an 'orthodontic' technique. With technical supervision by

Rishworth, a 'bridge' of rigid bars extended from a metal plate resting on the forehead to a complex splint fitted over the lower teeth. This was the fixed retainer against which force was applied to draw the upper teeth and jaw forward by a system of bars controlled by screws; these were adjusted daily and painfully to maintain traction.

This was not the refined orthodontics that uses minimal force to move teeth within the bone without damage to their roots. On the contrary, this was a 'brute-force' but controlled approach that deliberately opened up the fracture lines, releasing in some the pockets of infection that would have been contributing to the patient's debilitation. It was a painful procedure that took two months but, after a graft of rib cartilage to straighten the bridge of the nose, excision of scar tissue in the cheek, and re-contouring the most distorted cheek bone, the outcome was a much fuller face and a greatly improved relationship between the upper and lower jaws. Such was the lateral thinking that characterised the Sidcup approach to restoring a measure of appearance not achievable by the usual methods. Pickerill believed this application of force had never been used before, and that 'apparatus of similar design might be useful in civilian life'. The techniques used at Sidcup were indeed the foundation of modern plastic and maxillofacial surgical techniques.

Grafts using the patients' own bone and rib cartilage became common practice to replace missing segments of the facial bones and mandible. These had to be carefully shaped to fit into the space, then fixed into place by means of wires or screws. Combinations of splints linked to screws that protruded through the skin, splints inside the mouth wired into position, or teeth in the upper and lower jaws wired together, were used to immobilise the fragments and grafts sufficiently to allow union to occur.

A variety of skin grafts or flaps were used to replace lost soft tissues. The requirement to maintain the blood supply of large grafts meant that skin could not simply be lifted from one area and sutured into the new position. Rather, as previously mentioned, the donor skin had to remain attached to its original site at its base, and the free end sutured into place. The two areas, donor and recipient, remained connected until the graft had 'taken'. Once an alternative blood supply was established in the new position, the surplus tissue could be sutured back into its original position on the neck, chest, shoulder, or forehead. The model (illustrated) shows the range of skin grafts used.

Pickerill described in detail the use of the various forms of flaps and grafts in *Facial Surgery*, which, prior to publication, was the thesis for his Master of Surgery (MCh) at Birmingham.[45] Arbuthnot Lane included these words in his Introduction to *Facial Surgery*:

> I am very pleased to have been asked to write a short introduction to Mr Pickerill's work on the application of the principles of plastic surgery, much of which he evolved during a long and arduous experience in the Queen Mary's Hospital [*sic*] at Sidcup, to which I had the good fortune to be consulting surgeon. I mention this, since it shows that I had every opportunity of observing the very excellent work that was done in the New Zealand Section, which was in the charge of Mr Pickerill. The new methods which he devised and the improvements that he made in the operative procedures for the removal of disfigurement of the face and head, produced by bullets or high explosives, were most striking.

Pickerill returned to New Zealand as one of the leaders in the modern art and science of plastic surgery. He was undoubtedly in the same league as Gillies and the other surgeons, and he made several original contributions to the pool of knowledge and experience. Unfortunately, his contribution to the development of plastic surgery has frequently been overlooked in his adopted country in favour of Gillies and, later, Archibald McIndoe in the Second World War. Pickerill, however, deserves to be ranked alongside these other pioneers.

12

Sidcup in Dunedin, 1919–1920

The work at Sidcup continued well past Armistice Day, 11 November 1918. The flow of injured diminished, but the nature of the injuries meant that many servicemen required several operations, separated by enough time for fractures to mend and bone and skin grafts to stabilise. The authorities decided the New Zealanders should return home as soon as possible after the war ended, and Pickerill insisted on continuing in his role – if long-term favourable results were to be achieved, a suitable unit needed to be established in New Zealand. General Richardson was strongly supportive – he wanted the men to be able to get to their homes and see their friends, and to learn trades at technical schools, not to be, as he thought, 'wasting time' at Sidcup.

> The right policy to adopt is to do what is best for the men – and in my opinion there is only one thing to do – i.e. to take the whole Unit back to N.Z. with you in charge as soon as possible – if the N.Z. Govt can install the men in a hospital together.[1]

He acknowledged Pickerill's work, and spoke about it to the War Office, 'without result in the shape of a reward, but you can leave the matter in my hands to insist on your being rewarded for what you have done for our men. I hope the Imperial authorities will reward you for what you have done for their men'. Reward was eventually to come in the form of Pickerill being made an 'Officer of the Most Excellent Order of the British Empire for valuable services rendered in connection with the War', which was announced on 15 June 1919. The civilian CBE was to come later.

Before returning to New Zealand, Pickerill looked at an alternative proposition, for in January 1919 the Dean of the London Hospital Medical

College asked him to consider the new position of Professor of Dental Surgery. The usual salary for a professor in the University of London was £600, but was likely to be raised to £800. The Dean wanted an urgent answer.[2] Whether the offer was seriously considered is not known, but Pickerill probably wanted a position of higher status and probably a higher salary. He was, after all, the Dean of his own Dental School and already a full professor; further, he was also now recognised as one of the highly experienced, even elite, group of pioneers in the new discipline of plastic surgery. Acceptance would have resulted in a possible reduction in the scope of his work, and besides, there was still unfinished business with his own patients and, of course, the Dental School. Back in New Zealand he would have national recognition.

The Army moved quickly to establish the unit envisaged by General Richardson. In mid-February 1919, Colonel Falconer, the Medical Superintendent of Dunedin Hospital, sought the advice of the Otago Hospital Board on setting up a jaw hospital in Dunedin, specifically to provide for forty-three patients expected home from Sidcup in April. Various sites were considered, including the Knox Church Sunday School, the Knox Church manse, the Forth Street Maternity Hospital, and Allen Hall; all were thought to be too small.[3]

Close links between the Red Cross and the Otago Hospital Board during the First World War are no better illustrated than in the Dunedin Branch's association with this new venture. The Red Cross undertook to equip an establishment for twenty-five jaw patients.[4] Woodside, a large house on the corner of Cemetery Road (now Lovelock Avenue) and Clyde Street, formerly owned by Judge Chapman and at that time owned by Mr Richard Brinsley, was leased by the Red Cross for three years. It was designated the Woodside Auxiliary Hospital for Facial Injuries, more commonly known as the Jaw Hospital.[5] It would accommodate thirty-six patients, and another seven would stay at the Red Cross convalescent home at Montecillo (the Montecillo Veterans' Home and Hospital); later it was announced that the overflow would be in Dunedin Hospital, where the old Victoria Ward was temporarily renamed the Sidcup Ward.[6] The Red Cross Society agreed to spend around £1,000 to supply full equipment for twenty-five beds, and a further £600 for an annexe in the grounds of Dunedin Hospital to accommodate Pickerill's staff. The latter building contained rooms for the dental officer, mechanic, and photographer, and also plaster and dark rooms.[7] Woodside was formally handed over to the Otago Hospital Board at the end of April 1919.

Pickerill left Sidcup in March 1919, and arrived in New Zealand on the troopship *Tainui* on 30 April. A number of his patients also returned on the

Tainui and, after a month's leave, were scheduled for admission to Woodside on 28 May.[8] How the hospital was to be administered seemed not to have been considered – not until late June did the Hospital Board decide it should be run along the same lines as the Montecillo Convalescent Home, and the suggestion was made to the Red Cross Society that it should administer the institution.[9] The Red Cross and others consulted (including the Ministers of Defence and Public Health) agreed, and Woodside became the responsibility of the Red Cross from 16 July 1919. It was staffed by Red Cross VADs (members of the nursing-assistant group Volunteer Aid Detachment). The work of the Jaw Hospital was now spread between Woodside, the Sidcup Ward at Dunedin Hospital, and Montecillo; nursing staff were situated at Woodside, technical services in the Red Cross Annexe in the Dunedin Hospital grounds, and clerical staff in the committee room in Dunedin Hospital. Surgery took place in Dunedin Hospital.

Pickerill had expected to return to the University in June 1919. The Defence Department, however, could not yet release him from full duty: 'in a few months [he] may be placed on part-time service', but this would depend on how soon he could complete the treatment of the soldiers coming to Dunedin.[10] His arrival and the establishment of the Jaw Hospital certainly captured the attention of the local press and his extensive interviews featured headlines such as 'Wonders of plastic surgery', 'Marvellous results achieved', and 'Miracles of plastic surgery … an afternoon with Dr Pickerill'. The public learnt that 'A high explosive shell can make a wreck of a man's face, and the most sympathetic people find it difficult to repress a shudder at the sight of a man with his jaw or nose, or any of his features shot away … The late war brought wonderful developments in many departments of knowledge, but no development was more wonderful than that of the art of plastic surgery'.[11] Pickerill listed his patients as those whose treatment he had not yet completed, those he had sent home earlier to await treatment, and those who had returned 'without having passed through his hands in England'. He emphasised the importance of meticulous records for historical and research purposes and for future reference on methods of treatment. He commented that many of the records from Sidcup were incomplete because the work 'was of such a strenuous nature that the staff could not keep pace with it, with the result that there are several months of back work to overtake'. He spoke about the importance of restoring function to the affected parts, appearance being secondary. One advance he stressed was the repair of severely damaged lips so as to overcome the distressing condition of uncontrolled drooling;[12] surgical repair of cleft lip was a field in which he was to excel.

On 15 June he was appointed Officer Commanding Military Hospitals in Otago and promoted to Lieutenant Colonel. His staff at Dunedin Hospital consisted of two other officers – Captain Seed and the anaesthetist Captain Marshall – three nursing sisters, and four sergeants, the latter his technical staff. The services of the technicians (an artist, a photographer, a modeller, and a dental mechanic) were indispensable, but the Army initially failed to appreciate their worth – they had been demoted from the temporary rank of sergeant at Sidcup to private once they returned home. Their commanding officer came to their defence through the Returned Services Association (RSA), which learnt that these highly trained men were receiving just five shillings per day. The RSA secretary thought they should be paid at the specialist rate of ten shillings a day. Pickerill noted that the men had civil employment waiting for them, yet the Defence Department would not discharge them.[13] They were willing to remain in the service provided they were adequately paid, so Pickerill must have been relieved to see the situation resolved – the four of them are wearing sergeant's stripes in the staff photograph.

Despite assurances that all returning servicemen with facial and jaw injuries were to be sent to Dunedin, Pickerill became concerned that some such patients were retained elsewhere. One of these patients, in Auckland Hospital, refused operations there, and requested Pickerill to arrange for his transfer to Dunedin– 'You started on me, and I am to let you finish me. If not the jaw can stay as it is'.[14]

Except for the lack of 'fresh' cases, the work in Dunedin followed the pattern developed at Sidcup, and was well illustrated during a full day of seminars and demonstrations attended by selected members of the New Zealand Dental Association from throughout the country. This was New Zealand's first continuing education programme in maxillofacial surgery, and was jointly presented by the Association, the Dental School, and the Dunedin Hospital. Pickerill described the work at Sidcup, illustrating bone-grafting techniques using fixation by means of screws made from the patient's own bone; the repair or replacement of noses by grafting cartilage and skin; rebuilding lips; skin grafting to replace lost tissue in the mouth; and transposition of sections of muscle to restore function to otherwise paralysed muscles. Participants viewed the vast display of records, and Captain Seed showed the types of splints and surgical equipment used. After a ward round and a tour of the facilities, Pickerill demonstrated the placement of a bone graft and an intra-oral skin graft in the operating theatre. The methods of endotracheal anaesthesia used by Captain Marshall were described as 'peculiar and interesting'. This exhausting and concentrated day was relieved by an evening smoke concert hosted by the Otago Branch.[15]

Those attending this day course were understandably greatly impressed. Frank Armstrong later described it as 'a unique occasion in the history of Dentistry', and 'Colonel Pickerill's Jaw Section is undoubtedly the finest series of clinics this country is ever likely to get'. Armstrong was actually firing shots to have the next Association conference in Dunedin when the University would be celebrating its jubilee, but he had been very moved by what he had seen and heard. He also used the occasion to stress the need for a new Dental School, a matter that was soon to involve Pickerill's energies.[16]

The publicity given to the Jaw Hospital attracted the attention of civilians in need of plastic surgery, but the country's only plastic surgeon was fully committed to the military. The Hospital Board considered the possibility of making an appointment to the Dunedin Hospital in October 1919, but the matter was held over until Pickerill had been demobilised. In the meantime, however, he was authorised to undertake care and treatment of any civilian patients requiring plastic surgery of the face 'who may be referred to him by members of the staff'.[17] He could not simply start up his own civilian section, but had to work with the Medical Superintendent and a committee of honorary surgeons. This development resulted in some problems over allocation of beds, and Pickerill had to be conciliatory toward one of the other surgeons. He also had to rebut firmly any impression of Professor Ferguson, Dean of the Medical School, that his work was 'chiefly of academic interest'. He did this by sending photographs of patients currently under his care to show the 'necessity of such work amongst the civilian community'. Ferguson hastily made an about-face, replying that he was 'alive to the necessity of retaining [Pickerill's] experience and skill' but that he had a problem allocating limited beds between two surgeons. The photographs he found 'horrible looking things' and were a strong justification for him championing the view that 'plastic surgery of the face should be in the most skilled hands we can find'.[18]

This exchange influenced the Board to formalise the place of facial and plastic surgery in the hospital – just days later it resolved 'That a special Department be instituted for treatment of cases requiring special Facial and Jaw Surgery for Dunedin Hospital'.[19] Pickerill's dual role in the University and the hospital now had to be clarified. The University Council, recognising the breadth of his skills in oral medicine, oral pathology, and oral surgery and his teaching in these areas to medical students, had requested the Board some years previously to appoint him honorary stomatologist. In March 1920 he intimated that he wished to resign from this post. The Medical Superintendent discussed the matter with him, pointing out that this would have to be a decision of the University Council, unless he were willing to accept the alternative position of Surgeon-in-Charge of the Facial and Jaw Department.[20]

This would be exactly what Pickerill wanted, but before accepting he needed assurance that he would have first call on the eight beds for facial and jaw patients. He also wanted the title of the dentist who worked with him to be 'Dental Surgeon' rather than 'Assistant Dental Surgeon'. The Medical Superintendent agreed that the stomatology post should lapse by being absorbed into the new position, that the type of case to be submitted should be considered by the medical staff, and that Pickerill be appointed subject to agreement of the University Council. The Medical Committee of the Council, meeting on 29 June, agreed to recommend these proposals to the full Council. The only remaining matter to be resolved was the type of patients to be admitted. In July the Registrar was informed that the honorary medical staff had agreed that patients 'clearly defined as Special Facial and Jaw Case' be placed under Pickerill's care, but 'border-land cases' should be placed under a general surgeon and referred to Pickerill 'if necessary'.[21]

The Jaw Hospital relied on the surgical equipment brought from Sidcup – the Dunedin Hospital itself had no such specialised items. The obvious course was to transfer the Army equipment to the hospital, and the Board therefore asked the Ministry of Defence to donate to it all the equipment for the Facial and Jaw Department.[22] The 'very elaborate equipment' was thought to be beyond the finances of the Board, but if it were donated it would be for 'National use'. The Board would agree to admit any patients requiring special facial and jaw surgery that other boards wished to send, provided the costs of maintenance were guaranteed by the hospital board concerned. Dunedin, with its highly skilled surgeon, was destined to become, for the time being, the national centre for plastic surgery.

By this time, Pickerill was beginning to sever his formal ties with the Army, but the actual date for his return to civilian life and to the Dental School is unclear. The Minister of Defence informed the Chancellor of the University at the end of 1919 that Pickerill had asked the Director of Medical Services for his demobilisation at the end of February 1920, but had found the necessary work could not be completed by that time. If the Council could not spare him for a few months longer, the loss of his 'very special experience in this particular work …' would mean his department would 'suffer under great disability, and those wounded soldiers who still require this treatment would be at a great disadvantage'. If the Council agreed to this request, the Defence Department would be under 'great obligation' and the University would be 'rendering a very real service to the returned disabled soldier'.[23] The Council could not deny such an appeal, but it wanted the Ministry to live up to its obligation by meeting additional costs that would follow – the University was Paying Davies, the Acting Director, £50 per annum to cover the rent of his surgery rooms while he was at the Dental School, and Pickerill was receiving a retainer of £100 per annum.[24]

The Council naturally wanted a definite date when Pickerill would return to the School. The Ministry of Defence informed the University in March that it agreed to meet its obligation to make the payments requested, and would give a definite date when Pickerill would be released from service.[25] The Minister later informed the Council that Pickerill's duties would be complete about the middle of June, 'supposing no more fresh cases' were admitted. The University could assume he would be available by 1 July. The Minister noted there may still be occasional operations required for facial and jaw deformities, and asked whether the University would still allow Pickerill to perform these operations. The Council agreed with this request, 'as long as it did not interfere with his University work'. The University was getting impatient and wanted its Dean back full-time, but this was not all. At the end of June, the Medical Committee learnt from Pickerill that the Defence Department was now unwilling to relinquish his services on 1 July.[26] The Council, annoyed by this development, reminded the Minister of his earlier commitment, and said Pickerill's services were required at the Dental Hospital at the agreed time.

To add to the confusion surrounding his return to the University, Pickerill's military records show he was demobilised on 1 February 1920. It is therefore hard to see how the Ministry could hold on to him so determinedly.

The Sidcup Ward at the hospital was found to be in need of some maintenance before it could be handed back to the Board. In October 1920 the Medical Superintendent told the Board he had approved repairs, and the Minister of Defence had been informed.[27] The Officer Commanding the Otago District was directed to assemble a Court of Inquiry 'in the matter of repairs to the Sidcup Ward'.[28] Although this unusual course of action suggests the intriguing possibility that the 'cheery' patients Pickerill had previously boasted about had become over-exuberant and caused damage, the extensive inquiry, inspections, and correspondence reveal little more than some chipped paint in the ward's sunroom. The Court did not support Falconer's opinion that the amount of chipping was more than the result of fair wear and tear.[29] The total repair and cleaning bill was just £39 – probably significantly less than the cost of the inquiry and the correspondence it generated.

The annual meeting of the Red Cross Society in December 1920 learnt that only twenty patients were in care at Woodside, and spare accommodation was being used by 'several orthopaedic cases'. The military tasks of the Jaw Hospital were almost complete, but it did not close until 22 December 1921.[30]

Following the closure of Woodside and the Sidcup Ward, any military patients still requiring treatment were sent to Trentham under the care of T.D.M. Stout, and the order was made for all records to be sent to Defence Headquarters in Wellington. This command was, however, resisted in Dunedin, chiefly by Professor Ferguson, Dean of the Medical School, who was no doubt encouraged by Pickerill. The Director General of Medical Services pointed out very firmly that the records 'are not in any way the property of Pickerill' and that they belonged to the Department of Defence. It was eventually agreed that they should stay in the Pathology Museum at the Medical School, but any records required by Stout would be sent to Trentham. In 1926 Pickerill wanted the records to be housed in the new Dental School, then nearing completion. This initially did not go down well with Hercus, who accused Pickerill of being 'on the warpath' trying to secure half the models of facial and jaw cases for the Dental School.[31] Unfortunately, most of the records, with the exception of the patients' files, have now disappeared. No plaster casts seem to have survived, and only a small number of watercolours are included in the patients' files, which are deposited at Sidcup in the Macalister Archive, and in the Hocken Collections, Dunedin. Several files and also wax models graphically illustrating the nature and severity of the facial injuries are retained in the School of Dentistry.

Although Pickerill's distinguished wartime service had now ended, recognition of his expertise was transferred to his work with the civilian population. A feature article headed 'One gain from the War … Civilian cases now treated' extolled the achievements of wartime plastic surgery, and described the type of conditions now able to be treated successfully. The article concluded:

> [the] new surgery is wonderful, surpassing all the imaginings of our forefathers … surprising even the experts …
>
> Already we have the outstanding restoration of function and to hope and to health and usefulness of soldiers who in all probability would have been otherwise doomed to despair and misery, if not early death. Now the civilian population is getting the benefit of the experience. Uncomely women are made presentable, infants are rid of deformities, persons who are disfigured by accidents are made comfortable and able to resume work. It is one of the great wonders of the age. The practitioners following the tradition of their profession have said very little

> about their achievements. Let us, who receive their astounding aid, take care that their modesty does not cause the marvels to shrink out of their due place in our vision.[32]

Pickerill's status as a civilian plastic surgeon was firmly established, but events at the Dental School were to dominate his life over the next seven years.

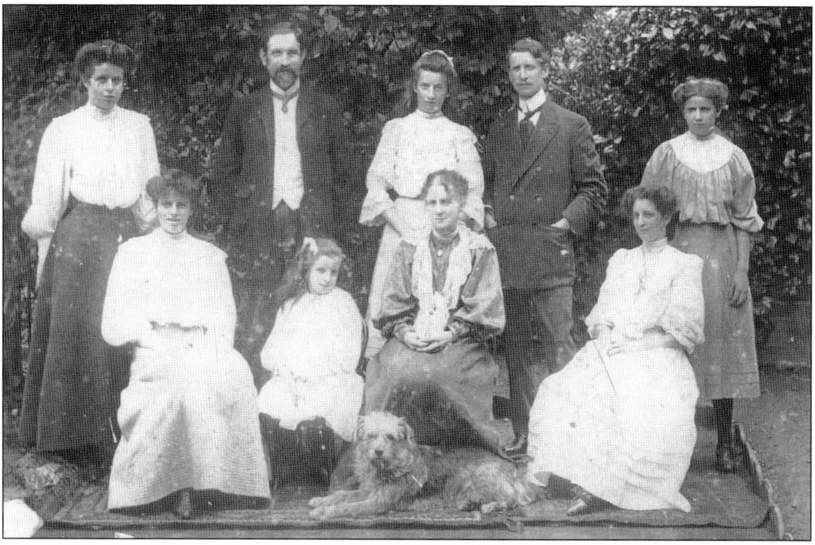

The Pickerill family, Hereford, c. 1905. Front row, from left, May, Doris, Mary Ann Pickerill, Gertrude; standing, from left, Ethel, Thomas Pickerill, Maud, Henry Percy, and Grace.

***Right**: The family home, No.1 Montrose Villas, 13 Harold Street, Hereford.*

***Bottom**: The Wye River at Holme Lacy, scene of much family enjoyment.*

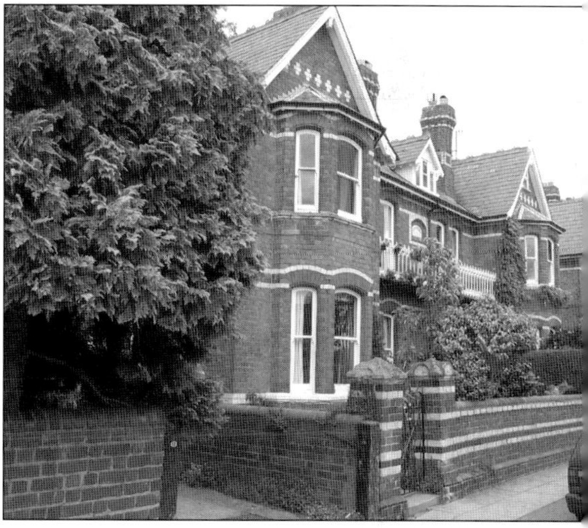

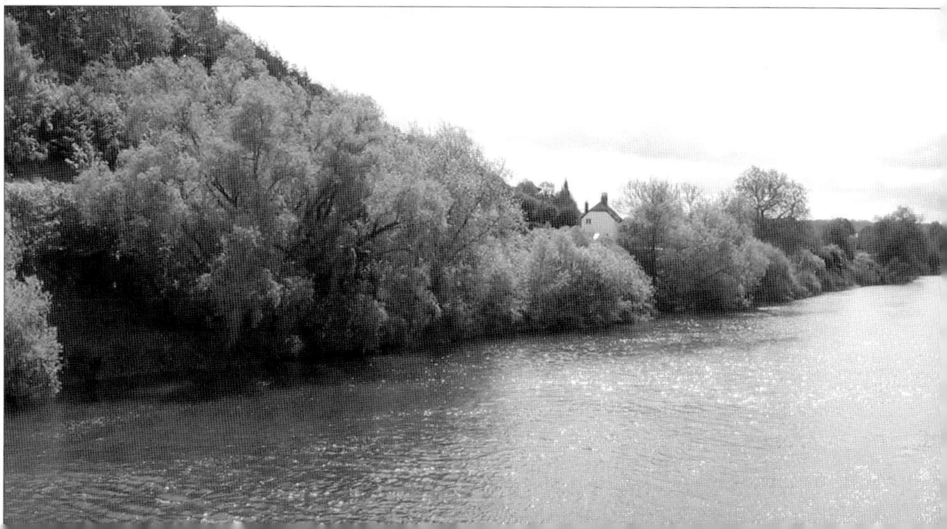

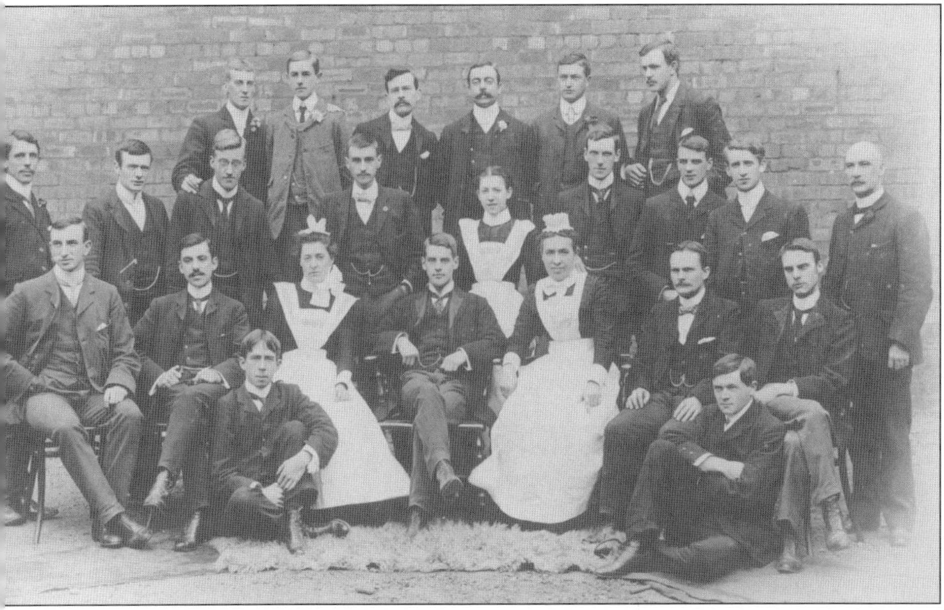

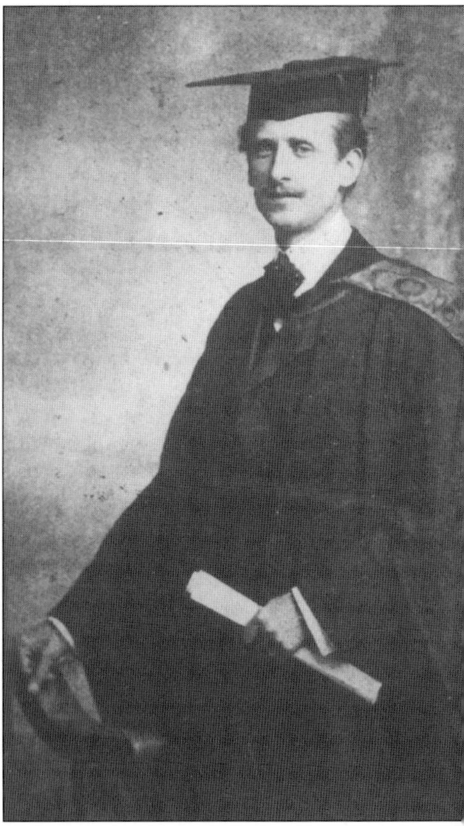

Top: *Students and staff at the Birmingham Dental Hospital, 1901. Pickerill is second from right in the second row. Future brother-in-law Jack Knott is on Pickerill's right.*

Right: *Dr H.P. Pickerill, graduating MB, ChB, University of Birmingham, 8 July 1905.*

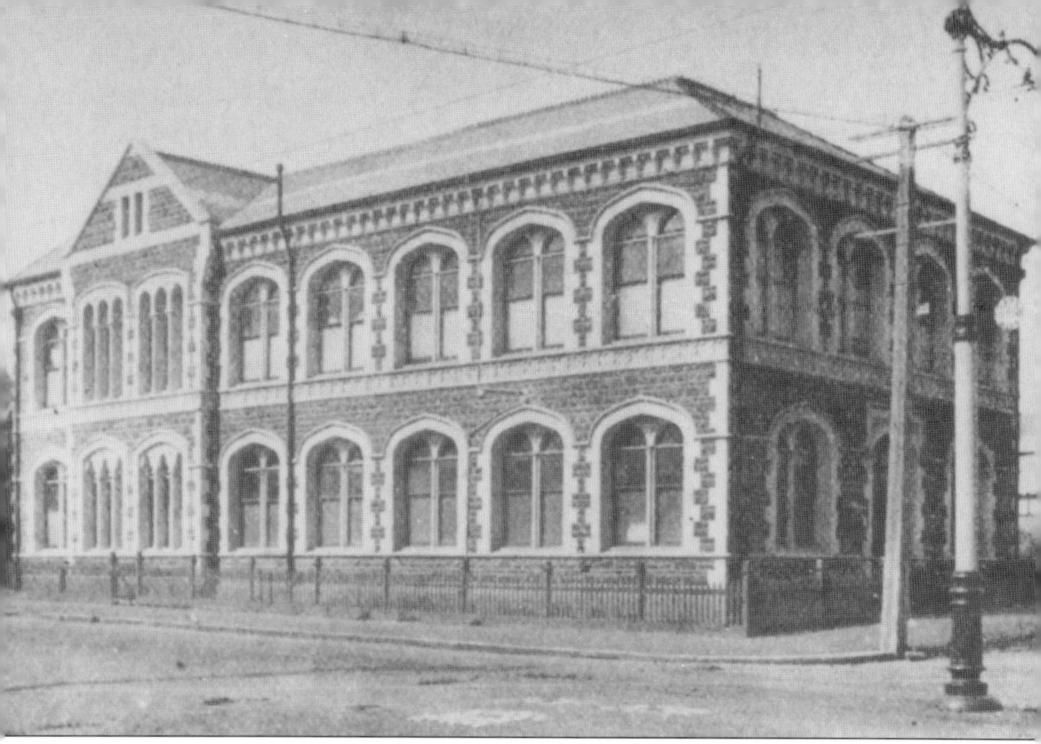

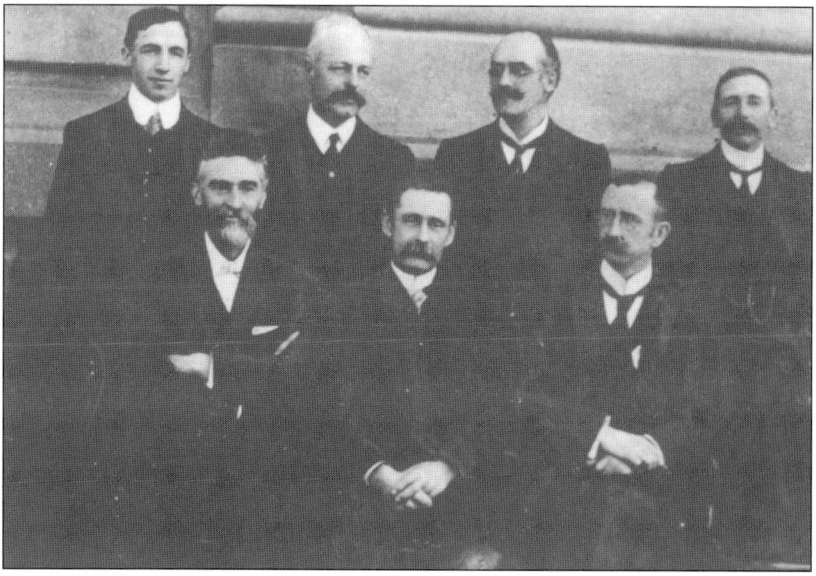

***Top**: The pride of the New Zealand Dental Association – the first Dental School and Hospital, University of Otago, corner of Union and Castle Streets, on the banks of the Leith Stream.*
***Bottom**: The first Executive Committee of the New Zealand Dental Association. Standing, from left, K Gilmer (Treasurer), F.W. Thompson, Herbert Cox, A.E. Smith; seated, from left, A. Hoby (Secretary and Vice-President), H.P. Rawson (President), T.A. Hunter.*

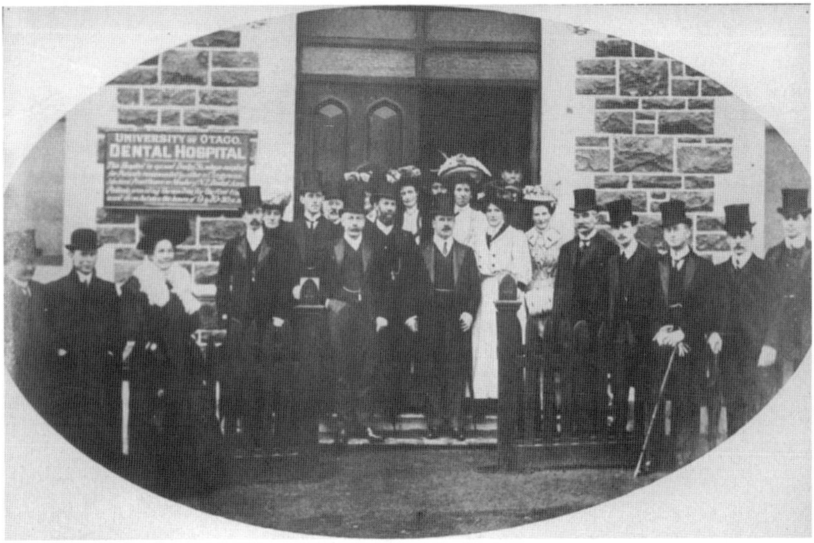

The official party at the formal opening of the Dental School, April 1908. The Prime Minister, the Right Honourable Sir Joseph Ward, is in the centre of the front row; second from his right is the Minister of Education, the Honourable George Fowlds, and T.K. Sidey is on Fowlds' right in the front row. The Vice-Chancellor, Sir James Allen, is immediately to the left of the ladies in the front row, and Pickerill is on his left. Otago Witness, *15 April 1908. Hocken Collections.*

Facing page, top*: The operative room on the first floor in the early days of the Dental School and before the gross overcrowding following the First World War. Bell Collection, School of Dentistry.*

Facing page, bottom*: The first graduates with the Bachelor of Dental Surgery, University of Otago. Left, C.E. (later Professor Sir Charles) Hercus; centre, W.S. Seed; right, A.J. Hansen. By permission of the Editor,* New Zealand Dental Journal.

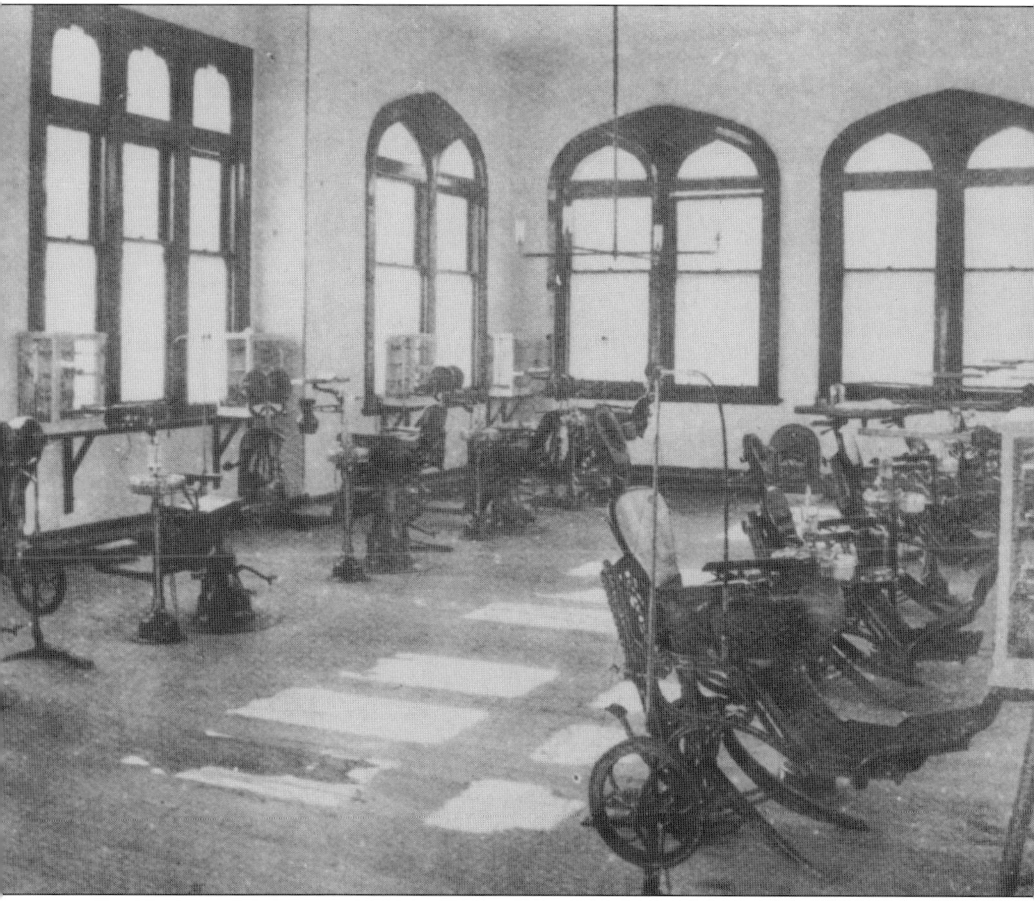

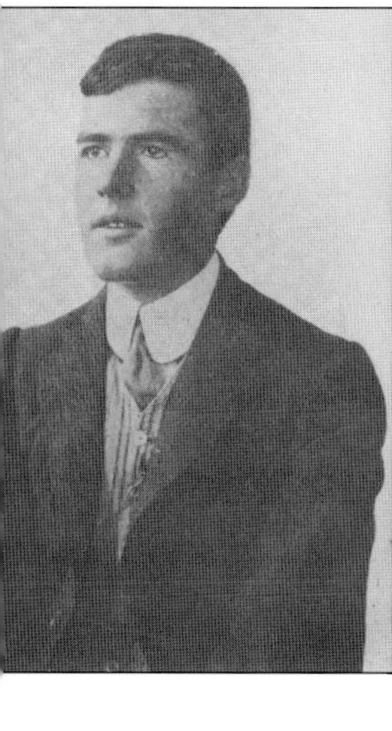

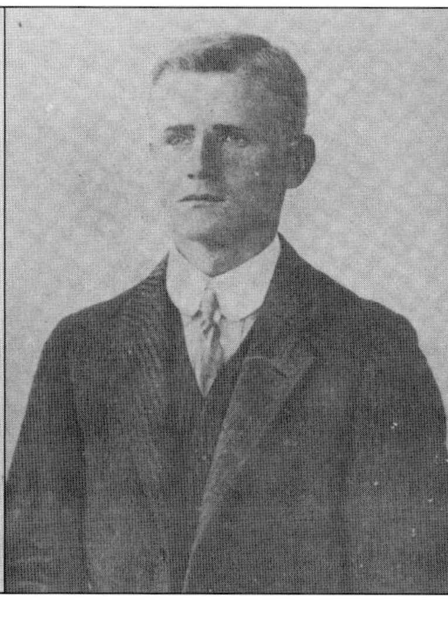

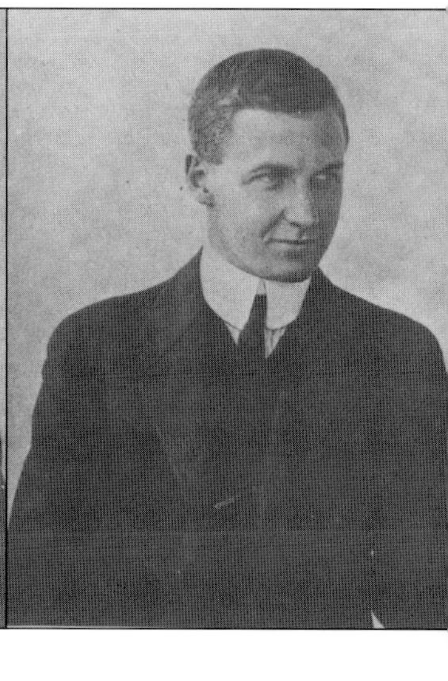

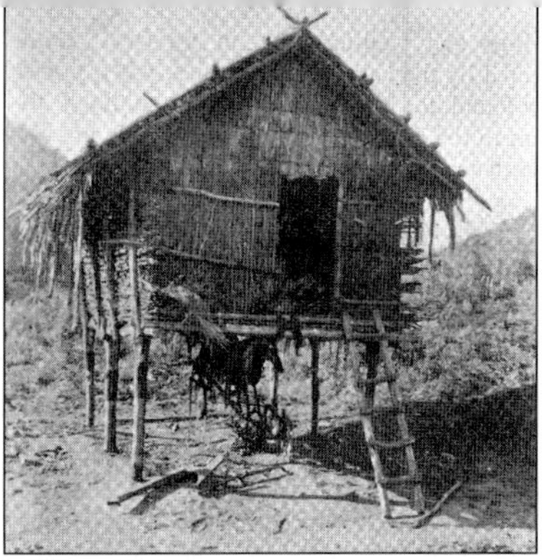

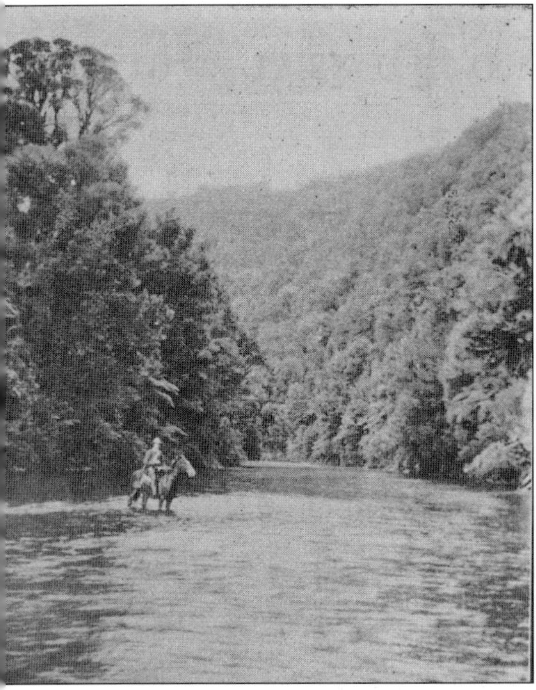

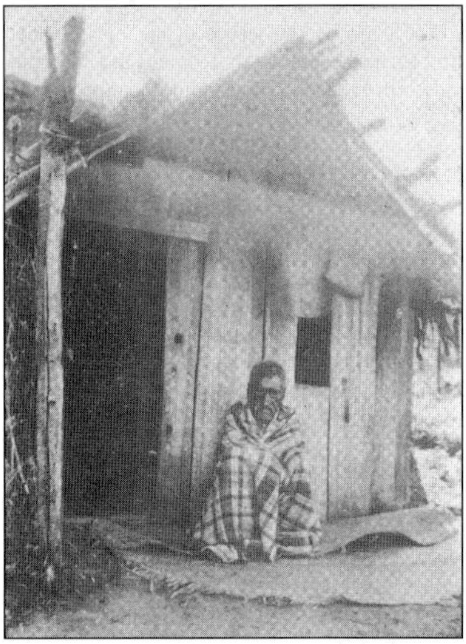

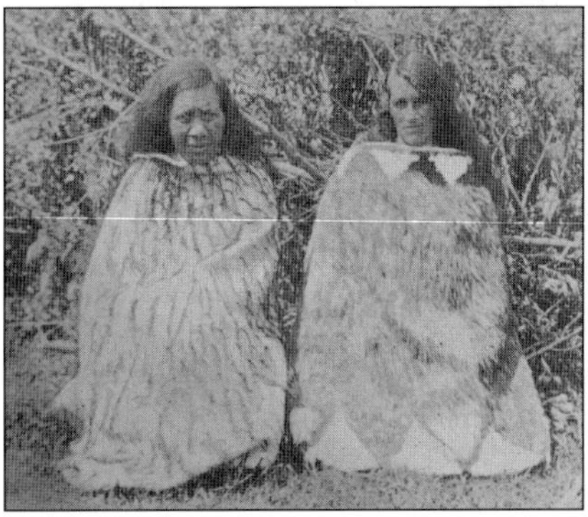

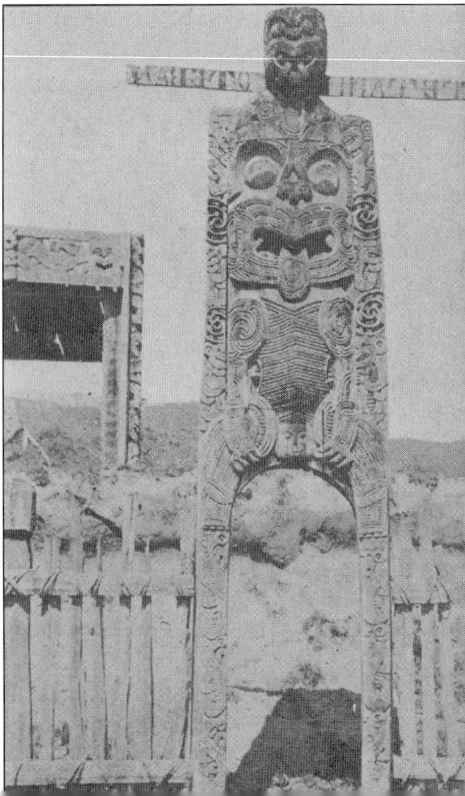

Photographs from the Urewera expeditions, 1912–13.

By permission of the Editor,
New Zealand Dental Journal

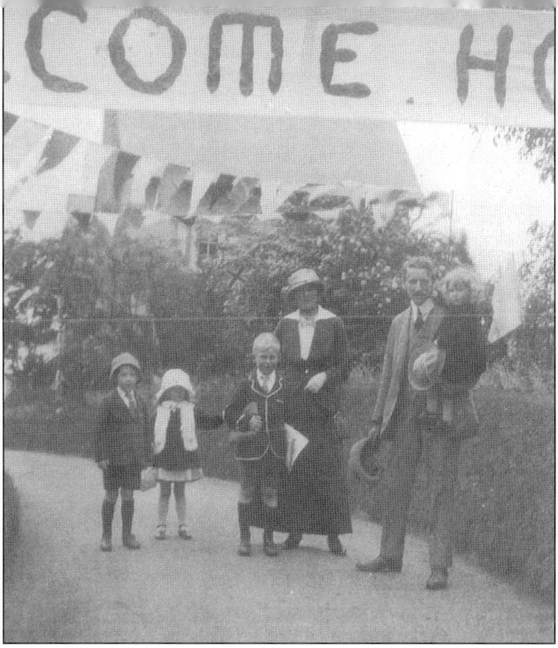

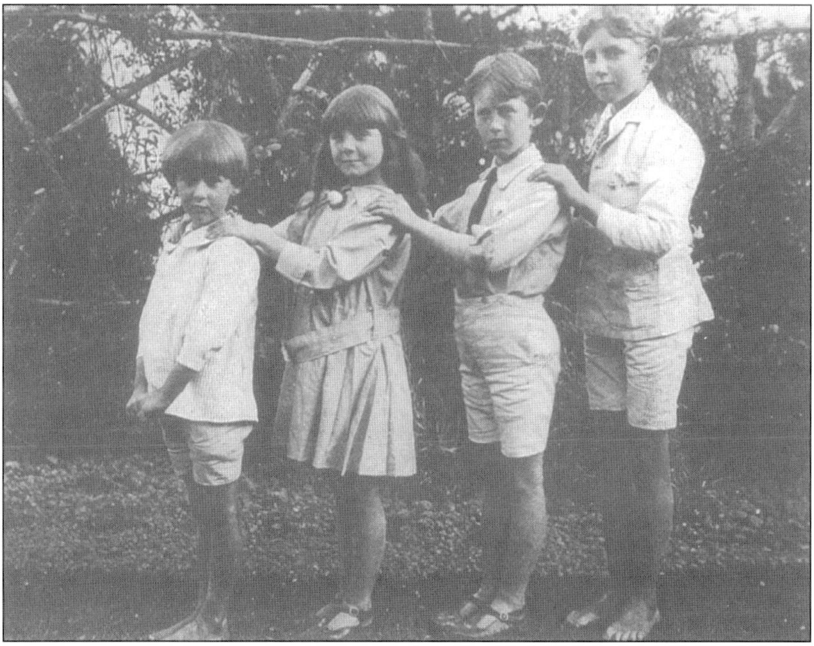

Top: *The family accompanied Pickerill on his 1914 sabbatical in England, where he presented his caries findings to the International Dental Federation. They received a very warm welcome back in Hereford. From left, Thomas (Kana), Kathleen (Kay), Val (John Percival), Mabel, and Percy holding Paul.*

Bottom: *The Pickerill children, c. 1919. From left, Paul, Kay, Kana, and Val.*

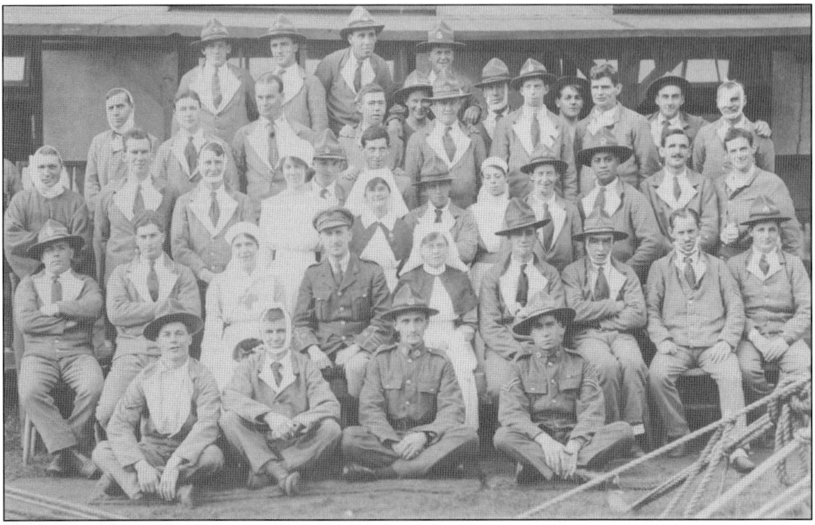

At the Second New Zealand General Hospital, Walton-on-Thames. Pickerill (centre) with patients and staff, 1917. *By permission of the Editor,* New Zealand Dental Journal.

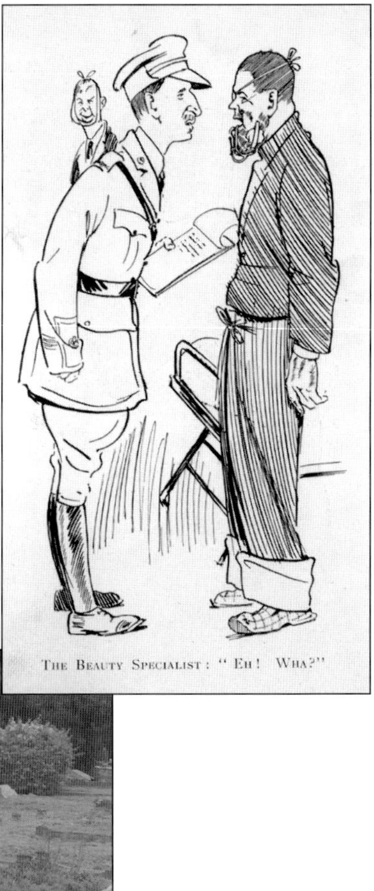

***Right**: The Major as viewed by his patients, 1918. With acknowledgement to Light Diet, a Collection of Sketches In and Out of N.Z. Hospitals by Sergeant E.H. Thomson. New Zealand War Records, 1918. Pickerill Papers, Hocken Collections.*

***Bottom**: One of the pair of monuments in the churchyard of St Mary's Church, Walton-on-Thames, memorials to the New Zealand soldiers who died at the Second New Zealand General Hospital.*

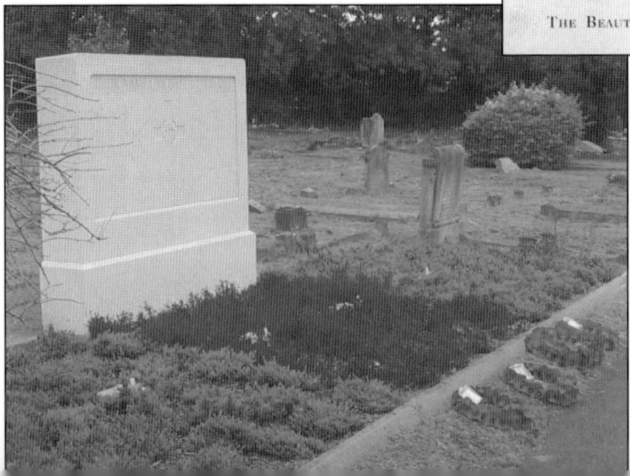

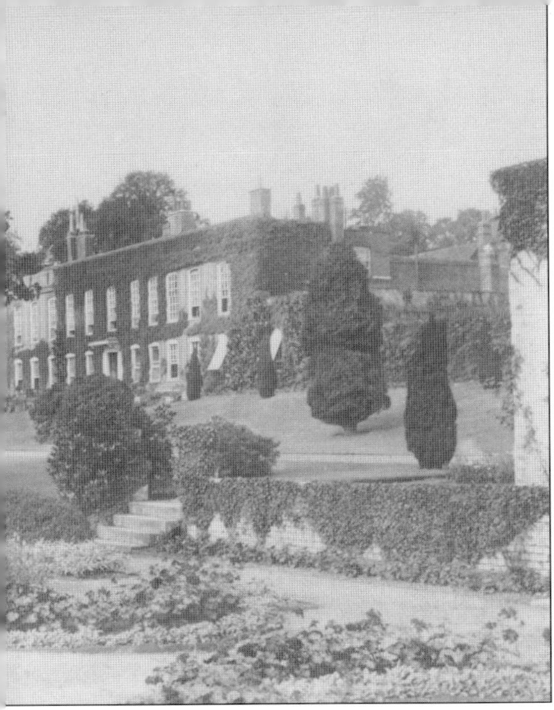

Frognal House, the central building of The Queen's Hospital, Sidcup. From The Queen's Hospital, Sidcup, Kent, 1917–1929.

***Below**: The visit of Her Majesty Queen Alexandra to Sidcup, 30 April 1918. Pickerill is third from right, and Gillies third from left. From The Queen's Hospital, Sidcup, Kent, 1917–1929.*

***Bottom**: Major Pickerill and his staff at Sidcup.* Otago Witness, *13 August 1919. Hocken Collections.*

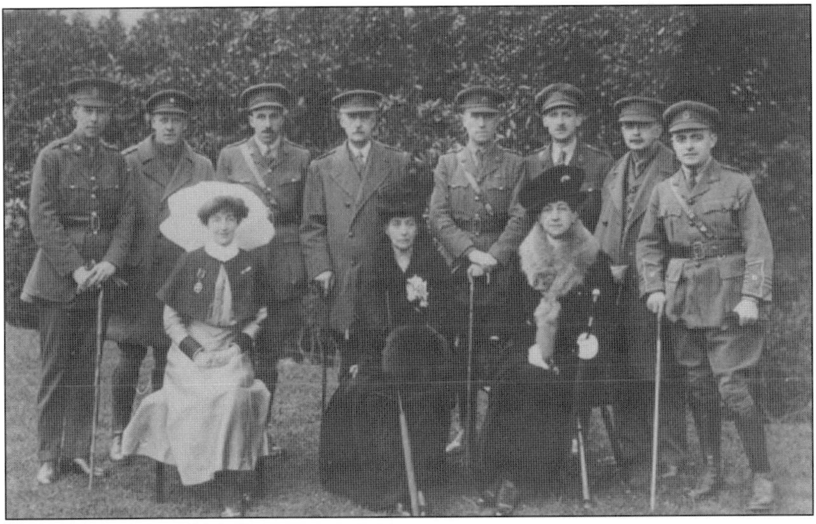

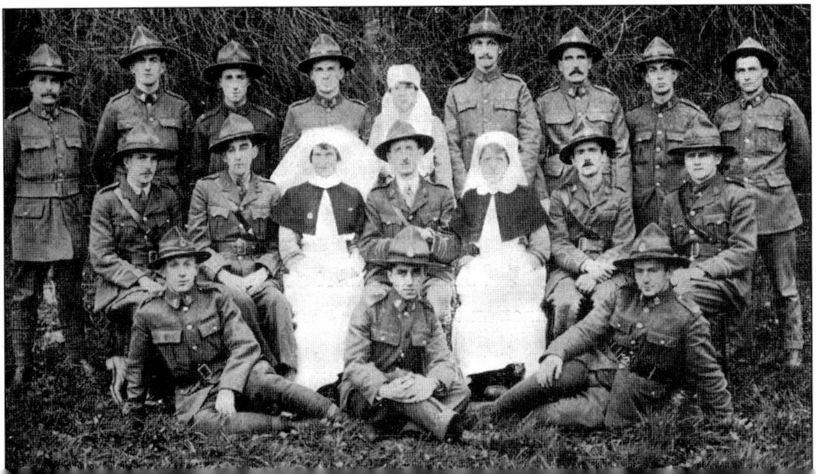

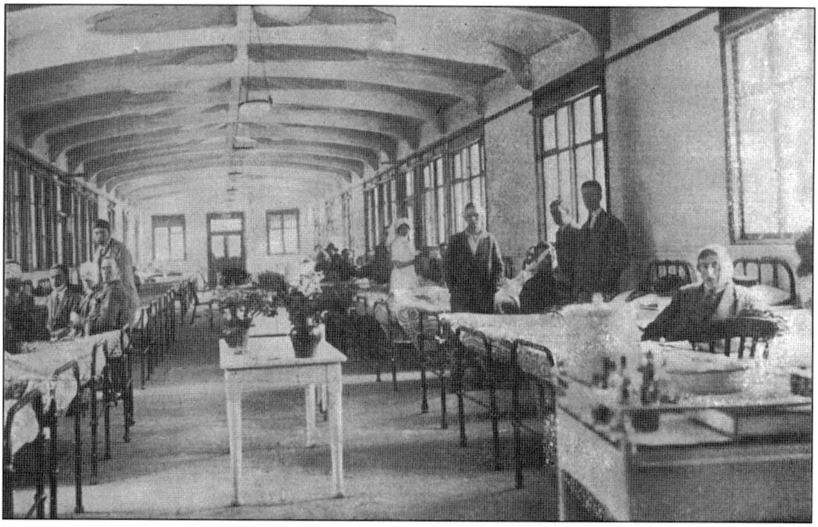

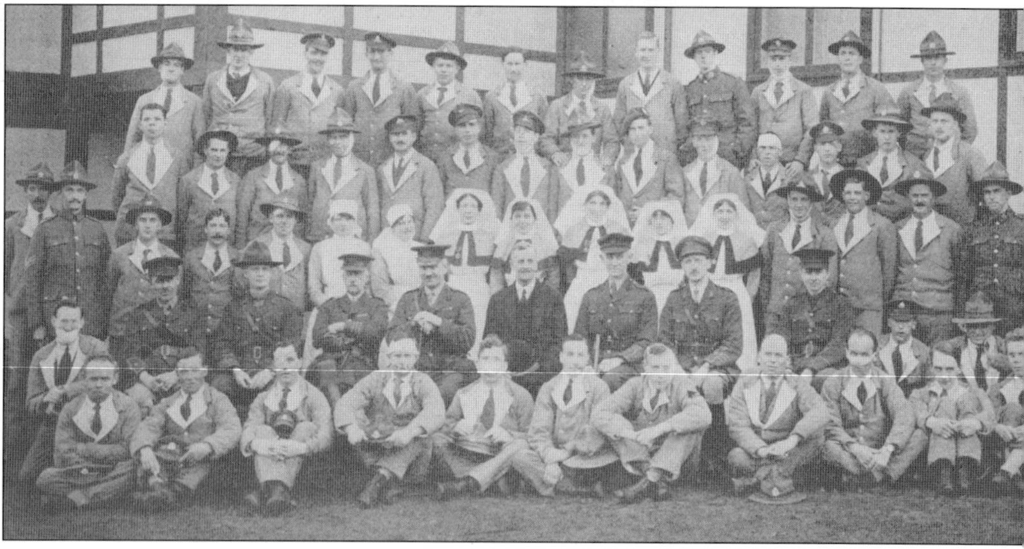

***Top**: The interior of Ward 15, New Zealand Section, The Queen's Hospital, Sidcup.* Otago Witness, *13 August 1919. Hocken Collections.*

***Bottom**: The visit of General G.S. Richardson and Colonel Heaton Rhodes to the New Zealand Section at Sidcup, 21 March 1918. Seated from left, Major B.S. Finn, DSO, NZDC (Deputy Director of Dental Services); Major J.N. Rishworth, NZDC; Lieutenant Colonel J.R. Colvin, Hospital Superintendent; Brigadier General G.S. Richardson, CB, Administrative Office of the New Zealand Forces; Colonel Heaton Rhodes, Special Commissioner of the New Zealand Branch of the British Red Cross Society; Colonel Parkes, CMG, NZMC, Director of Medical Services; Major Pickerill; Lieutenant Birt, RAMC.*
By permission of the Editor, New Zealand Dental Journal.

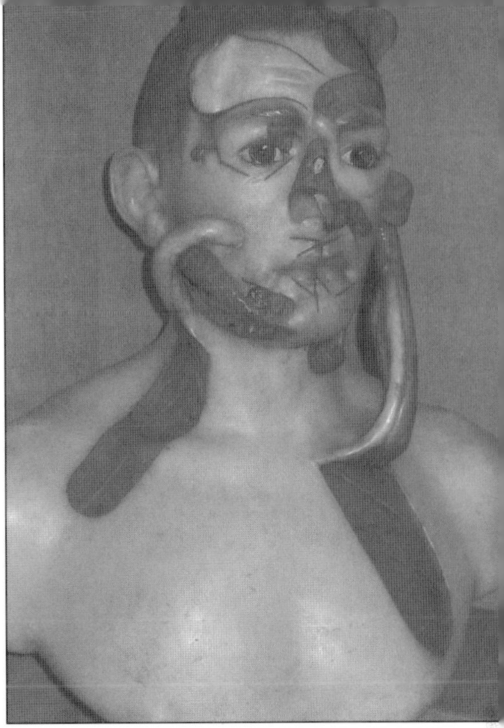

Wax model showing the types of tubed and other grafts used by the units at Sidcup. Published by kind permission of the Curator of the World War I Archives at The Queen Mary Hospital, Sidcup.

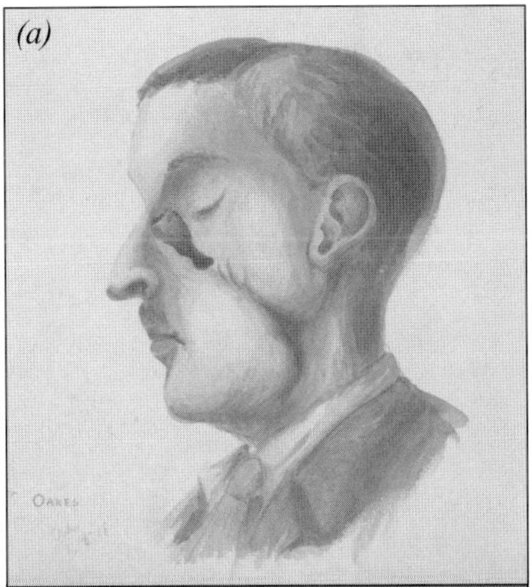

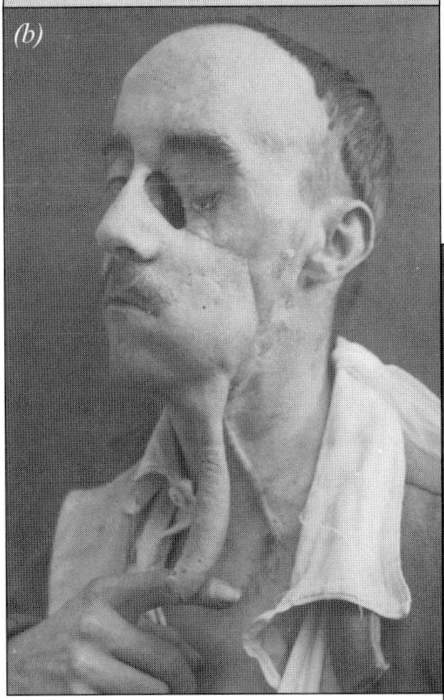

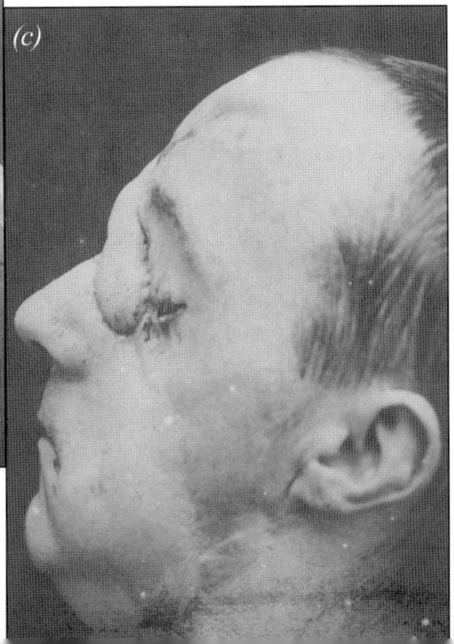

***Left**: An example of the surgery by Pickerill and his team at Sidcup.*
***(a)** the water colour illustration of a soldier with an 'old' facial wound, on admission to the New Zealand Unit; the left eye has been lost;*
***(b)** the cheek has been partially repaired by a tube graft from the chest;*
***(c)** a tube graft from the forehead is being used to repair the defect in the side of the nose.*

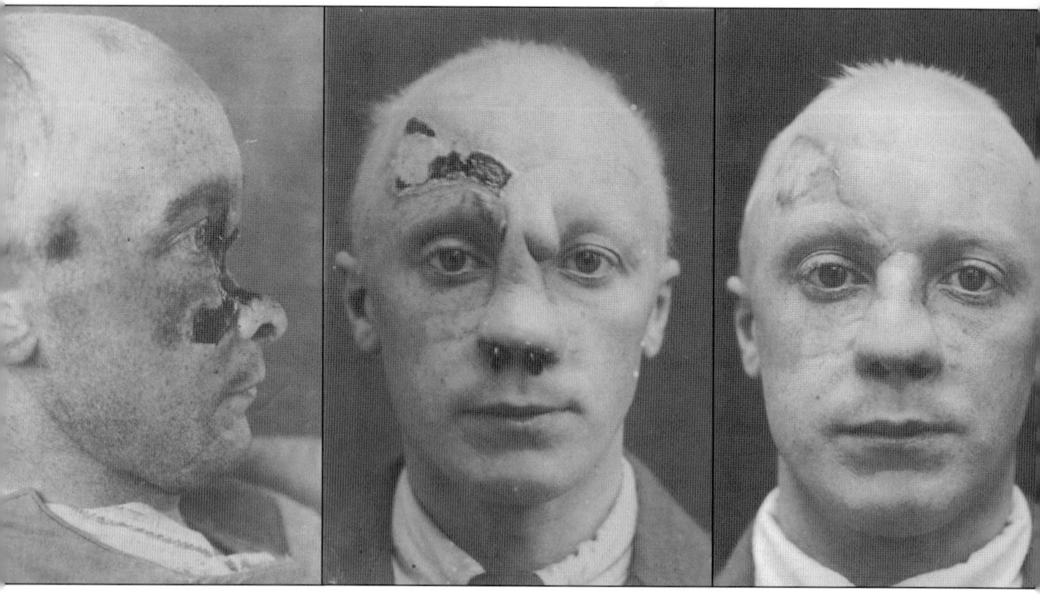

An example of a Pickerill specialty – the repair of the nose.
***Left**, showing loss of the central part of the nose. **Centre**, graft from the forehead completing the replacement of lost tissue. **Right**, during the later stages of healing.*

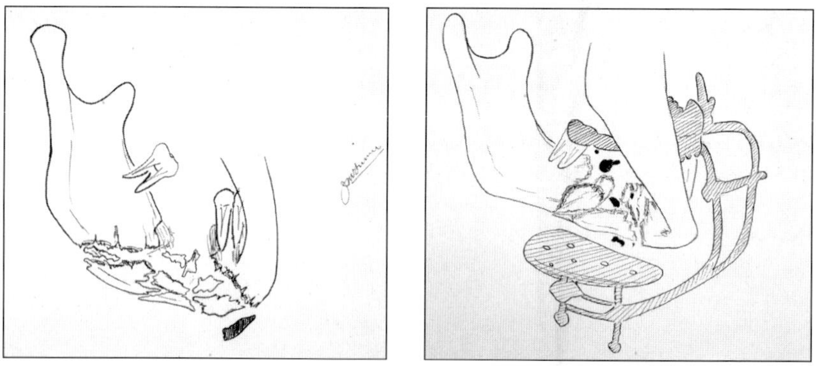

Examples of the tracings of radiographs of the mandibles of two patients with severe comminuted fractures. The tracing on the right shows a splint in situ designed to stabilise the two sections of the mandible. From the folder by Captain J.M. Turner, NZDC, Jaw Records Queen's Hospital Sidcup 1918 held at the Defence Dental Directorate, Wellington.

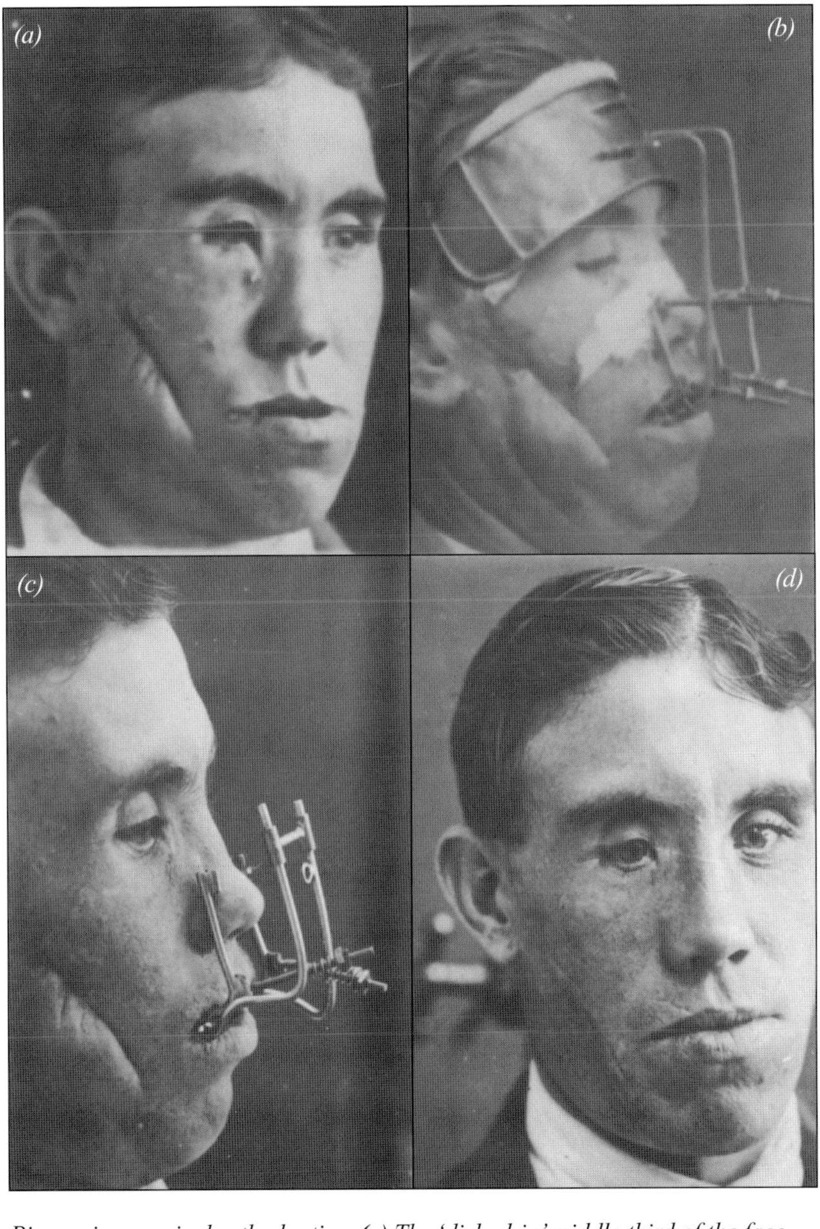

Pioneering surgical orthodontics: ***(a)*** *The 'dished-in' middle third of the face following suturing without replacement of lost bone by grafts (patient on admission to Sidcup), the scar proved to mask deeply seated infection;* ***(b)*** *the 'orthodontic' appliance is anchored by a metal plate on the forehead with bars and a splint attached to the teeth; a splint is also attached to the upper teeth, and this draws the maxilla forward by a system of bars and screws;* ***(c)*** *splints stabilising the new position of the maxilla;* ***(d)*** *the patient at completion of treatment, including removal and repair of the scar, showing greatly improved appearance. The splints display the technical expertise of Major Rishworth.*

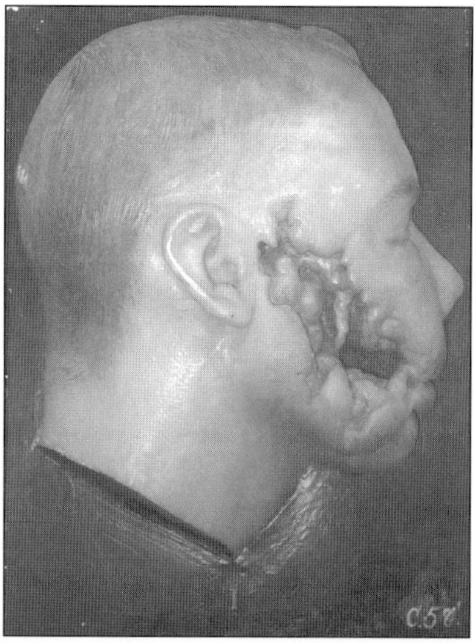

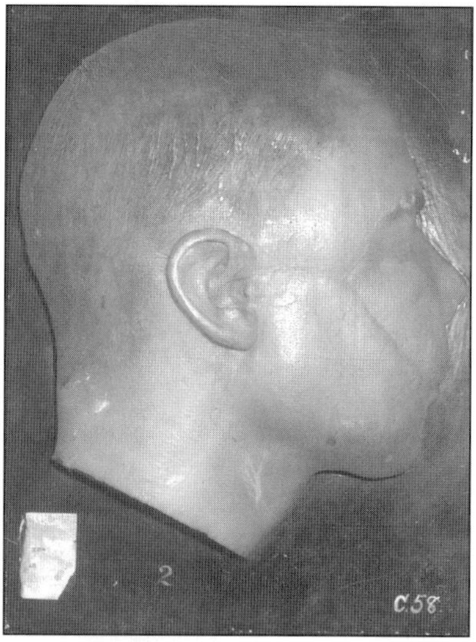

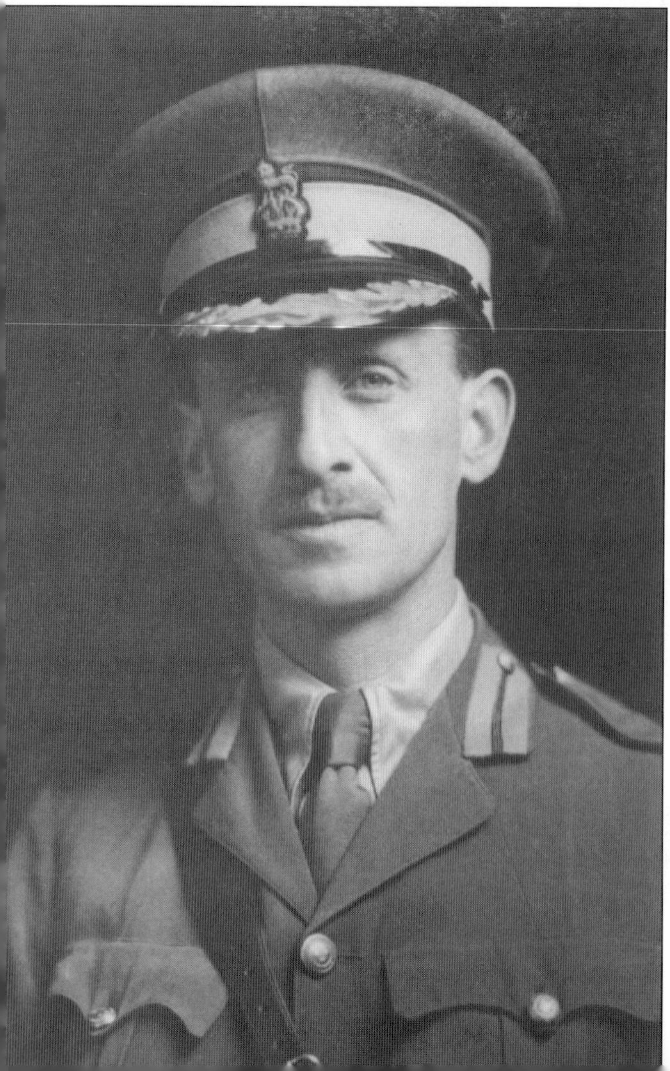

Top: *Examples of the wax models of patients with facial injuries.* ***Left***: *pre-operative, showing the deep wound to the right side of the face;* ***Right***: *post-operative, showing minimal scarring.* *School of Dentistry, University of Otago Collection.*

Left: *Lieutenant Colonel Pickerill, Officer Commanding Military Hospitals Otago, 1919.*

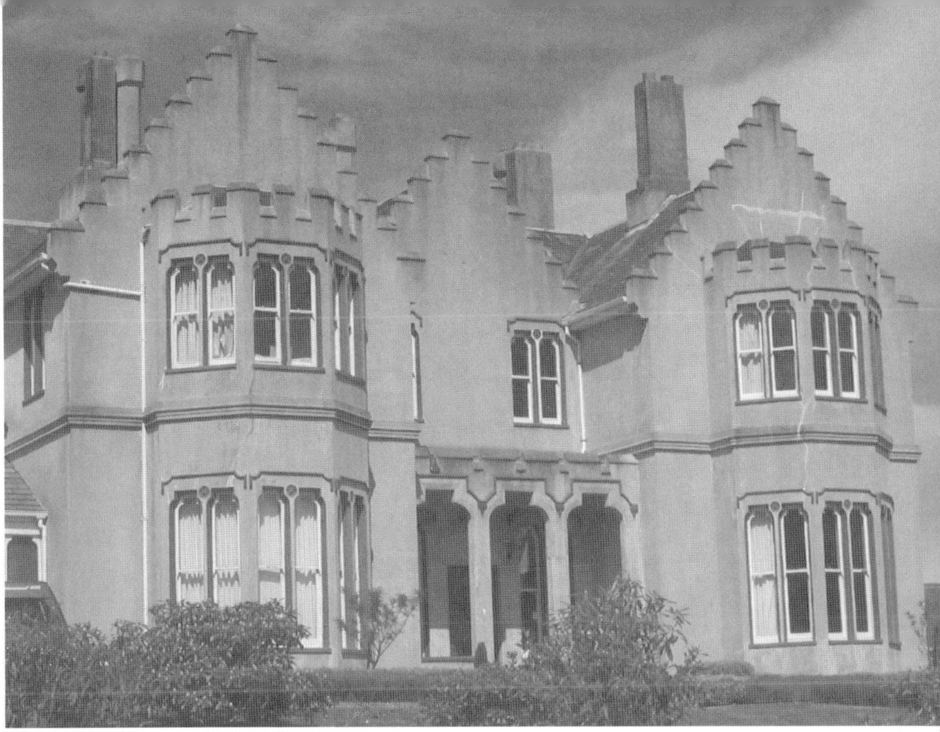

Top: *The large home in Lovelock Avenue, Dunedin, designated as the Woodside Auxiliary Hospital for Facial Injuries, 1919–21.*

Bottom: *The hospital staff pictured outside the technical annexe in the grounds of Dunedin Hospital. Standing, from left, Sergeant Ferguson, Sergeant Thomson, Sister Erwin, Sergeant Cole, and Sergeant Meltzer; seated, from left, Captain Marshall (Anaesthetist), Sister Millar, Lieutenant Colonel Pickerill, Sister Finlayson, and Captain Seed (Dental Officer).*

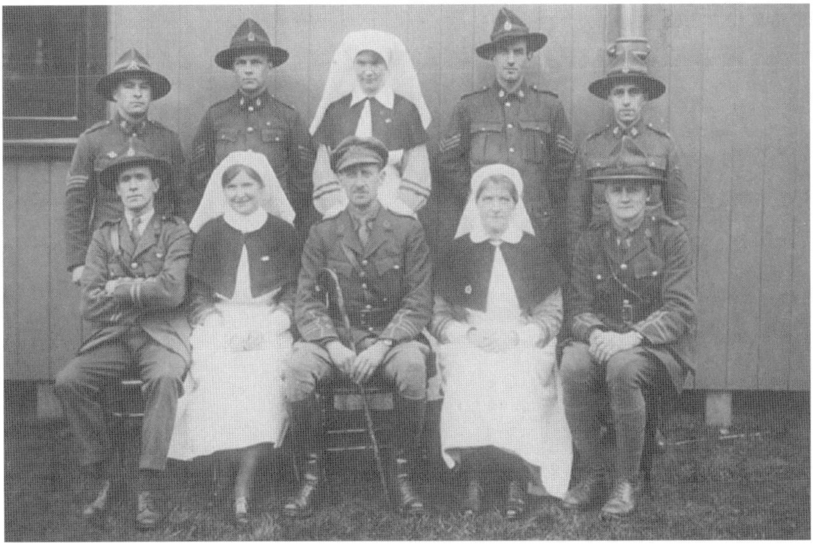

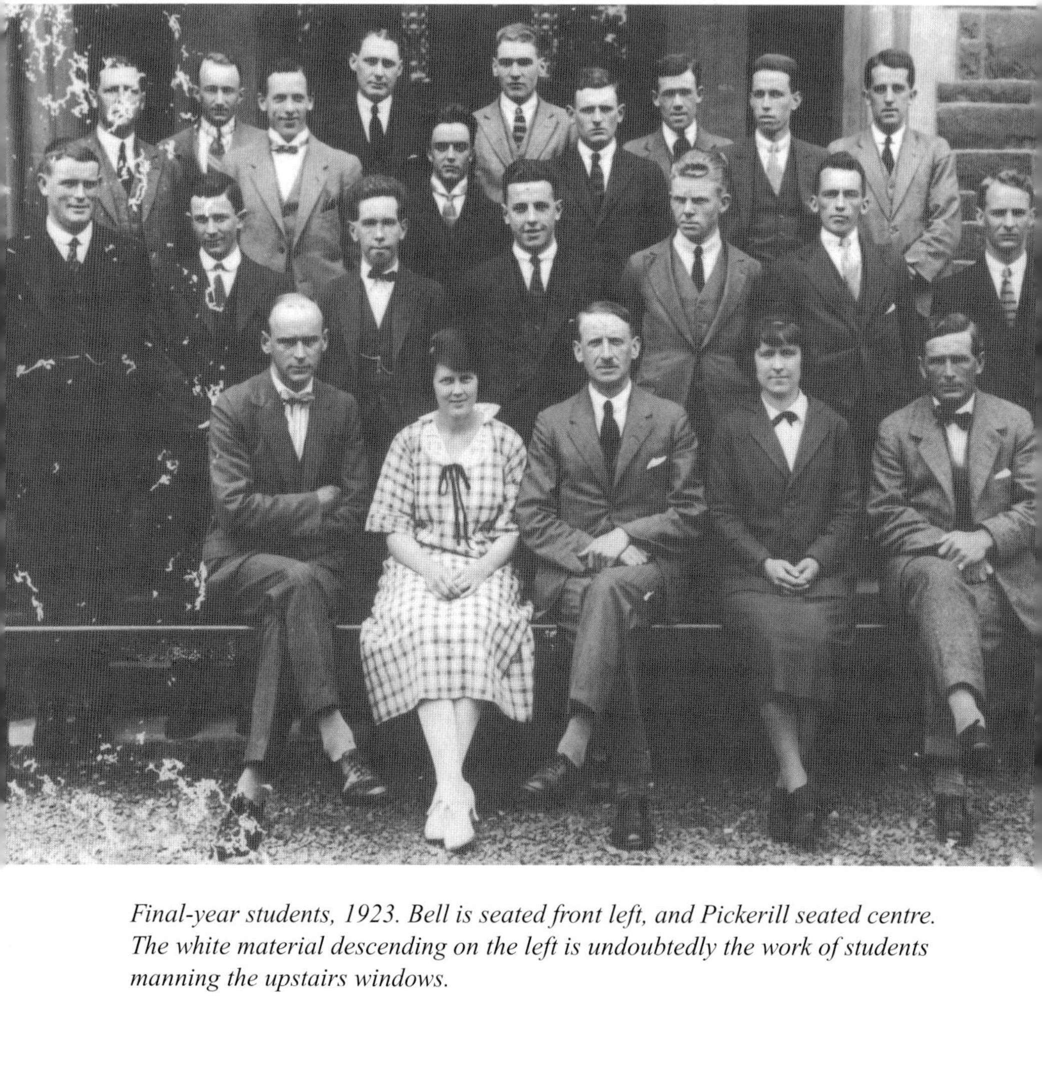

Final-year students, 1923. Bell is seated front left, and Pickerill seated centre. The white material descending on the left is undoubtedly the work of students manning the upstairs windows.

13

Back to the Dental School, turmoil and trauma

The low number of dental students before the war was very worrying. In a curiously unfocused editorial in March 1915, Pickerill had mused on several possibilities for overcoming the problem, asking whether the expense and the difficulty of the course were discouraging applicants, whether the course was too much like the medical course, or whether the preliminary examination might be too challenging. He sought the opinions of members of the Association, asking if the time was now right for the introduction of 'some qualification of a lower standard, such as is provided for in the 1906 Act, [to be] put into operation'.[1] This seeming indecision was in contrast to his words delivered the previous year when he proposed the toast to the University of Birmingham at a meeting of the Central Counties Branch of the British Dental Association. Discussing the shortage of dental students in the United Kingdom, he proclaimed 'I am not suggesting for one moment that from an academic point of view the present course is either too difficult or too lengthy, indeed I am the last man to suggest any such thing, for I regard it as desirable that every dental student should also take a medical degree'.[2]

O.V. Davies quickly found a solution to the acute shortage of students he inherited when he became Acting Director at the end of 1916: bursaries to cover the cost of living in Dunedin and university fees. He proposed payment of £50 per year to non-resident students, and for Dunedin students an amount to cover the fees. A 'Bursary Collecting Committee' that included staff and members of the Otago Branch of the Association was formed, and the Chancellor was invited to be a member.[3] The scheme was soon very successful, although the committee was over-enthusiastic in one critical area – the Faculty and the Branch had canvassed all dentists, including non-members of the Association, without the Association's approval. Charles Hay, a member of the committee, managed to sort out the problem,[4] and the Executive approved the actions early in the New Year, albeit after some opposition from the Christchurch Branch. By September 1917, dentists had donated £270, and Sidey generously contributed £400;[5] £929 had been collected by April 1918 and by then the School had thirteen BDS bursary students and three non-bursary students, one of whom was taking the COP course.[6] Davies was delighted with this extremely healthy outcome, noting that nine bursary applicants were entitled to the Higher Leaving Certificate – the School was now attracting '… the type of men that is needed, those who will keep up the standard and who had a good preliminary education'. He wanted to increase the value of the bursary to £200.[7]

The 1918 Annual Report focused on the success of the bursary scheme, Davies stressing the need to keep it going. The Association lobbied the Government, resulting in the Minister of Public Health providing ten dental bursaries annually – their purpose was to lay the foundation for a School Dental Service. Thirty-two students were taking the full BDS course, including ten Public Health Bursars.[8] When Pickerill returned as Dean on 1 July 1920, he found the School in a much healthier situation than when he left early in 1917. The tenure of Davies had been remarkably successful.

The relationship between Pickerill and Davies had been an uneasy one for many years. An explosive exchange that was to involve the Chancellor occurred at a meeting of the Faculty back in 1910; Pickerill complained to the Registrar that 'one of the junior members' (Davies) had criticised his teaching in a 'very vulgar and impertinent manner', saying that he taught 'with no method at all'. Pickerill had been unable to obtain an apology or withdrawal. 'It is obvious that unless such withdrawal is made either the member referred to or myself must cease to be a member of the Dental Faculty of this University'.[9]

The Chancellor sought specifics, and although Pickerill could not give a verbatim report of the exchange, he quoted Davies using the very curious but highly abusive terms that Pickerill was 'a beauty' and a 'shuffler'. Pickerill said Davies was not in a position to criticise the Director's work or conduct, and doing so made him unfit to be a member of a university faculty. As Chairman of the Faculty, Pickerill again demanded the withdrawal of the remarks, but Davies refused. Thus 'an impasse is reached which can only be overcome either by Mr Davies not being elected to the staff in the future or by my being relieved of my duties as chairman of the faculty'.[10] He also casually mentioned that he was being head-hunted by the University of Sydney to be Dean of its Faculty of Dentistry, and was having difficulty coming to a decision. The

Chancellor must have calmed the situation, as Davies subsequently claimed: 'the matter ended in my favour'.[11] Both remained on the staff, but in a very strained relationship.

A public disagreement in teaching methods occurred at the Association's conference in 1911. G.V. Black, a prominent American dentist, advocated a system of restoring decayed teeth by placing the junction of tooth and filling in places believed to be less susceptible to further decay. This concept of 'extension' of the margins for 'prevention' had its ardent disciples, members of the G.V. Black Club. Opponents decried the method on the grounds that the tooth was greatly weakened as a result of excessive and unnecessary removal of healthy structure. Davies displayed his enthusiasm for the method in his conference paper,[12] and Pickerill was one of those who were harshly critical – the Dean strongly opposed the techniques that presumably were being taught in his own school at the time. It seems, however, that Davies prevailed, as the method was still being taught at the School as late as the 1970s when it was finally discredited. At that time the greatly reduced decay rates meant a more conservative approach to preparing cavities for restoration could be adopted.

The rift surfaced again in 1912, when once more the Chancellor had to intervene. Davies had suggested to Pickerill that the lighting in the main teaching clinic was seriously inadequate and suggested how it could be improved. Instead of considering the matter, Pickerill said he did not think anything was wrong, and that bringing the matter up was a 'shibboleth'. The reply, and the manner of the Dean, provoked Davies to say: 'You do not know what you are talking about'. Davies said that other staff members agreed with him. He was subsequently astonished to receive a letter from Pickerill, and subsequently commented: 'Apparently Dr Pickerill considers it impudence in a member of the staff to venture to make a suggestion; as for rudeness, if you should think my retort was rude, I hope you will make allowance for the provocation, and for the fact that the action of the other members of the staff shows that Dr Pickerill was wrong, and I was right'. Davies copied Pickerill's letter for the Chancellor's information, quoting the extraordinary words: 'Your impudence and rudeness is evidently so innate that I wish you to understand that in future I refuse to know you. I exceedingly regret that I consented to your re-election to the staff'. Davies also enclosed a copy of a resolution passed at a meeting of the honorary staff at the time: 'That the staff consider the light as difficult and recommend that experiments be made with a view to improvement – Mr Hunter to consult with Dr Pickerill re the above'. Pickerill was upset that the Chancellor had been involved. He thought the dispute must remain a 'purely private and personal communication, as indeed I have all along regarded it'. The very diplomatic Chancellor informed Davies that Pickerill had considered the letter indeed to be private and personal. He was sorry there should be misunderstanding and unpleasantness between the Director and Davies, and hoped that Davies could also look on it as a personal matter and continue his good work as honorary dentist.

This was not acceptable to Davies. At another meeting of the honorary staff he moved that Pickerill's letter be received. Hunter, the chairman of the meeting, gave his casting vote to ensure it was not received, and then promptly left the room. Davies had intended, should his motion have been carried, that the matter would not go any further. He told the Chancellor, Sir James Allen: 'My reason for bringing it up before the staff was to show that Dr Pickerill could not insult a member of the staff with impunity'. As far as he was concerned the matter was now dropped and he thanked the Chancellor for his good intentions.[13] And no doubt Sir James sighed with relief.

The effect of all this sniping on the students is not known, but the atmosphere around the School must have been electric. The animosity was to prevail for many years after both had left the Dental School. In the lead-up to its fiftieth jubilee, Davies wrote a paper for the *Journal* purporting to be a history of the Association.[14] It was, however, in the main a history of the School, and it offended Pickerill greatly on numerous fronts. Amongst these he complained to the Secretary of the Association that it 'belittles or ignores my work for the N.Z.D.A.'. He outlined his achievements as Secretary and Editor, and criticised Davies for the lack of any equipment at the school when he arrived in 1907. 'Mr. Davies as a member of the staff and former acting director should have stood by me but did not. He made no secret of the fact that he regarded me as the wrong man for the job.' He went on to describe Davies as 'the only man available with any experience or interest …' to be his *locum tenens* while he was overseas during the war. He stated that it was an open secret that Davies wanted to continue in the role. 'I could have stayed in England, for 2 of the plums in my line were more than offered to me – Dean of the London Hospital Dental School and/or Chief plastic surgeon at Sidcup, but I was determined to finish my job in N.Z. … You may make what you like … of these facts but I think most [of] my past students would not care for their former and first Dean of their Dental school to be handed down as a misfit and a failure. I finally handed over with a new Dental School (as good as could be bought with the money) … and brimful of students'.[15] The Davies' article was indeed a curious mixture, and certainly Pickerill did not receive the acknowledgement he so clearly deserved, although he himself never acknowledged the role Davies played in increasing the number of students during the time of his locum.

The Secretary, Maurice Priestley, supported Pickerill's complaints, harshly criticised Davies, criticised the Editor for accepting a paper dealing mainly with the School and not the jubilee of the Association, and praised Pickerill's contribution, pointing out that it was Pickerill who was awarded Honorary Life Membership on the occasion of the jubilee.[16] As will be seen, however, Pickerill's relationship with the Association had not always been so amicable.

Davies himself had some problems with staff loyalty when he became Acting Director. He complained to the Registrar that an assistant nurse was inefficient, and that she had not kept her department clean. He would have overlooked her inefficiencies 'but for one thing' – she had questioned his authority '… in an impertinent tone, insinuating among other things, that as I was only here temporarily, she practically only held herself responsible to Pickerill. She kept her impertinent attitude up … and went out of the room with a melodramatic air'.[17] He sought her dismissal, which was declined, and he had to request her dismissal again several months later.[18]

With Pickerill's resumption of his duties imminent, Davies would have been considering his options for the future. An obvious one for him would have been the post of Director of the proposed School Dental Service, and Pickerill supported the application: 'Although we should feel his loss in Dunedin very considerably, yet I feel he would make an excellent Head …'.[19] The application was, however, unsuccessful, as Hunter was appointed. Pickerill's support of Davies would have been a strategic move – the appointment of Davies would have removed him from consideration for the pending appointment of a new member of the staff. It would also have checked the progress of Hunter's career – by this time Hunter was promoting a structure of the State Dental Service that was to embroil the two in bitter disagreement.

An aspect of the relationship between Davies and Pickerill that on the surface worked amicably, albeit with one exception, was the complicated arrangement for Davies' remuneration while Pickerill was overseas. The exception was payment for the period January–February 1918. Davies must have sought payment through his bank, only to be informed by the manager that Pickerill had given the following instructions: 'If I should not return by the end of 1917, no payments will be made to Mr. Davies for the months of January & February of 1918, but payment will recommence at the end of March, 1918'.[20] This suggests that Davies was receiving no pay for the 'holiday' period, during which he would have been deeply involved in preparing for the substantial increase in student numbers. Davies would have interpreted this as scant reward for the huge effort he was making to keep the school viable. The Registrar intervened and Davies was paid the outstanding amount of £83.6s.8d.

The University was, however, beginning to worry about the financial arrangement. In July 1919, some three months after Pickerill arrived back in Dunedin, the Registrar asked him whether he should still be paid, given that he was engaged full time on military service, with the salary of Lieutenant Colonel. Pickerill thanked the Council for its support while he was on active service, and warmly thanked Davies for the '... very able and enthusiastic way in which he has run the school'.[21] He suggested that, until he resumed his duties, he be paid £100 per annum. Even while still in the Army he said he would be increasingly devoting time to the teaching of medical and dental students in new methods of treating fractures of the jaw and plastic surgery of the face. Further, he would, of necessity over the next six months, be devoting time and thought to the reorganisation of the Dental School in view of the increased number of students. The Council agreed to pay the retainer 'in the meantime', but then was successful in its request that the Ministry of Defence cover these costs.[22]

Before Pickerill resumed his position, the University sought his advice on staffing in view of the increased number of students.[23] An important outcome was the appointment of an additional senior member of staff. This resulted in yet another very unpleasant disagreement between Pickerill and Davies. In a letter to Vice-Chancellor Sir John Roberts, Davies claimed that Pickerill had offered him the position, as associate professor.[24] In an attached note, written many years later, he further claimed that Pickerill had invited J.L. Saunders to apply, but without telling Davies; Saunders declined on the grounds, according to Davies, that it was a ruse to get him away from Hunter and the School Dental Service. Davies also believed Pickerill invited Raynor Colin Bell to apply, and that, at the appointment meeting, Pickerill stated his preference for Bell, who was elected by one vote. Davies complained that new members of the appointment committee had been elected 'without knowing what I had done'. Davies recorded that the Vice-Chancellor had sided with him, and did not 'mince matters' in subsequent discussion with Pickerill.

R.F. Stockwell, a colleague of Davies in his later years, believed Davies would 'have welcomed the chance to remain in academic dentistry but it was not to be, and so swallowing his disappointment manfully he returned to private practice in his own rooms'.[25] This was a sad ending to the academic career of a man who had served the School with distinction. The two men just did not get on. Pickerill was used to getting his own way, a style no doubt successful in the Army; Davies seemed to be much more of a team player, but able to stand firm on matters of principle or when he felt he was being demeaned. Clashes were inevitable, with unfortunate consequences. Davies, however, continued to serve the Dental Association with honour, including election to President in 1922–3, and chairing the 1924 conference in Dunedin. He died in 1970.

Raynor Bell, Pickerill's choice for the new position, was in charge of the Christchurch Dental Hospital for a short period after graduation and served in the New Zealand Dental Corps between 1915 and 1917. When he successfully applied for the Chair in Clinical Dentistry, he was in private practice in Masterton. He was considered a brilliant student as an undergraduate,[26] this promise being fulfilled when he became the first person to gain the New Zealand Doctor of Dental Surgery degree. His thesis, *The Development and Histology of the Teeth of Some New Zealand Fishes* was published in a series of articles in the *Journal*, and brought him international recognition.

The school and its patients

From the early days of the School, local dentists maintained a close interest in the nature of the patients treated at the School – an interest that continues today – there being a natural concern that the School would 'poach' patients away from private practitioners. The School needed patients for the education of the students, and there was general agreement that these would be drawn mainly from the indigent population. The demands on the School's resources was great, and Pickerill, supported by Professor Scott and the University Council, had sought increased funding from the Otago Hospital and Charitable Aid Board in 1911[27] – a procedure familiar to all subsequent Deans of the Faculty. A special committee of the Board received a deputation from local dentists and further information from Pickerill and Scott. The outcome was a recommendation that the Board grant £2000 per annum, provided that inmates of any of the Board's institutions receive free dental treatment, and other applicants for treatment submit a recommendation from a registered dentist and declare in writing their inability to pay for private treatment. The School could charge a 'nominal' fee for materials used in the treatment of the latter category of patient. For teaching purposes the School was permitted to admit ' a few patients annually' for more advanced work, such as gold work, crowns, and bridges, the material to be paid for by the Board. Half of all fees collected were to be refunded to the Board,[28] but this was reduced to the more acceptable level of 10 per cent. The Council and the Board negotiated the fine details, but Pickerill complained that the 10 per cent return of fees to the Board was too stringent, particularly as the University was saving the Board a large sum for dental care.[29]

The nature of the patients was also a problem. The patients treated free on behalf of the Board actually cost the University £96, and were almost all denture patients. 'From a teaching point of view too, these patients are a very undesirable class'. The School also found it difficult to get patients to pay for material for students' advanced work and noted that they were 'largely that class who insist on having all their teeth extracted which is not what we want here in great numbers'.[30]

The agreement between the University and the Board was modified in 1917 after the hospital Board met with the Otago Branch of the Association. The School was to continue to provide treatment for people unable to pay the fees of private dentists, but the subsidy from the Board was increased to £400. The School would also be required to treat all patients that normally would be treated by the Board, subject to the Board providing a dental chair (and presumably the necessary associated equipment); the Board would have the right to inspect the School 'when necessary'. The School was to provide treatment for 'inmates' of all the Board's institutions without extra cost to the Board.[31]

This was the unenviable situation Pickerill inherited on his return to the School, and he was soon involved in advocacy on two fronts – a better return for the School and University for the treatment provided for the Hospital Board, and ensuring a better flow of patients suitable for training his students, especially in the more advanced types of procedure.

He first argued that the subsidy from the Board should be £600, close to the sum paid by boards in other centres for dental services,[32] and this information resulted in the Council sending a deputation to the board.[33] The Dental Hospital's debit balance for the year was £1,658, which had to be covered by the University. Expenditure for purely hospital purposes was £3,385. Patients' fees amounted to £1,698 which, with the grant from the Board, left a debit of £1,287. The Council was therefore paying out of its own funds a contribution to charitable aid. The deputation pointed out that the North Canterbury Board had appointed a dental officer at £800 per year for the treatment of children, and the officer was to be sent to England for further study. Pickerill added information on the number of people in hardship and the recent increased workload in the School. The board declined the application, but resolved to take it into account when framing the next year's estimates.[34]

At this point the students complained that the majority of their patients could not afford to pay for more advanced dentistry and they were getting insufficient experience. Pickerill argued their case to the Registrar, comparing the Otago situation of relying on charitable patients with that of schools in the United States where 'practically without exception [they] are open to all persons irrespective of income or social position … [The school at] St Louis points out that unless the middle classes are admitted it is impossible to give

Dental Students a proper training'. He believed that if any well-to-do person demanded treatment at the Dental School 'we could not legally refuse it'. He felt that any objections by private dentists would be slight. Dunedin also now had only twenty-seven dentists compared with nearly forty before the war. He argued that an 'open door' policy would enhance the finances of the School and provide the necessary experience for the increasing numbers of students.[35]

The dentists were uneasy with this suggestion and wanted assurance that only patients unable to pay for private dental treatment would be admitted. At a meeting of representatives of the Council and the Branch, the Branch sought more time to consider the matter, and would bring it to the forthcoming conference of the Association.[36] At the same time, the Faculty proposed that: 'in order to preserve the interests of resident dentists and at the same time provide material for teaching and practice of higher branches of operative dentistry, admission be extended to students in all faculties and to parents of dental students'; and further, that Hospital Board nurses be admitted upon payment of the School's fees – the latter being the practice in the North Canterbury Board.[37] These moves resulted in more of the 'better class of patients', and were to prove crucial when the School came under threat from Auckland interests.

Meanwhile, after a reminder from the Registrar, the Board had increased its grant to £500.[38] Pickerill was rightly unhappy with the agreement for the School to provide treatment for all Board in-patients. This meant staff had to travel to Wakari Hospital, where no facilities for treatment existed. He argued that only those Board patients who could come to the School should be treated, but the Registrar declined to support him.[36]

A further development occurred when the Board appeared to initiate a proposal for Bell, as Professor of Clinical Dentistry, to assume control of dental treatment for in-patients.[40] Supporting the proposal, Pickerill noted that outcomes would include clinical experience for students, especially in operating under general anaesthesia. The present situation was unsatisfactory as the University was really responsible for a service it did not control – far better for it to be under the direct control of a senior member of the Dental School's staff. The work would be undertaken at the request of honorary physicians or surgeons. Pickerill considered Bell should be entitled to additional remuneration, payable by the Board.

Bell, however, had reservations about how the scheme would work. Previously, the Dental Hospital's own dental surgeon and assistant dental surgeon had provided dental treatment for in-patients. Now the responsibility would be transferred to him; he or one of the staff of his department could be expected at any time to attend to in-patient needs when requested by the Medical Superintendent. He refused to accept the proposal, as the terms of his appointment did not include the treatment of in-patients, either personally or in providing supervision of others. He believed such work should be the responsibility of an officer of the Public Health Department. He then offered, however, provided it would be on his own terms, to 'arrange and see that the dental treatment of the in-patients of the Otago Hospital Board's institutions was carried out to general satisfaction'. He pointed to his previous experience at Christchurch Hospital, and noted that this new role would involve considerable extra duties, for which he should receive an increase in salary.[40]

Who would pay for dentures for patients unable to pay fees was the subject of a testy debate between the Council and the Board that continued for over a year, and must have been a considerable distraction for the Dean.[38] His final word on patients at the School occurred in 1927 when he sought clarification on the payment of fees for children living in orphanages – some orphanages paid fees but others did not. The Council, by this time no doubt tired of discussing Dental School fees, responded that all orphanages should pay fees.[39]

Yet another aspect of who could be treated at the School was much more personal for Pickerill, and must have disturbed him greatly. The matter had rumbled on for many years, but came to a head in 1922. Although there is no suggestion that the relationship between Pickerill and Bell was other than cordial and respectful, Bell's name was raised during an interrogation that Pickerill endured with the Medical Committee of the Council in 1922. The subject of the interrogation suggests some form of resentment by staff, or perhaps by other Dunedin dentists. The problem first surfaced in 1911 when Pickerill sought guidance from the Council on the treatment of patients referred to him personally by doctors and dentists. Many of these patients had medical or surgical conditions of the jaws that were valuable for teaching purposes. He suggested he should see such patients in consultation, and to operate if requested by the referring doctor or dentist. He sought advice on the payment of fees.[43] The Medical Committee recommended that the matter be referred to the Faculty of Dentistry, which approved the proposal after lengthy debate.[44] Pickerill had to raise the matter again in 1915 when he heard rumours that he was engaged in extensive private work and was doing so without the approval of the Council. Not only were the rumours contrary to the facts, he pointed out, but the implications were against his principles and did him a serious injustice. He added that eight years earlier he had left a very remunerative practice in England 'because I recognised that a man cannot do

University teaching and private practice. I prefer to devote my whole energies to the former'.[45] Rumours must have risen again in 1921, for he outlined his timetable to the Registrar – attendance at the School from 9.30 am to 5.15 pm, and in the evenings '... numerous Faculty, Professorial Board, and staff meetings'. He operated at the hospital one afternoon a week, the sessions attended by medical and dental students as part of their required courses in clinical surgery, and he attended the Woodside Facial Hospital for about an hour each week.[46]

This response must have been unsatisfactory, for members of the Medical Committee of the Council closely questioned him. He stated that he never saw anyone not referred by doctors or dentists, and the patients were usually those whom nobody else wanted to treat. In the past 10 years he had seen no more than 100 such patients, and he tried to see them at 'odd moments' so as not to interfere with his regular duties. Seeing private patients allowed him to keep an interest in clinical work, and he noted that Sidey knew that the Dean in Sydney was allowed private practice. He observed that he had been offered that post, but had dedicated himself to the School; he could earn much more if he did go into private practice. Remarkably, he was then cross-examined. To Professor Hewitson he denied he had ever seen a patient not referred from a dentist, reaffirmed that he had seen only 100 patients over a period of 10 years, and that the consultations had been at odd times. Dr Fitzgerald then asked a very curious question – would he report assistants to the Council if they were not fulfilling their duties, to which Pickerill replied in the affirmative. Sidey then asked whether he had been absent in the past twelve months, receiving the reply that he, Pickerill, had been very busy during the past year, and did operations one afternoon a week. Sidey then asked another odd question – whether he had any reason to find fault with Bell, which Pickerill denied.[47]

This extraordinary episode, which must have been extremely traumatic for Pickerill, suggests someone was out to undermine his standing in the University by persisting with serious allegations about his activities and commitment. Whether Hewitson, Fitzgerald, and Sidey were his allies, wanting to clarify the situation to ensure his reputation was unsullied, or whether they were genuinely suspicious of inappropriate activities, is not known. The outcome of the inquiry was, however, that the committee reported the same day that Pickerill 'had honourably kept his agreement with the Council'.

Why Bell came into the questioning is intriguing – his appointment seems to have been successful, and he was respected as a researcher and teacher. His career was tragically brief, however, for he died in 1926.

'Dental School in danger'

This was the headline greeting readers of the *Otago Daily Times* on the morning of 24 April 1924.[45] Torrential rain resulted in the normally placid Leith Stream becoming a torrent. It seriously damaged the School, sited as it was on the stream's banks, unprotected by the concrete channel that exists today. An extension consisting of an old Mining School building was completely swept away, and pieces of it were found in the harbour at Ravensbourne. The main building was seriously undermined. A case containing a full set of instruments was found on the Peninsula side of the harbour, and other material had been 'fished out of the Leith by boys'. The Dean subsequently reported the damage to the Council. About an eighth of an acre had been lost; the foundations of the recently completed permanent extension on the north side were seriously undermined; on the morning of 23 April, one of the foundation piers of the main building was exposed for its whole depth, and the north-east corner of the building had been saved only by sandbagging; movable equipment had been removed. The loss included the mechanical laboratory and its contents; the students' common room containing chairs, students' coats, and personal belongings; the dark room and its contents, including all Pickerill's research records, the negatives of Bell's research work – 'no money or trouble can ever replace them' – and dental materials had been swept away with the store room. The Dean closed the School for three days. He proposed converting the lecture room into a mechanical laboratory and dark room, and converting two-thirds of the upstairs section of the new extension into the students' cloak room and lavatory. To overcome the shortage of thirteen operating chairs and the lecture room he had negotiated to use a room in the old Physics Department and asked for the loan of the Maheno and Marama Halls. The latter buildings had been erected as a result of public subscription as memorials to the war-time hospital ships of those names, and he felt their temporary use for the treatment of children would be fitting. He sought immediate attention by the University's architects and its Works Committee to these emergency alterations, repairs, and replacements. He also took the opportunity to appeal further for the building of a new school, which had been authorised in 1920.[49] The flood proved to be a major impetus for this important development.

'Back-door' ructions

At the 1917 conference the Association had flirted, under ministerial pressure, with supporting an amendment to the Dentists Act to allow courses leading to the Certificate of Proficiency to be taken wholly or in part outside Dunedin. This was not pursued, and the University of Otago, through the University of

New Zealand, retained its sole right of awarding the BDS degree and the COP. But pressure from unregistered 'dentists' for amendments to the Act to allow eventual registration continued to plague the Association and the School after the war. The alarm was raised when large numbers of unregistered practitioners were able to register in Great Britain. A major fear was that such persons would seek admission to the New Zealand Register. Although Pickerill thought the Senate had sufficient power under the act to refuse to register anyone who could not produce a diploma, the Association wanted the senate alerted to the possibility.[50]

In 1920 the Auckland Unregistered Dentists' Association sought the Dental Association's support for an amendment to allow its members to take an examination leading to registration, but the request was declined. The admission of such persons, who were mainly dental mechanics but worked directly on patients, ostensibly under the direct supervision of a registered dentist, would be unfair to those qualifying through the BDS and COP courses and 'still more grossly unfair to succeeding mechanics who might also seek admission'.[51]

Pickerill took a different view, totally at odds with the principles he had espoused since his arrival in New Zealand. His action appalled the Association. Hunter, by this time the Chief Dental Officer, sent to the Executive Council a copy of a letter Pickerill had written quite independently to the Minister for Education, the Honourable C.J. Parr. He had pointed out that many of the unregistered dentists had been on active service, and were therefore exempt from matriculation if they applied for admission to the School before March 1921. The remaining 'fifty or sixty' could be granted similar exemption and then, while continuing their dental work, take the first two years of study in any town where physics and chemistry were taught. Under the bursary system, they could then complete the course in Dunedin free of cost. 'In this way, at an exceedingly low cost to themselves, they could properly qualify as dentists, for which they would ever be grateful … These "fifty or sixty" men could then be available for the School Dental Service'.[49]

This was Pickerill's answer to Hunter's plans to employ school dental nurses in the School Dental Service. Although it would be a moot point that these men would turn out to be the 'fully-trained' dentists Pickerill was advocating for the Service, at least they would have had more than the two years' dental education proposed for the dental nurses. The Executive could not support the suggestion – it considered that all men who had been on active service were adequately provided for; it could see no reason why such special privilege should be accorded to the favoured few and withheld from regular students; and that the requirements of the School Dental Service had already been met.

The situation of these operating mechanics was vigorously debated at the 1921 conference, strong cases being made for and against the employment of operating mechanics. The Association wanted to be fair to the mechanics and to its members who employed them, but some speakers recognised that 'the profession had itself largely to blame, because these men were given the opportunities which naturally led into the surgery'. The Association was also aware of the delicate relationship with Members of Parliament – precipitate action might materially assist the dental mechanics in securing from Parliament the right to register. Some speakers supported the operating mechanics being allowed to take an examination, but their intent differed from Pickerill's proposal to the Minister: the new suggestion was that a searching examination, taken without completing some formal courses, would have been difficult to pass, and the implication was that the work of these people would then be limited to laboratory work only.[53]

Pickerill, however, was proposing a new course, and the concern of the conference for the welfare of the students and of the good name of the School was understandable. His proposal would have totally undermined all the effort and struggle, by him and by the Association, to raise the standard of admission to the BDS course. The conference was furious over this matter as well as being furious over the way he had, by this time, opposed school dental nurses. Hunter vehemently took advantage of the situation and informed the conference that: 'he [Hunter] was astonished that Professor Pickerill should have put to the Minister a scheme so grossly unfair to the dental students', and more was to come. Under the heading 'Dr. Pickerill's action condemned', the *Journal* recorded the unanimous passing of a motion, moved by J.N. Rishworth, a former close but now estranged colleague from Sidcup days:

> That this meeting expresses its emphatic disapproval of, and protests against, the action of Dr. Pickerill in approaching the Minister for Education in the manner set forth in his letter of December 3rd, 1920, in direct opposition to the expressed views of the New Zealand Dental Association; and that a copy of this motion be sent to the Minister for Education, the Chancellor of the University, and to Dr. Pickerill.

Hunter expressed further astonishment 'that a proposal so destructive of the interests of the Dental School students should actually have come from its head'. The President, Nelson Mitchell, declared that 'Professor Pickerill's suggestion was iniquitous, therefore no condemnation could be too strong'.[54] This was without doubt the strongest public rebuke ever received by a member of the Association.

The Registrar duly replied to the Association's letter to the Chancellor, hinting that Pickerill had been further rebuked – on receipt of the Association's letter, the Council resolved: 'That the New Zealand Dental Association be informed that the Council is requesting that letters to the Minister from the Dean of the Dental Faculty affecting questions of University policy shall in future be sent through the Council'.[55]

The Association was now greatly alarmed at the wording of the current Dentists Act – 'Every adult person shall be entitled … to be registered as a dentist who is registered, or is entitled to be registered, in the United Kingdom'. Any of the 'many thousands' of previously unregistered practitioners in the United Kingdom were now able to register there, and the Association believed the Senate of the University of New Zealand would be unable to prevent their registration in New Zealand. The Executive Council resolved to seek amendments to the legislation to prevent those now registered without proper examination in England from registering here, and further, to stop unqualified assistants (the operating mechanics) doing any surgical operations at all, which would solve the problem of these practitioners endlessly seeking registration.[56] A full meeting of the Executive Council was held in November 1921,[57] to which Hunter, J.A. Young, MP, and Sidey were invited, as was Pickerill, even though distinctly out of favour, but he apparently did not receive his invitation.

Events then moved quickly – the Act was amended in 1922, and was warmly received by the Association. The chief features were: the prohibition of all dental practice by anyone not on the Register, even if supervised; special provision by means of an examination for 'certain persons who, although hitherto unregistered, have been carrying on, for not less than a specified period, routine dental practice …'; and allocation to the Senate power to discriminate in the case of applicants whose names appear on the British Register as to who shall be eligible in New Zealand.[58]

The syllabus for the Special Examination, to be held in December 1922, included written and practical examinations and recommended texts for study. No special courses were proposed. The names of persons claiming eligibility for and registered to sit the examination were also published, accompanied by an appeal for members to supply the Association with any information about any person whom they considered ineligible – the 138 names listed proved that the 'fifty or sixty' previously quoted was grossly underestimated.[59] The examination was duly held, and Pickerill was an examiner in dental surgery.[60] Davies conveyed the Association's view on the examination standard to the Prime Minister, the Right Honourable W.F. Massey, when he proposed the toast to the Government at the annual dinner in May 1924 – in no way were the standards equal to those of the BDS or COP courses, and a sixth-standard certificate was sufficient preliminary education. 'A syllabus was arranged that anyone of ordinary intelligence could master in the time allotted'. Of the 138 applying to take the examination, 79 sat and 42 passed. Davies appealed for the Government to 'stand firm' against further attempts to amend the Act.[61]

Despite Pickerill's problems with the Association, the Executive Council graciously congratulated him when he received in the 1923 New Year Honours the award of Commander of the Order of the British Empire (CBE).[62] The *Journal* stated:

> We congratulate Professor H.P. Pickerill, of the Otago University, on the distinction His Majesty the King has seen fit to confer upon him … Professor Pickerill well merits the honour. Among those labouring in the field of remedial and plastic surgery of the jaws and face, it is probable no one has attained a greater measure of success than he, and the recognition his work has received will be marked by pleasure, not only by his confreres, but even more so by those whom, by his skill, he has rendered life once more possible.[63]

The Association also warmly acknowledged Pickerill's role in lobbying against yet another liberalising amendment to the Dentists Act, but this was dropped by the Government in 1924.[64] His name was not, however, mentioned regarding the failed efforts to defeat a further Act passed in 1926.

So the back door remained open, aided by a commission set up in 1925 to deal with specific cases of hardship. Despite desperate lobbying by the Association's Secretary, Maurice Denniston, and others, the commission recommended a further amendment. The outcome was the Dentists Amendment Act 1926, which provided for yet more examinations, with candidates to continue practising until 1929 under 'supervision'; this was virtually a continuation of apprenticeship. Between 1908 and 1925, the *Journal* editorial of September 1926 pointed out, 147 'back-door' entrants had gained admission to the *Register*, compared with a mere 35 entrants through the School of Dentistry.[65] The Editor compared derisively the much higher entrance standards of school dental nurse students (either matriculation or Public Service Entrance Examinations) with the low standard required for admission to the dental qualifying examination, set by no less a body than the Senate of the University of New Zealand. The 'one-portal' entry to the profession Pickerill had hailed so long ago as the end of back-door entry had been made a mockery, not by omissions of the Association or by Pickerill and the University, but by pressure of vested interests on short-sighted politicians and an indifferent public.

Caries, surgery, and stomatology

Pickerill's post-war term as Dean of the Faculty of Dentistry was an extremely difficult time for him. He no longer had the responsibilities of Secretary of the Association or Editor of the *Journal*, but his opposition to the form of the School Dental Service, along with staffing problems and the flood, must have been enormously stressful. Nevertheless, this was an extremely productive period for his research and writing. For a lesser individual, it would have been an overwhelming workload.

Pickerill's interest in dental caries was on hold during the war, but it soon reawakened, to the extent that a third edition of *Prevention of Dental Caries and Oral Sepsis* appeared in 1923.[66] It contained new diagrams that would 'render the wonderful adaptability of the salivary secretion to be better and more quickly grasped', and it contained additional information on the 'immunity' of Maori children. Its review in the *Dental Record* was very favourable – 'As a presentment of the problem of dental caries it takes rank amongst the best work of this kind ever done'. This in-depth review comments on the author's research on the susceptibility of enamel to attack by acid, the importance of saliva in modifying the intensity of the attack, and Pickerill's advocacy of the need for health promotion through Government legislation to regulate the quality of the diet. The only criticism was the curious omission of Pickerill's dental qualifications: 'For whatever reason … we deplore it'. Pickerill was again recognised internationally as a leader in dental research.[67]

The care of returned servicemen had extended seamlessly into his appointment as Surgeon-in-Charge of the Facial and Jaw Department of Dunedin Hospital. In a major paper to the 1924 conference of the Association (from which he had by now resigned), he described the surgical correction of malformations of the jaws due to trauma and infection and repair of cleft lips and palates in children.[68] The patient he described to illustrate the latter condition was, as he explained many years later to Sir Charles Hercus,[69] the first case in which he used mother-nursing, this in 1923. Surgeon Stanley Batchelor, when handing over the baby to him, said: 'He will die, he's bound to die – but do as you like'. Pickerill described the baby as 'certainly a weakling, and in a public hospital I think he would certainly have died, but the mother found suitable lodgings … where I visited them daily. The infant had three operations and not only did he not die, but continued to gain weight … He is now [1954] pulling his weight as a Canterbury farmer'. Mother-nursing was to be an important feature in the subsequent success of the surgery practised at Bassam in Lower Hutt.

In addition to such presentations and papers, and all his other duties and distractions, he somehow found time to prepare his thesis for his Master of Surgery (MCh), Birmingham, which he was awarded in 1923. Out of this came his major text *Facial Surgery*, published in 1924.[70] The first part of the book covers wartime injuries, centred on his Sidcup experiences. He then applied the lessons of war to civilian practice, and illustrated the type of conditions he was treating in Dunedin. These included reconstruction of facial tissues following the surgical treatment of malignancies; reconstruction in patients with congenital syphilis, including the complete replacement of a nose; repair following acquired syphilis; excision and the subsequent skin-grafting of the lesions of *lupus erythematosis*; treatment of birth marks, moles, burns, excessive scar tissue (keloid); treatment of cleft lip and palate; and treatment of protrusion of the upper or lower jaws. Some of this civilian section is presented in virtual note form, but it is nevertheless an authoritative work by an experienced, highly skilled, and versatile surgeon who worked closely with other surgical colleagues, notably Batchelor and Barnett at the Medical School and Dunedin Hospital. In applying the lessons of war to civilian surgery, Pickerill's work differed from the lavishly illustrated book produced by Gillies which, published in 1920, concentrated almost exclusively on wartime injuries.[71] The review of *Facial Surgery* in the *Lancet* is fascinating and decidedly sexist in comparison with an American text on plastic surgery:

> Two books have recently appeared on cosmetic surgery. The one deals with surgical trivialities, little alterations in the form of lips or eyelids which might appeal to a woman of fashion or vanity. The other [Pickerill's] plunges straight away into the most ghastly injuries that even civilised warfare has been able to achieve … the dimensions of a defect bear no relation to its effect upon the patient, and that to a woman with nothing but herself to think of a slight droop of an eyelid may seem as terrible as the loss of half his face to a healthy man.[72]

The reviewer acknowledged the quality of Pickerill's photographs and drawings, and commented on the 'new and interesting method' of treating cleft palates – 'Though we may not agree entirely with the methods advocated, the book is full of interest and suggestions, and we can strongly recommend it to the notice of all surgeons who aspire to deal with facial deformities'. Although not a resounding endorsement, the review nevertheless reinforced Pickerill's international standing in plastic surgery.

Stomatology, first published in 1912, was a further major work, and its revised second edition appeared in 1925.[73] It covered essentially the same material as the original, but with additions 'derived from experience in the late war, on the treatment of fractures and cleft palate'. It also contained a new chapter on the relationship between oral and alimentary secretions. The book was favourably reviewed in the *Journal*.[74] Although the review was general rather than detailed, the reviewer ('JLS', probably Saunders) had 'expected to find a fuller reference to apical infection, a subject which, of recent years, has come to loom large in the public eye, and is probably the most frequent cause for consultation between the [medical and dental] professions'. (The reviewer was here referring to infections or abscesses in the bone surrounding the teeth, and their perceived role in causing infections or other symptoms elsewhere in the body.)

This was a very minor criticism compared with those of the *British Dental Journal*'s anonymous reviewer who, acknowledging the revision and new material, described the changes as being 'insufficient to redeem the book from a dating which a book published at a time as relatively remote as 1912 must inevitably bear 14 years later … instead of having that touch of originality which characterised Professor Pickerill's … *Prevention of Dental Caries* [it] is only a meritorious and somewhat dull example of a machine-made book'.[75] The reviewer felt there were many omissions, and that 'in so many parts of the book, the revision seems to have been insufficient, with a result that though the date on the title page is 1925, the matter of the book still retains, to an undue extent, the dating of fourteen years earlier'. Such a critical review, even if only partly justified, may have indicated Pickerill's serious overload – it seems an impossible task for him to have kept abreast of modern knowledge and to advance his own research amidst everything else that was going on at the time.

But Pickerill soon fired right back. He was 'amused' that the reviewer, after complaining about a lack of originality,

> then slates me unmercifully for expressing my personal views in preference to those of other writers.
>
> I do not expect the book to have any sale in England, for unfortunately, and to the disgrace I think of the dental profession, no proper courses in dental and oral surgery or stomatology form part of the medical curricula in any of the universities or medical schools.
>
> … The course is compulsory [here] and no medical student in New Zealand can sit for the final examination until … he has satisfied me as to his knowledge in stomatology.

After outlining his course in the subject for medical students, he concluded: 'It is high time the dental profession in England woke up and insisted on compulsory courses of this kind'.[76] This vigorous protest shows he was still at that time deeply involved in teaching at the Medical School, yet another facet of his demanding schedule. Not everyone was so dismissive of *Stomatology* as the *British Dental Journal's* reviewer – it was still listed as a recommended text for Otago dental students until the early 1950s.

By this time Pickerill had received two overseas accolades. In 1921 he had been made a Member of Honour of the Belgian Society of Stomatology,[77] and the Stomatological Clinic of the Royal University of Budapest sought a photograph for enlargement and framing to be placed in its gallery – 'Your most admirable experimental works on Dental Caries … as well as your excellent book on Stomatology in General Practice have raised you into the first ranks of scientists in Stomatology …'.[78] A further distinction was election in 1923 for a term as Vice-President of the Odontological Section of the Royal College of Medicine.

This post-war period at the School was marked by achievements and turmoil. In addition to what is recorded in this chapter, Pickerill had two other major challenges that tested his endurance even further – the development of the School Dental Service and the pressing need for, and eventual achievement of, a new Dental School. Both involved him in bitter controversy.

14

Services for children, 1907-1927

Pickerill's deep concern for the health of children was apparent as early as 1902 when, as a student, he submitted his treatise on the treatment of caries in the primary teeth.[1] Much of his early research on dental caries focused on children, and he soon became deeply involved in plans for a public health service for their dental care. His involvement fell into two distinct phases. Before the war, as Secretary of the Association and Editor of the *Journal*, he worked within the policies of the Association and contributed greatly to their development. But immediately after the war he bitterly opposed the form the service was taking, resulting in a complete break with the Association and its affairs: his leadership declined into anarchy.

From its inception, the Association recognised the enormous health issue of caries in children, and wrestled with means to prevent and manage the problem. This concern eventually led to the formation of the School Dental Service. Although its establishment was accompanied by controversy and dissent, it eventually settled, in the main, into a service in which the Association has taken pride. Despite this, the Service has been subject to varying degrees of criticism since its inception – by the Association and individual members – and has received praise and also harsh comment from overseas. Today, despite serious problems with funding and a greatly reduced and aging workforce, it remains an important component of New Zealand's child health services.

The oral health of adolescents has also been an ongoing focus of the profession. A source of friction between the Association and the Government over a long period, the State-financed Dental Benefit Scheme has experienced a decline in support by dentists in recent years largely because of a general dissatisfaction with the scale of fees.

Current decay levels bear little resemblance to those persisting in New Zealand through to the 1970s and 1980s, when decay declined dramatically. But there are now ominous signs that the prevalence of caries is creeping upwards, and higher rates are of concern in Maori, Pacific Island, and low socio-economic families generally. But the Association, by its forceful advocacy of fluoridation, the use of fluoride toothpaste and, less successfully, dietary reform, can rightly claim a great deal of credit for the improvements that have occurred.

F.W. Thompson, to be the third President of the Association, was one of the first in a long line of presidents, researchers, and editors to point out the dreadful state of children's teeth, and to implore the Government for help in overcoming the problem.[2] At that time, the process of caries and how it might be prevented was only vaguely understood, as shown by the editorial in the January 1907 *Journal*: teeth were considered not strong enough to survive repeated restoration when decay re-occurred.[3] Although at that time there were no doubt instances of hypoplastic (poorly formed) teeth, which can be difficult to restore satisfactorily, the modern view is that the 'strength' of the teeth would not be the problem; rather, it is that caries, the cause of the breakdown, has not been controlled. Understanding of caries was greatly advanced when Pickerill published the results of his research; a clearer direction for the development of a public service for children emerged.

The Association wanted to stress the importance of prevention, and had spent a lot of energy developing a 'lecturette' for the instruction of schoolchildren in oral hygiene. This had been presented and fully discussed at the 1909 conference. Although supporting its general style, Pickerill did not support the proposal that it be delivered by dentists. For the scheme to be effective, he claimed, the message would need frequent reinforcement, and it would need to be presented at levels suitable for different age groups; implementation of the plan would have placed a huge burden on dentists, especially in the cities. His alternative was for the lectures to be given by teachers, not dentists. While the 1909 conference was discussing the matter in Wellington, he coincidentally was addressing the annual meeting of the 'Teachers' Institute' (possibly the New Zealand Educational Institute) in Dunedin, where he advocated that all teachers be instructed in oral health by dentists, preferably during teacher training, and in special classes for teachers already practising. If the teachers were to provide oral health education, they would be able, he believed, to tailor the material specifically for each age group. He also advocated for teachers to be examined in the subject during their training, and schoolchildren tested on their knowledge. 'In this way, and in this way only, can this much desired instruction be made both universal

– systematic and adaptable'. He thought his proposal had been well received, members of the Institute wanted to include oral health in the curriculum, and already in one district a dentist had instructed local teachers. Large, simple, coloured diagrams he had displayed were now with the Education Office for printing. He was convinced that health education was the responsibility of the State, not the Association.[4]

He was also very much aware of the importance of the newly created Plunket Society, whose nurses were in a strong position to promote sound health practices of diet and hygiene to the parents of newborns and young children. He addressed the Society's first annual meeting in 1908, and spoke on 'The proper development and care of the teeth and masticatory apparatus' in 1912.[5] He was honorary dental surgeon to the Society from 1908 to 1927, so it is likely that he and the Society's founder, Truby King, had mutual respect for their roles as allies in health promotion.

In addition to this public health approach to health education, Pickerill brought a similar approach to treatment. His first *Journal* editorial, July 1909, was an impassioned call for action on children's teeth. Although appropriate for dentists to do some charity work, he suggested, dentists could not and should not be expected to be responsible for turning around the current serious situation. He advocated the English system of local authorities appointing medical officers to examine all children in the district and to report on, amongst other things, the condition of the teeth. Subsidised care was sought if parents could not pay for extensive treatment. If a similar scheme were not possible in New Zealand, he at least wanted dentists appointed to examine and advise on treatment. For universal application, dentists should be appointed in every town to undertake treatment at reduced fees. These dentists 'would receive either a fixed sum annually from the Government, or payment in proportion to the number and character of cases treated'. He proclaimed that the situation had to be addressed if New Zealand was not to 'lag hopelessly behind the governments of other countries'.[6]

Thomas Hunter, so long a close colleague, but eventually to be an adversary, soon endorsed the public health approach. His presidential address to the 1910 conference drew the connection between oral and general health. 'How long, O Lord! How long will this apathy continue?' He stressed the importance of good diet during pregnancy, feeding infants the 'natural way', that 'sweets should be avoided as much as possible, that infants' food should not all be pap, but hard as soon as the teeth appear, and that cleanliness of the mouth is of the utmost importance'. He called on the medical profession to use its influence more effectively, and praised the efforts of Dr Truby King in his advocacy of improved methods of child rearing. He also praised Pickerill for introducing dental pathology into the training of medical students, a suggestion he claimed to have made just before Pickerill arrived in New Zealand 'fully imbued with the same idea'.[7]

Hunter went on to suggest how the Government should assist, asking why dental disease is not included in the health services, despite oral ill-health leading to other serious health conditions. Economic benefits would accrue if the Government assisted in providing oral health services, such as employing a dentist in every general hospital. To ensure early detection and management of caries, he reiterated an earlier suggestion he had made that 'the authorities should have an organised examination and efficient treatment of the children in our public schools'. He continued:

> On a former occasion, I lamented the fact that we had been very lax, that for want of cohesion, our efforts had been spasmodic and futile. I am pleased to be able to say that never before in the history of the dental profession has there been such a general awakening to an appreciation of the importance of the mission which dentistry can, and ought to perform, in a humanitarian way, for public health, and it is interesting to note that for some time past there has been a growing interest in medical circles regarding the same problem.

Hunter was, in effect, advocating a school-based, universal dental service for children. Much needed to be done, and many years were to pass, before he and others in the profession were to bring this to fruition. But Hunter's vision never flagged, despite his own diversion into leadership of another form during the First World War.

Alexander Paterson's 1911 presidential address resurrected Pickerill's proposal that dentists should teach the teachers, not try to teach the children. Paterson wanted the pamphlet on the care of the teeth to go to every parent and teacher, that teachers be required to 'see that every child receives a proper course of teaching on the subject …', and that each dental society should select members to give lectures to teachers in all public schools. He regretted that recommendations for examining the teeth of schoolchildren seemed to 'have died a natural death'. He wanted every child to be examined and the results sent to every member of Parliament for them to have an appreciation of the gravity of the caries problem, 'without which we shall have little hope of getting dental wards established in our public hospitals'.[8]

Paterson, although not advancing Hunter's suggestion of a school-based treatment programme, spurred further action. In the subsequent discussion of the address, Pickerill thanked him for again raising the matters of teaching the teachers and the dental inspection of children in schools. He moved that the Executive Council send a deputation to the Minister of Education 'to press upon the Government the urgent need for the dental inspection of school children, and for the necessity of primary teachers receiving instruction in the teaching of dental prophylaxis'. The Executive Council was also instructed to prepare a pamphlet on 'Dental Prophylaxis and Oral Hygiene' for distribution to the public and to dental patients.

At that time Pickerill was deeply immersed in his research on the aetiology, pathology, and prevention of caries, extending this to advocate an epidemiological and public health approach to the problem. Without an understanding of the size of the problem, he reasoned, there was little hope of attracting either the interest of the public or commitment to action by the Government. This was the reason for his paper at the 1912 Association Annual Meeting,[9] in which he proposed a method of charting teeth, and for his repetition of the suggestion that the Department of Public Health's medical officers extend their examinations of schoolchildren to include dental health. The conference instructed the Executive Council to convey these suggestions to the Government.

A delegation met with the Honourable R.H. Rhodes, Minister for Public Health on 19 July. Hunter opened the discussion by advocating that children's teeth be examined as part of the medical inspections of school children currently being planned.

> If the four inspectors who had been appointed took a short course under Professor Pickerill at Dunedin, they might easily become qualified in the dental branch of their work. They knew very well … that the state of teeth at the present time represented a great evil, but the public did not know it as yet, and it was very desirable that the facts of the case be made generally known.[10]

Pickerill noted that ideally dentists should be the examiners but, as this would be expensive, he would be happy to provide a course at the University of Otago of a fortnight's duration at very little cost. The Minister responded favourably, and stated 'they had made it very easy for the Department and the Government to accept it by offering to give the necessary instructions to the medical officers in a fortnight. He would put the matter before his colleagues, and recommend that they fall in with the suggestion'. The Minister must have felt it all sounded too simple, as he subsequently asked whether a more thorough inspection might be necessary. Pickerill acknowledged this might be so, but indicated he would be satisfied to await the results of the proposed scheme – at this stage he was happy with a pilot study. The Minister added that he:

> could see the importance of the proposed [Urewera research of Pickerill] from what he had heard recently. [The delegation] had impressed him as he had never

> been impressed before as to the evils that arose from dental defects. They would of course, have the sympathy of the Department in their research work.[11]

Hunter and Pickerill, a formidable team of lobbyists, undoubtedly won the support of the Minister.

Pickerill's July 1912 editorial revealed his excitement about progress being made. He claimed, somewhat extravagantly: 'the aims of the New Zealand Dental Association, as regards the public health, have now the full sympathy and support both of the Government, the Education Commission, and of the officials of the Public Health Department'. He regarded the dental inspection of schoolchildren by medical officers as a *fait accompli*, and that it would 'commence in less than a month's time'. Money saved by not having dentists examine the children would now be available for treatment. The Minister had promised that four medical inspectors of children so far appointed would undertake a 'special short course in dental work, involving diagnosis and methods of charting etc., before commencing their work'. He suggested the 'scheme will prove efficient and economical; and moreover the statistics obtained will possess the inestimable value of being given by absolutely unbiased observers. They therefore will hardly fail to convince the authorities of the necessity for the institution of the means of treatment.'[12] Pickerill's imprint on the proposal was clear: he would be training the medical officers using both his clinical criteria and method of charting caries.

The medical inspectors subsequently attended a short training course in Dunedin, after which Pickerill noted:

> The necessity for the course was not at first, perhaps, quite apparent or recognised by all the inspectors, but fortunately now, after the conclusion of the course, that is not the case. For it may be said that not only are the medical inspectors quite efficient in the examination and charting of the teeth, but they are also quite enthusiastic.[13]

This suggests he had some difficulty convincing the inspectors that teeth were sufficiently important for another task to be added to what would undoubtedly be a busy schedule.

With the examination scheme under way by the medical inspectors and by various branches of the Association, the method of payment for treatment was the subject of his November 1912 editorial. He once again supported the developing English system whereby children of parents not able to afford the fees of dentists would be treated by salaried dentists working in clinics in schools in the larger towns. In the smaller towns, he suggested, a dentist could be paid a retaining fee and agree to treat 'certain children for a reduced and fixed scale of fees and to do extractions free.'[14] He believed the body responsible for the scheme would be the various hospital and charitable aid boards, with the cooperation of the Education Department. Although hiding many pitfalls, the proposals were a practical basis for further discussion and development of a school-based treatment programme for children.

A major problem in health education was well illustrated in the debate at the 1912 conference on the nature of information to be included in the public health education pamphlet, which had been having a difficult gestation. It had undergone various modifications, the latest by the Executive Council. As Secretary and as researcher, Pickerill had a large input. His research challenged old concepts, so much so that President-elect A.M. Carter appealed for those with views contrary to Pickerill to:

> withhold any expression of their opinions until they have read his book. Personally I may say that the views expounded are quite contrary to those that I have hitherto entertained ... Nevertheless, after going into the matter with Dr Pickerill for some three hours, I have come to the conclusion that my former views on the subject of dental caries were quite wrong, and those of Dr Pickerill are quite right ... the principles set forth in the book are unanswerable, and they justify all that is now expressed in the pamphlet.[15]

Norman Cox promoted some radical views in his presidential address to the 1913 conference. He powerfully argued for a universal system of State dentistry as the only solution to the caries problem in children. He proposed establishing clinics in schools and two classes of dentists – stationary in the large towns, and travelling to service the small towns. These dentists, however, would not be fully trained:

> I have no doubt that at the Dental School in Dunedin a fairly short course could be arranged specially adapted for state oral hygienists, or state dentists, which of course would not entitle them to the right of private practice, but would be amply sufficient to make them thoroughly equipped for this particular branch of dentistry.[16]

Here, in effect, was the blueprint for New Zealand's School Dental Service, and the first hint of how the Service might be staffed: the issue which was to provoke enormous controversy in the future. Cox was convinced that using fully trained dentists to provide a satisfactory service was wasteful:

> The idea of utilising the services of dentists in each branch of the New Zealand Dental Association has so many drawbacks, and would under the most favourable conditions be so inefficient, that I have been forced to the conclusion that only by some universal scheme organised by a central authority, that is, the Government, would any complete and satisfactory result ensue.

Major players in the controversies surrounding the eventual establishment of the School Dental Service were quick to respond to these radical proposals.[17] The first was Hunter – the future first director of the Service – who endorsed the President's approach, but advised caution and the setting up of a sub-committee to outline a scheme to be put to the Government. J.N. Rishworth, later to become a strong supporter of school dental nurses, believed Dr Cox had greatly underestimated the number of dentists required in such a scheme, and criticised the level of training proposed: 'Will the public, when they are educated in the way we all desire, be satisfied with men of mean attainments? Will they not want men who are skilled as high as the country can make them?' W.R. Hursthouse criticised the scheme on the basis that prevention needed to be paramount – 'much progress is hopeless unless we can get the patients to eat proper food. We fill their teeth, and perhaps in another twelve months they come along again with twenty or thirty cavities' – a prophecy that would haunt the eventual School Dental Service for decades.

Pickerill, after thanking the President for his 'excellent and stimulating address', endorsed the concept of State dentistry, which, he stated, he himself had been advocating for some time. But he felt it quite inappropriate for the Association to suggest relying on dentists with lesser training, and strongly advised the President to delete such references from his address before it was given to the press:

> I think it would be very undesirable for the public as a whole to get the idea that we were offering as a University to train men at a lower standard for children than we are training them at present. To train men who were not so skilled and properly trained as other men would be very undesirable. What is to become of those men with a sort of semi-training? They are not going to stay in the service all the time! After four or five years they would be practising as 'quacks'. We must face the facts. When we are going to have a State Dental Service we must have properly trained and qualified men. – (Hear, hear, and applause.) In that service there must not be anyone who is not on the New Zealand Register.

This was a dramatic moment in the history of the New Zealand Dental Association when, despite the calmness of the reporting, feelings must have been running extremely high. One can picture Hunter meditating on the proposal of the President and imagining the School Dental Service as it subsequently became: a universal, school-based programme staffed by operators of a 'lower standard' than fully qualified dentists, but female rather than the males naturally expected at that time. One can also visualise the horror and embarrassment of the Dean of the Faculty of Dentistry at the suggestion that he might be required to train such people, after all the effort that had gone into the establishment of a respected degree course of high quality. And the despair of members, typified by Hursthouse, who recognised that restoration of teeth without concurrently lowering the decay rate would be a recipe for disaster – a theme also echoed by Pickerill, who resented the President's assumption that his own theories on prevention of caries were really just a pipe-dream.

The President was not, however, without his supporters. Goodwin Cox echoed his brother's pessimism on prevention of caries because of the indifference of parents. He also defended the concept of using people trained specifically for the tasks of filling and extracting, not trained in the more complex aspects of dentistry:

> It is a practical work-a-day world now, and it is a scheme we can put into practice pretty soon. I do see a little danger in what Professor Pickerill says in regard to turning out 'quacks', but I think that in years to come that if those dentists had to be properly trained in every department it would be many years before their services would be available.

The discussion on the President's brave and visionary address eventually concluded with the President undertaking to revise parts of the text before it was submitted to the press. Debate had been vigorous and thorough but, as Pickerill was to note in his July 1913 editorial, not one voice had been raised against the concept of a State Dental Service. The oral health of the 'poorer classes of the community' was a genuine concern of the Association and, although opinions differed on how dental services might be delivered, the meeting was unanimous that something had to be done.[18] The problem was too great for the resources that could be provided in private practices – new approaches to the problem were necessary.

Proposals for 'the establishment of a system of State Dentistry' were conveyed to the Minister for Public Health, the Honourable R.H. Rhodes, and the Minister of Education, the Honourable J. Allen, by a deputation of Norman Cox, Hunter, and Pickerill.[19] The ever-supportive T.K. Sidey introduced the deputation to the Ministers, pointing out that the contents of a pamphlet 'The Care of the Teeth', which the Association had worked hard to bring into being, needed to be widely known. He thought it would be fair if the Public Health Department either undertook the reprinting of the pamphlet or paid for sufficient copies for circulation throughout the Dominion.

Cox emphasised the 'grave state of affairs' revealed by the finding that almost 90 per cent of 10,000 children examined in the last few years were suffering from dental caries. He claimed that 'The question of unclean mouths in children overshadowed all other physical defects', and went on to ask for 'consideration of a scheme with a view to remedying the evil'. They realised that a 'comprehensive scheme' was not possible given the present 'state of Public opinion'; but what they were proposing was really a pilot scheme 'whereby the results of State Dentistry could be ascertained in a small way, so as to discover its effect on the efficiency of the pupil'. In the United States, he pointed out, statistics had shown gains in 'efficiency' of primary school children of 15 per cent from the system of dental inspection. Presumably he was implying that treatment of disease after its identification by the inspection resulted in improved behaviour and learning in the pupils – a reasonable outcome given the serious nature of the dental problems of many children. The deputation sought one State dentist to be appointed in each of the four main centres, working in:

> a thoroughly-equipped room at one of the schools, and probably the services of an attendant. The estimated cost at each centre was something like £1500. They believed that State Dentistry must come sooner or later. It was the poor people who had to be considered, because well-to-do people looked upon dentistry as a necessity. After such an institution had been working for a time they could judge whether a larger scheme should be gone on with.

Pickerill noted:

> the magnitude of the disease was so great that they could not hope to eliminate it at present, but if the efficiency of the children, both mental and physical, was to be maintained, it was necessary that some relief should be given from this national epidemic. Nevertheless, prevention as well as remedial measures should be instituted.

The proposal for a pilot scheme was sound and well presented: although not over-ambitious, it was directed at high-caries-risk children from low socio-economic families, a target likely to appeal to the politicians and to the public. The emphasis on prevention was also a sensible message.

The deputation was received with cautious support: the Ministers seemed impressed with the idea of wide distribution of the pamphlet to schoolteachers and parents, and the deputation assured them that it was 'simple enough for the teachers to understand it'. Allen said they might 'ask Cabinet to allow a small sum of money for the purpose'. Although sympathetic to the main proposal, the Minister noted that already the Government was supporting a system of physical training 'which they hoped would be effective, and had adopted a scheme of medical inspection in schools'. The latter was 'merely an experiment' but, if proved effective, it should be extended: 'it was not enough to inspect the children; they had to go further'. The Ministers undertook to raise the matter in Cabinet and discuss it with the public health officers. Allen wanted the first step to be in the 'right direction'; what was proposed 'would only be experimental, and it loomed before their minds as a scheme that would eventually cost a great deal of money'.

The press was much more enthusiastic about the Association's proposals. Pickerill summarised reactions in his July 1913 editorial.[20] He began with a quote from the editor of a Wellington daily: 'The New Zealand Dental Association has earned the gratitude of the country by the persistence with which it emphasises a grave public danger, and urges the adoption of the necessary measures to avert it.' Pickerill commented on the Ministers' acceptance of the seriousness of the problem:

> The Ministers, too, recognised that children with unhealthy mouths could not be physically fit. Therefore, we logically conclude that it is essential that their unhealthy mouths and teeth should be made healthy, that the gateway of their bodies should be rendered clean, and further, that for what is *essential*, money can and always will be found, and no party, section, or class of the community can in any possible way cavil at it …
>
> It is most gratifying that both the Opposition and the Government press in Wellington have strongly supported the inauguration of such a State dental service. The *Dominion*, in a leading article, states 'When it is borne in mind that many forms of disease are … due to dental defects, it becomes manifest that effective measures should be taken to ensure that the teeth of the children attending our schools shall receive proper attention … There can be no doubt that the provision by the State of medical and dental attention for the children of the poor will mean very considerable expenditure, but the national health is a matter of supreme importance, and from this point of view the proposals of the Dental Association are deserving of most careful and sympathetic consideration …'
>
> The *New Zealand Times* is no less emphatic when it says: 'The only objection of the educational authorities was of the expense …' The objection is futile: the care of caries is not a luxury … It is a vital national matter.

Pickerill smugly concluded the editorial by commending 'these eminently rational and business like remarks to our readers, to the general public, and also the Ministers of the Crown concerned'. The public response was certainly remarkable: it is doubtful that the Association has ever had such positive endorsement. The result was a team effort in which Pickerill was a dominant figure because of his roles as the Association's Secretary and Editor, and his status as a world authority on dental caries. He was certainly determined to place his imprint on the scheme, as he included in the editorial the proposal that 'each clinic should be provided with the means of application of *prophylactic treatment* on modern scientific lines, and that if necessary, each state dentist should attend the University of Otago for a short course in this subject before taking up his duties'.

Hunter and Pickerill went to England in March 1914,[21] Pickerill on sabbatical leave for six months, and both were at the International Dental Conference in London when war was declared. On their return, they devoted their combined talents of organisation and their status as the senior officers in the Association to the establishment of the Dental Corps.

But just because two of the major players were otherwise engaged during the war did not mean services for children were forgotten. They were certainly prominent in the mind of Wanganui dentist Richmond Dunn. He had a paper ready for the 1915 conference and it would have caused a sensation had it been delivered – that conference was cancelled – but the paper was eventually published in 1917.[22] He graphically described the appalling state of oral health of children, and the hopelessness of 'repairing the ravages of dental disease instead of striking at the causes of it'. Increasing the number of dentists would allow the repair of more teeth, but do nothing for prevention. He reached the startling conclusion that:

> we spend our lives in great measure in bolstering up the unfit … only the dentally well provided should survive in the struggle of existence … Dentists, doctors, chemists, and nurses are all at the same game to some extent, diluting the vigour of future generations by nullifying Nature's attempts to weed out the weaklings. The only person perhaps who does real service to the race is the Plunkett [*sic*] Nurse, although she is not above suspicion.

What Dunn wanted was a new category of dental worker, the dental nurse, 'to be the same real help to the dental profession as the Plunkett [*sic*] Nurse is to the medical.' She would serve an apprenticeship with a dentist and face a board of examiners who would license her to practise as a 'Dental Nurse', and the State:

> might assist successful candidates by granting a few months training at a Dental School … She would then be qualified either to practise privately as a Dental Nurse or to be appointed by the State or by a local body as a 'District Dental Nurse'. Her duties should be strictly limited to advising parents with regard to the dental wants of their children; to teaching them the evils of improper feeding and foolish luxury; to tactfully instil into their minds the rudiments of oral cleanliness; to warn them of the infective nature of dental disease, and of the danger of 'letting the first teeth go'; to examine the teeth of very young children, and to treat the teeth and perform certain simple operations on them when necessary.

Dunn did not elaborate on the nature of 'certain simple operations', leaving the details for others to pick up and for the Executive Council to take further if it thought the plan had merit. He addressed a major potential objection by suggesting that this 'better class of girl' would experience a 'natural thinning-out of their ranks by marriage and maternity [that] would prevent the new profession from being flooded'. They would relieve the dentist of a 'good deal of child-work that many of us find so trying to the nerves …'. He felt that, as New Zealanders were 'apt to pride themselves on their country being a laboratory for social experiments', it could be an example for other countries to follow and might even 'lead to the extinction of the dentist altogether'.

Pickerill was overseas during the 1917 conference, which was perhaps just as well, as he would no doubt have been angered by much that was discussed. Norman Cox made specific proposals in a major paper.[23] Whether he knew what Dunn was proposing is not known, but he argued that the task of providing necessary treatment for children was far beyond the supply of fully trained dentists; the solution lay, not with the partly trained dentists he had advocated in his 1913 presidential address, but with female dental nurses who, after working with a dentist for two years, would spend a further two years at 'the Dental College' receiving instruction that would include fillings and extractions.

Cox's paper, however, did not specifically feature in a lengthy debate at the conference, which focused on extending facilities for the training of dentists. The meeting had before it Pickerill's proposals to institute the Certificate of Proficiency at Dunedin as a lesser alternative to the BDS. But the mood of the meeting was to take away from the University the sole responsibility for training dentists. The vigorous debate therefore centred on how courses leading to the Certificate of Proficiency could be made more accessible, and be taken either fully in centres outside Dunedin, or by a combination of two years' study in outside centres followed by two years at the Dental School. Opinions on the School varied. One revealing comment was:

> at Dunedin there was an excellent school, with excellent teachers, but it was a national failure. Why? The real answer was that parents looked over the situation when deciding on a career for their sons, and found that dentistry did not pay. The course differed but little from the medical course, the social status of the doctor was higher, and he entered upon remunerative practice earlier.

The debate ebbed and flowed, between support and criticism of the School, between lowering admission standards and supporting the current admission requirement of matriculation, and between needing to enhance the perception of dentistry and the risk of lowering public perceptions, but always with the knowledge that something had to be done.[24] Two matters were absent from the debate: Norman Cox's suggestion for school dental nurses, possibly because he gave his paper after the debate; and means by which enrolment at the School could be increased. O.V. Davies stated his belief that a scheme of bursaries would be forthcoming, and he also cautioned against a panic response. It is likely he came away from the conference determined to make his bursary scheme work.

The outcome of the debate was that the Association supported a two-year dental course at any centre where teaching facilities were provided, followed by two years at the Dental School. The Minister of Hospitals and Public Health, the Honourable G.W. Russell, made the most of it when six months later he met the committee appointed by the conference to report to the Government on 'preventive and corrective dentistry for the children of the primary schools'. Of its four recommendations,[25] three were constructive: that the Government should immediately inaugurate a Dental Department to establish a 'thoroughly comprehensive system of State School Dentistry'; that the scheme should begin in a small way in the four main centres, extending gradually so that eventually all children would be included; and that applications be called for a Director of the Department. The final and remarkable recommendation went even beyond what had been debated at the conference and directly against many of the principles that the Association had fought for years:

> To ensure a sufficient supply of school dentists, the Committee suggests that students may receive free education at the Dental College [of two years' duration following two years' mechanical training in the students's 'own town'], together with a living allowance, in return for which they will serve the State, under bond for five years as School Dentists, at a stated salary, after which period they would have the option of continuing in the State service or of entering into private practice.

This free, abbreviated dental course would provide a supply of 'school dentists' who had to work for the State only for five years, and then were free to enter private practice with no apparent restrictions. No mention was made of dental nurses and Dunn's 'natural thinning-out by marriage', nor of Norman Cox's own support for nurses, even though he was a member of the three-man committee.

If the report had been adopted in full, it would have led to disaster. The 'Dental College' mentioned presumably meant the Dental School, which would have been expected to provide an entirely different and lower quality course for an entirely different category of student: not only would education be free, but also the students would be paid allowances. During its meeting with Russell and the Honourable J.A. Hanan, Minister of Education,[26] the committee endured Russell venting his dissatisfaction with the supply of dentists graduating from Dunedin and his views on liberalising their training. He threatened to amend the current Dentists Act in order to take sole responsibility for educating dentists away from the University altogether; he wanted a clause that would allow the Minister of Public Health to prescribe a separate course of study, and would establish training centres in Auckland, Christchurch, and Wellington. Hanan emphasised the importance of prevention, and praised the efforts of the school medical inspectors and school nurses in promoting better dental health. He concluded that although the scheme proposed was unique, the Ministers could not support it as the costs were prohibitive under the current circumstances. The committee – Norman Cox, Major E.C. Winstone, and Maurice Denniston, now the Association's Immediate Past President – received Russell's tirade meekly, without any protest, and thanked the Ministers for 'their sympathetic reception'. The committee made no attempt to defend the Dental School that it had so carefully nurtured and still regarded as its own.

Subsequent editorial comment at the time was similarly muted:[27] delays in implementing the committee's report were deplored, but no comment was made on school dentists or the proposed new training pathway. Many members of the Association must have been outraged, including Davies who, as Acting Director at the time, was enthusiastically and successfully promoting his bursary scheme.

Agitation for a school dental service continued to build, supported by medical inspectors and parents of children afflicted by advanced caries.[28] But no progress was made until early in 1919, when the first tentative steps were taken with advertisements appearing in the press for four 'School Dentists'.[29] A minor furore occurred a year later when Hunter learnt to his embarrassment that the Association had not been consulted over his appointment to the position of Chief Executive Dental Officer.[30] The Executive overruled his intention to resign from the position, including in its resolution that it was satisfied his motives were 'thoroughly honourable and straightforward', but the Government had failed to uphold the Association's rather pompous 'principle' that it be consulted over such matters. The decision of the Executive, however, did not please the members who raised it at the conference later in the year and who thought the appointment should have been discussed at a general meeting of the Association. The subsequent debate revealed that Denniston had also been an applicant.[31] (Pickerill had supported the application of

Davies.) Hunter took this debate as a personal attack against him, but he remained secure in the position.

He moved quickly to establish a school-based scheme staffed by female operators, the school dental nurses. He wrote persuasively to the Faculty of Dentistry, and presumably to the executive and branches of the Association:

> As a result of long and earnest consideration I am suggesting that a scheme such as the following should be put into action.
>
> … From observation and experience gained during the war, I am convinced that a proposal to utilise the service of women in this work is one that should receive earnest consideration …
>
> I consider a concentrated course of eighteen months to include Dental Anatomy … and at the chair all spare time. Of course this would have to be arranged by the University Dental School Authorities.
>
> … the services of these women operators would be limited entirely to simple extractions and plastic fillings.
>
> The advantages to be gained … would be:-
>
> 1. It would lead to an earlier solution of the problem of shortage of dental service for this work …
>
> 2. Women are instinctively better fitted to deal with children than the average man.
>
> 3. … whereas much of the skill of the fully qualified practitioner would not be utilised and would be lost to the general public, the training received by these women, having been directed solely to this special class of work, would be utilised to the fullest extent …

He also covered means for ensuring the female would not be able to compete with dentists, and was confident their introduction would not adversely affect the status of the profession.[32]

The response when the faculty received Hunter's letter was firm but completely negative. Although it recognised the need to establish services for children, the Faculty considered the full dental training was necessary for the 'arduous and difficult work'. The Faculty also believed that 'such students being ill-trained would bring nothing but discredit upon the University and would probably by reason of their necessarily insufficient training for their work bring the Education Department into discredit also'. The Faculty did offer, however, to train women to assist the fully trained dentist working in the Service, and suggested that if twenty dental bursaries were granted as originally requested, staffing needs in the Service would be met and, if employment conditions were made sufficiently attractive, a large proportion of other degree and COP graduates would also enter the Service. The Faculty predicted that the fully trained dentist would do 'three times as much work in the same amount of time as the partially trained nurse'. It asked the University Council to 'give effect to its protest on this matter'. In his subsequent covering letter to the Registrar, Pickerill noted: 'if the Education Department's proposals are carried out it would result in the further overcrowding of our class rooms, and it would be necessary to provide special lectures and practical courses in the subjects involved. It is also obvious that the present proposals would if they become effective kill the present bursary system.'[33] The first shot had been fired.

The Faculty was not the only body to oppose Hunter's scheme. The Association had received responses from fourteen branches and, as the majority were opposed, the Secretary was instructed to write again asking branches to submit proposals 'that would adequately deal with the matter, and to state that the Association were in honour bound to supply the Government with some scheme to meet the requirements of the service'.[34]

The proposals soon aroused the interest of the press and public, and it was then that full-scale battles commenced. The *Otago Daily Times* (*ODT*) was worried about the 'unusual and quite unnecessary amount of secrecy' surrounding the scheme and, as shown by opposition by the profession, the impression was gained that 'the Government is acting along unsafe lines'. A legal opinion suggested employment of the partially trained nurses was in breach of the Dentists Act.[35] Three days later, Pickerill issued a public statement that began with tongue-in-cheek praise for the Minister of Public Health and Education, the Honourable C.J. Parr:

> I have read Mr Parr's statement … and entirely agree with much of what he has to say, and I consider New Zealand is to be congratulated on having a Minister of Public Health and Education who takes such a keen interest in such an important matter as the dental treatment of school children. It is, as he rightly says, a vital matter affecting the health and welfare of the rising and succeeding generations. A State School Dental Service has been urgently needed for some years past, and now that it has been inaugurated it behoves all concerned to see that it is developed on lines which will deal adequately, justly, and fairly with the situation.

But then came the barbs:

> Does the Minister realise that what at present is the great menace to the health of New Zealand children is oral sepsis? Septic infection from advanced dental caries which bids fair to poison their systems and undermine their constitutions? The trivial and simple cavities for the present do not matter: the duty of the State is to treat the most urgent cases first. But this is not to be done: all the bad cases, all the scholars in the standards throughout New Zealand, are to be

> 'jettisoned'. Their health and welfare … are to be intentionally thrown to the winds – neglected. And only those children with little holes in their teeth are to be treated … I am satisfied that no medical man in New Zealand who has had experience of the effects of oral sepsis – and few have not – would sanction such a scheme.[36]

Children, in his view, should receive only the best, and he repeated his suggestion that women be trained to assist dentists; he also appealed for the smaller centres to be included in the Service at an early stage. His statement was accompanied by an editorial highly critical of the scheme, and supportive of his alternative. The *ODT*'s Editor was appalled at the prospect of 'half-trained and poorly equipped women' being let loose on children, and considered the scheme is 'fraught with the most lamentable consequences'.[37]

The Minister was quick to respond, through a lengthy statement no doubt scripted by his Chief Dental Officer:

> Dr Pickerill's statement is as misleading as it is inaccurate … he does not scruple to be unfair … Within the last couple of months we have established clinics not only in the four main centres, but in several of the boroughs as well … Emphatically I must state that it is not proposed to neglect all the serious cases of dental disease as Dr Pickerill suggests … No one knows better than Professor Pickerill the insidious rapidity of dental caries. To concentrate on the serious cases would mean no preventive dentistry …
>
> Professor Pickerill's attempt to arouse enmity against the scheme from other districts is unfair. If the Dunedin critic were wholly disinterested and sincere, he ought to be pleased that the department has already been able to establish facilities for dental treatment in the centres in which half the population of the dominion lives.

The Minister quoted the Association's President, Nelson Mitchell, as stating: 'it was a fact that after two years of intensive training in simple filling, the extraction of temporary teeth, and dental hygiene, these nurses will have a higher training in their own branch than the average dental student. Qualified dentists would direct the nurses' work …'. He also refuted the legal opinion obtained by 'a little Dunedin coterie'.[38]

Pickerill responded forcefully point by point in the same issue of the *ODT*, and was supported by Frank Armstrong. The arguments went on, the scheme being condemned by the Women's Citizens' Association, and the Dunedin Branch of the New Zealand Educational Institute. Opposition statements from the Otago, Canterbury, and Wanganui branches of the Association were also published, and opposition also came from the Wellington, Hawke's Bay, Taranaki, and Southland branches. The Minister, Hunter, and Pickerill presented new and old arguments: Hunter stating that Pickerill had offered to support the scheme if it were approved by the Association, an assertion Pickerill strongly denied, and Pickerill deploring the proposal for the nurses to receive a salary of £250 per annum after only two years' training, whereas dentists entering state service were to be paid just £275 after four years' training. Pickerill also claimed that equipping a school for the nurses in Wellington, the proposal for training to occur at the Dental School having been quickly dropped, would seriously jeopardise prospects for a much-needed new building in Dunedin.[39]

The Minister's statement of Mitchell's support arose from a special meeting of the Executive Council in September,[40] attended by Hunter, Pickerill, and the Chief Medical Officer of Public Health by invitation. Unfortunately the proceedings of that meeting were never published, but some branches deplored the outcome, claiming their representatives had voted for the scheme against the wishes of their branches – hence the public statements of opposition. These branches were criticised by the Chairman of the Executive, Norman Rishworth, as being disloyal to the Association, which had reached its conclusion after long discussion.[41]

Davies was one who was deeply hurt by his branch's opposition to the Executive's decision, and he resigned from the committee of the Otago Branch. Claude Moses, Secretary of the Association, commended him for this decision, and told him that Pickerill had originally stated he would support the scheme if the Executive approved it. Moses was appalled by Pickerill's subsequent actions.[42]

Up to this point, personalities had been largely excluded from public discussion, although one editorial had quite unfairly and judgmentally criticised the appointment of Richmond Dunn to head the training of the nurses: 'a man who, whatever his capabilities in his profession, belongs distinctly to the old order of dentists and who can scarcely be conversant with the modern methods so essential on the part of a dentistry instructor'.[43] Worse was to follow, however. Speaking to the Women's Citizens Association in Dunedin, Pickerill 'ventured to say that had he [Hunter] had the requisite training he would never have advocated the employment of unqualified women'.[41] This was a direct attack on Hunter's qualifications, experience, and abilities and was bitterly resented. The Administration Officer to the Director of Dental Services (Hunter still held this military position) promptly reported the insult to the Chancellor:

> It is well recognised fact among members of the Corps and the profession generally that the present Director of the Dental School obtained what practical experience he possesses in operative dentistry under the tuition of a number

> of Dunedin dental surgeons among whom Col. Hunter held such a prominent position.
>
> I would respectfully submit that for a member of your Professorial Board to pursue unchecked a course of public vilification of one of Col. Hunter's standing and reputation is a direct negation of that spirit of British justice and fair play which institutions such as yours throughout the Empire have ever held in cherished possession.[45]

The Chancellor was understandably disturbed by the insulting and patronising tone of the letter:

> The Chancellor recognises that it is regrettable that any reference should have been made to Mr. Hunter's qualifications. At the same time he is bound to point out that the statements as reported cannot be regarded as 'public vilification' of Mr. Hunter, and, indeed, are much milder in tone than are the statements contained in your letter with reference to Dr. Pickerill.

The current editor of the *Journal* (A.M. Carter) attempted to calm this chaos by clarifying the issues:

> it is fit that some record go down of what may justly be regarded as a crisis in dental history of the Dominion. Moreover, many individual members, as well as some Branches of the association, have seen fit to seize the occasion to freely air their opinion and to initiate a propagandism directly antagonistic to the action of their own Executive.

He then traced events to that point, including the Government's acknowledgement of the appalling nature of the caries problem; the appointment of Hunter, and his presentation of plans for the embryo service; the subsequent full discussion by the Executive leading to the Association's support of the scheme, albeit not unanimous; objections raised by individuals and branches, each of which the Editor addressed; and the inappropriateness of opening the matter for full debate again now that the Association had made its decision within its Rules. The editorial eloquently concluded:

> The Executive gathering in Wellington was composed of men selected by their fellows as representatives, presumably on account of their fitness for this position. Many of these men approached the discussion with a strong feeling, we might almost say, bias, against the proposed training of dental operative nurses; yet, after the most exhaustive enquiry, they came to the conclusion that no alternative suggestion was advanced to meet the case, and that no course was open to them but to support the scheme brought forward by the Chief Dental Officer. The scheme is yet in its infancy, and Mr. Hunter himself will be the first to admit that it may have imperfections which time alone will reveal, and experience remedy. We have the greatest respect for those who cannot view this

> matter as we ourselves do, yet, without sacrificing their own principles, remain loyal to their chosen leaders, but we frankly confess we have no sympathy at all with those who, by unconstitutional methods, seek to overthrow the expressed voice of their chosen representatives, and who, in so doing, imperil not so much the security of a proposed school dental scheme, as the welfare and cohesion of the body to which they belong.[46]

The same issue of the *Journal* reported the Executive's anger and frustration with the opposition to its decision. The Chairman (Norman Rishworth) deplored the 'Press campaign' and

> felt keenly the position in which several Branches and members were placing him and the Executive generally through their disloyal actions. It was a most improper and unconstitutional procedure, and, if not stopped, must result in the disintegration of the Association … He [Rishworth] trusted that better counsels would prevail, and that the offenders would express their regret … thus again bringing about that happy spirit of unity and comradeship which had always characterised the New Zealand Dental Association.[47]

The meeting denied the call of Pickerill and others for a special general meeting of members to re-open the issue, and it adopted a series of statements to be sent to him and to branch secretaries.

Hunter moved quickly to start the scheme. By March 1921, thirty-five 'nurse probationers' had been selected from 120 applicants and were serving a two-month probationary period. A suitable building had already been equipped in Wellington. In his brief article in the *Journal*, he reiterated the arguments for the scheme, including the delays that would have arisen if it were to be staffed by dentists.[48] In the same issue, the Editor also enthused on what he had seen at a clinic at an Auckland school, one of the first to be established, and staffed by two dentists, 'one of whom was a member of the fairer sex … We examined mouth after mouth, presenting in a clean and healthy condition, and in which the little owners took obvious pride'.[49]

Calm was prevailing, but the bitterness, especially against Pickerill continued. Nelson Mitchell's 1921 presidential address reviewed with pride the achievements of the Association, but subsequent discussion opened the gates of criticism against Pickerill. Norman Rishworth was scathing. After expressing his astonishment that Pickerill was not at the conference, despite him being made aware that 'the question of his disloyal actions would be discussed', he accused Pickerill of misleading other members of the profession. Referring to accusations that the Executive, based in Auckland, was seeking to build a rival dental school there, he stated: 'the only enemy the present school could have was its present Director, who, by his attitude of antagonism to the association, was forcing them to consider the possibility of having to establish a school which would train up the young men to join it in harmony, with ideas similar to its own'. Davies criticised his own branch, stating that although he had opposed the scheme at the meeting of the Executive Council, he supported the final decision. He felt his own branch had acted unconstitutionally, hence his resignation from its Executive. Rumbling criticism of the Executive continued, but defence of Pickerill's actions was non-existent – he was *persona non grata* in the Association.[50]

Good feelings to the point of smugness prevailed at the 1922 conference in Nelson, where Hunter presented a progress report that outlined the nurses' first-year course and summarised the treatment procedures completed in training.[51] The conference was impressed with progress and impressed, too, with the mouths of children treated at the Nelson school clinic. Previous opponents were won over, such as Lionel Sherriff of Wanganui, who moved the motion, passed unanimously: 'That the Conference, having had an opportunity of inspecting some of the good results obtained by the State Dental Hygiene Service, wish to convey to the Hon. The Minister for Public Health, its hearty appreciation of the work being done by the Department, and only hope that further financial support will be forthcoming to extend the good work'.

Progress continued, and the first clinic staffed by school dental nurses opened in Hawke's Bay in 1923. Local dentist Herbert Ziele was profoundly impressed with the clinic and with the statistics Hunter presented to the gathering of local dignitaries and Members of Parliament. After earlier opposition, 'the dental profession in Hawke's Bay was going to back up Colonel Hunter and his scheme to a man'.[52] By November that year, school dental nurses were stationed in twenty-five clinics.[53] The School Dental Service was now a reality, and firmly embedded in New Zealand's health services.

Pickerill's relations with the Association continued to decline, to the extent that he failed to pay his subscription for three years through to the end of 1923, despite several letters being sent to him requesting payment. If payment had not been received by November, the Association reluctantly would be forced to hand the matter to its solicitors. Assistance sought from the Otago Branch to resolve the situation was unsuccessful. He resigned in April 1923 under the threat of proceedings against him.[54] Although not the complete ending of his links with the Association, it was a sad conclusion of his formal connection with a body he had previously served with distinction as its Secretary and Editor, and from which he had received much praise and well-deserved accolades. But he still had a final, long-range shot to fire against the School Dental Service. In 1927 he wrote a letter to the Editor of the London *Spectator* in which, as was reported in the *New Zealand Dental Nurses Journal*, 'he severely and, it is considered, very unfairly, criticised the New Zealand Dental Service.' Hunter wrote a harsh and vigorous rejoinder to the *Spectator*, 'in view of the indignation and resentment that were aroused throughout the Service …'. It covered the old arguments and claimed that many visitors and experts had admired the system, whereas Pickerill had never observed its achievements at first hand. G.L. Taylor, then Association President, also responded to Pickerill's criticism, as reported in the *New Zealand Herald*, by reinforcing the Association's support of the scheme.

Pickerill considered a school-based dental service was essential for children's health, and campaigned vigorously for its establishment. But he failed to channel the School Dental Service into the form he considered to be the best possible for New Zealand's children. Rather than accepting the situation with grace, he stood by his opposition even to the extent of sacrificing his membership of the body he had served so well for some sixteen years. The Pickerill connection with the School Dental Service did not end there, however: perhaps ironically, three of his granddaughters were to become school dental nurses.

15

Defeating the Auckland challenge, 1919–1927

An early indication of serious overcrowding in the School came from anaesthetist Dr Emily Siedeberg (incidentally the first woman to graduate in medicine in New Zealand, in 1896), when in 1918 she alerted the Acting Director, O.V. Davies, to the problems of accommodation for patients recovering from general anaesthesia – sometimes she had five patients in an area designed for two. If the workload increased, as could be expected when the dental inspection of children in schools began, the facilities would be 'absolutely useless'.[1] Davies first complained to the Council about the School's shortage of space early that year, strongly recommending 'that, on the grounds of economy and efficiency a fresh building should be erected elsewhere'. He followed this up early in 1920, saying that temporary accommodation would relieve congestion for a while, giving enough breathing space to plan a new building. Pickerill took over the crusade when he returned to the School in July 1920, calling for an entirely new building as the only way to overcome the ever-increasing difficulties.[2]

He was progressively more forceful in subsequent complaints. He reminded the Registrar that his 1922 Annual Report had included: 'The overcrowding is daily becoming more acute and renders our work at times so difficult as to be almost impossible. No other University Department is so overcrowded and congested as we are'. He then listed the problems with each part of the School – the laboratory, the nurses' cloakroom, patients' waiting room ('utterly and absurdly inadequate'), museum and teaching specimens ('dismantled and dispersed'). … I beg to urge that an endeavour be made, in view of the urgency of the situation, to obtain authorisation for a new building to be proceeded with, the plans and site for which were approved last year'.[3] At this time the country, after a period of prosperity, was in recession,[4] and Government expenditure was severely curtailed. Pickerill recognised the financial difficulties of the times, but would 'be failing in my duty to the Council, to the students and patients if I did not make this urgent recommendation'. It was, he reminded the Council, no longer possible to give students an efficient training.

He later produced evidence of atmospheric pollution that could explain the frequency of throat infections in students and staff, including himself. He added two further arguments for a new building – although quite young, the School had already provided the University with two professors (Bell and Hercus) and that it was now providing, through patients' fees, 10 per cent of the University's revenues.[4]

A very distressing event then occurred – the death of a boy of fifteen years after he had had teeth extracted under general anaesthesia. Dr Siedeberg described to the coroner the dreadful conditions she was working under: lack of heating in the waiting room, instruments sterilised over a gas heater, lack of ventilation, and out-dated equipment. Pickerill praised her skill as an anaesthetist but, although this was the first mishap after over 3000 anaesthetics, she was carrying an 'unfair responsibility under the existing conditions'. The coroner concluded that neither the anaesthetic nor the surgery caused the patient's death, but 'the defects pointed out are such as should not exist in a school performing such important work. I hope that the representations which have been made and the evidence which has been given here will convince the authorities of the urgent need of these defects being remedied'.[6]

Further publicity on the conditions appeared the following day, after the *ODT* sent a reporter to the School. The article and associated editorial painted a grim picture of total inadequacy in all areas. The article concluded:

> Dr Pickerill has made the University Council fully aware of all the facts about the school – indeed his papers have frequently figured on the order paper. Plans for a new school, a three-story building, were approved … last year, when the Minister … after a look through the present school, described the conditions as 'ghastly'. The building was to cost £30,000, but it shared the fate of the other schemes when the axe was applied … if the conditions were 'ghastly' then they are certainly no better today.[7]

An impasse had now been reached: the School had neither sufficient space nor enough operating chairs to train the current third-year class. Pickerill passed the crisis to the Council, asking for advice on what he should do, especially with the class that was presently buying, at a cost of £30, instruments required for the following year, yet these students might not have been able to continue with their courses. Bell reinforced the pollution problem by complaining that, because of sickness, he rarely had a full complement of students and staff for clinical work.[8]

But the months went by with, despite deputations of the Council to the Government, still no signs of improvement. At the start of the 1923 academic year, Pickerill was 'surprised and much disappointed' to find that no funds were available even for temporary increases in accommodation: if additional space were not found in the next fortnight, at least fifteen students would have to be sent away. He recommended the temporary use of Marama and Maheno Halls.[9] The Chancellor reported that the Director of Education had authorised an architect to prepare plans and specifications for temporary extensions to the filling room and the Dean's office:[10] a short-term but modest gain, although the benefits to come were threatened by the flood the following year, which severely undermined the extension.

Further complaint to the Council and the subsequent discussion were widely publicised. 'Shocking conditions' was the headline of the *ODT*'s extensive report of the Council's meeting of 17 April. The School had been built to accommodate 26 students; now it had 106. Added weight was provided by remarks of external examiners, who included Nelson Mitchell, the Association's immediate Past President, and G.C. Tripe, the President-elect. Their criticism was scathing, and contained comments such as 'absolutely fossilised' and a 'disgrace'.[11] Once again the *ODT*'s Editor gave support, quoting a Council member as saying that 'the staff and students were simply "pigging it" at the present time at the Dental School'.[12]

At that particular Council meeting, a member had described the comments of the examiners as exaggerated. Pickerill jumped on this suggestion; he quickly telegraphed the remark to the examiners, who replied very firmly that their comments were factual. Tripe, for example, confirmed: 'you will find that you are hopelessly crowded and wanting in equipment'. Pickerill also responded to criticism that the problem was the Director's fault, reminding the Registrar that he had reported problems at least nine or ten times over the previous four years, and that in 1920 the Council and the Government both agreed a new building was essential.[13]

The Council was certainly sympathetic to the situation. In May 1923, a special committee recommended that the Council appeal to the Government for new Medical and Dental School buildings but, if the Council failed to receive a grant to allow both, Dental should be accorded priority.[14] The frustrated students also added their voices: 'After suffering in silence for over two years, in the hope that conditions generally would be improved, we have now reached a stage where we find it utterly impossible to carry on our work at the Dental School with any degree of satisfaction'. After presenting their detailed list of individual complaints and comparing the rosy picture described in the *Calendar* with reality, the students felt sure 'the true state of affairs will be appreciated and something definite will be done to remedy it'.[15] Pickerill used the opportunity to further his call for action: 'unfortunately the [students'] statements … are in the main correct. … Each year we have been hoping for a new building which could be equipped in a modern and efficient manner. Each year we have been doomed to disappointment and each year facilities and equipment have become more makeshift.'[16] He was to bring other student complaints to the Council the following year as two students informed him that, under medical advice, they had temporarily abandoned their course due to chest trouble: 'and to what extent the crowded vitiated [*sic*] atmosphere of the Dental School may be responsible for this … is a matter of serious suspicion'.[17]

The case for the new building had been well and persistently argued, and preliminary steps had been taken by reserving a suitable site in King (later Great King) Street and by preparation of plans. But the accommodation problems at both the Medical and Dental schools now spawned an alternative proposal: in the case of the Dental School, for a new school to be built in Auckland. This idea was advanced in an attack on Otago's dominance of the special schools by the Honourable G. Fowlds, a former Minister of Education and at that time Chairman of the Auckland University College Council. Wanting New Zealand to have four full universities,[18] he accused the Medical and Dental Schools of unfairly drawing the majority of their students from Otago, so discriminating against students from other centres. The Chancellor, the Reverend Dr Cameron, quickly pointed out the fallacies in his figures.[19]

Nevertheless the Government appointed a committee to report on the 'Provision of accommodation for the training of dental students'. It was convened by Dr E. Marsden, Assistant Director of Education, and included J.N. Rishworth, representing the Dental Association; Hunter, the Director of Dental Hygiene; and Mr R. Savage, architect to the Education Department. In view of events over the School Dental Service, the presence of Rishworth and Hunter might have been alarming to Pickerill. Hunter, however, was to continue his loyal support of the Otago School.

In the introduction to its long and complex report to the Minister of Education, the Committee noted its inquiries 'led to a general survey of the whole question of Dental training in the Dominion, and certain suggestions are respectfully submitted for your consideration'. This greatly exceeded the original purpose of the inquiry; the outcome was a very angry University and enormous public controversy – in the press and within the New Zealand Dental Association. The Committee interviewed Sidey (then Vice-Chancellor), Pickerill, the Registrar, the University's architect, and the Sub-dean of the Faculty of Medicine. It also met with representatives of the Otago Branch of the Association, including Davies, a deputation from the Auckland University College that included Fowlds, and several dentists, including Moses (like Rishworth, not a friend of Pickerill's), listed as representing the Auckland Branch.

Following its review of the current dental workforce, population trends, and demand for care, the Committee concluded that twenty-five dentists should be trained each year for the following ten years, preferably with the BDS degree rather than the COP. After its visit to the School and interviews with Pickerill, Davies (incorrectly spelt 'Davis' throughout the report), and students, the Committee reported that 'Conclusive evidence was placed before the Committee to show that graduates have not received, and the students are not receiving, sufficient training in either operative or mechanical dentistry. The situation is a very serious one', and was due, the Committee concluded, to lack of accommodation and facilities, lack of sufficient and proper supervision, and lack of clinical material. The Committee was concerned over the time many students were taking to complete their courses – the failure rate in examinations was considered 'unnecessarily high'. Members were 'alarmed' at Pickerill's proposals to increase the length of the course, and recommended shortening it by increasing the admission standards so that students could cope with its demands in the minimum time.

The report then assumed a more threatening tone: 'so long as the Dental School is situated in Dunedin only, in the interests of students, it will be necessary to arrange that they should obtain clinical practice at the hospitals of the three other main centres, where more clinical material is presenting, both during vacations and during at least six months of the fourth year of the course'. It then reviewed building options, including taking over a part of the Medical School soon to be vacated, but concluded that only a new building could meet the training needs of dentists for the Dominion. That section of the report then concluded: '… if no Dental School is to be built elsewhere than in Dunedin for the next ten years, the Beverly Trust site [King Street] should be used'. It also felt the plans for the new building were 'not excessive', but some economies could be made.

Moving on to the evidence received from the Auckland contributors, the report stated that the evidence and proposals presented:

> are so important and have such far reaching consequences that your Committee feels compelled to deal with the larger question, as to whether or not Dunedin is the most suitable place for a Dental School, and whether the time is opportune for the establishment of a second Dental School in Auckland to supplement or even supplant the training given in Dunedin … It has become necessary to

> consider whether the money might be used to better advantage, for the same purpose, elsewhere.

The report stated that Auckland University Council wanted a new school there, with practical and mechanical work to be done at the public hospital. Lectures and 'non-professional subjects would be taken at the University', and the COP would initially be the end qualification. Evidence submitted 'satisfied the Commission' [as the Committee was sometimes described] that Auckland had more clinical material available than the other three major centres combined, a large school-leaving population, no other local opportunities for professional training, and the cooperation of the Hospital Board, which would provide £15,000 toward initial and ongoing costs.[20]

Rishworth and Hunter added their own views to the main report. Rishworth was scathing of the hopeless overcrowding at the School:

> Instead of a well considered, supervised and meticulous training with due regard to Asepsis which, in the public interest … is essential, we found confusion, lack of cooperation and almost an entire absence of supervision.
>
> The Dean must be held blameworthy for this situation. Obviously he should have refused to allow his School to be so grossly misused and should have strictly limited the influx of students to the capacity of the building and the size of its staff.

After hearing the Dunedin evidence, Rishworth had concluded that a new, well-equipped school should be built on the King Street site. But he also praised the Auckland evidence and, against his 'better judgment to compromise', recommended moving the Dental School into the part of the Medical School becoming available (a matter disputed by the Medical School's Sub-dean), and establishing a second school in Auckland. Hunter acknowledged the unsatisfactory situation at the School, but did not support the suggestion of a new school in Auckland. He did favour, however, a reorganisation of the curriculum to allow students to take their first year 'in any big centre and at least six months of their last year together with their long vacations in centres where there is more clinical material than in Dunedin'.

Marsden, Rishworth and Savage then gave a cautious summary that seemed to conclude that the School should be taken away from Dunedin, and a new school established in Auckland. They rejected, however, suggestions that the course there be limited to the COP, even though such graduates 'would probably be better trained in the practice of the profession than the present Dunedin students'. The full BDS, with its greater emphasis on the medical aspects of dentistry, was the preferred option.

Hunter presented a powerful dissenting opinion, also included in the report. He considered the establishment of another school would be a waste of public funds, and the joint responsibility between the Auckland Hospital and the University College would be difficult to manage. He believed association with the Medical School was essential: 'The Medical School being in Dunedin is a point which cannot be overlooked and is decidedly in favour of the policy of retaining the Dental School there. Further, living conditions are cheaper in Dunedin and the climate is more suitable for work'. He continued to favour some work being undertaken by students in centres outside Dunedin, but recommended 'a new building at Dunedin equipped and staffed in such a manner that should ensure efficiency'.

Pickerill naturally was quick to respond. He noted that the Committee had initially recommended unanimously the erection of a new building on the King Street site – 'the request of the Council and our contention of the utter inadequacy of the present building is entirely upheld'. He was scathing of the second portion of the Committee's report:

> … the majority addendum [is] by the Assistant Director of Education (a Professor of Physics), an architect and a dentist, none of whom has had personal experience of University Dental Training. This second portion suggests, without any adequate reasons advanced at all, that the Dental School should be transferred to Auckland. The only reason … advanced is that more clinical material would be available. In all other facilities the report admits that Auckland is entirely lacking.[18]

He continued by endorsing Hunter's conclusion, which was based on both economic and academic grounds, against removal of the present school to Auckland. Not surprisingly, he disagreed entirely with the majority report. He questioned whether the Committee had been empowered to extend its deliberations to consider a school in Auckland, and stated that its personnel were entirely unsuited to make such a report. He enlarged on the breadth of knowledge required for the modern dentist – far beyond the operative and mechanical aspects – and noted that no proposals at all were made for the teaching of the range of subjects required. 'To establish a Dental School apart from a Medical School is unthinkable'. He then, as have later deans, defended the amount of clinical material available in Dunedin. There was, he claimed, more than the School could handle, but the problem was, as it would also be in Auckland, the lack 'of a class of patients who could afford to pay for gold and precious metals for crown and bridge work'. The situation had, however, improved with the Dental Association's agreement for the School to treat University students and hospital nurses. He agreed with Hunter, however, that, with a view to future needs or to provide greater variety of work, the curriculum might be arranged to allow students to do clinical and surgical work in other centres during their final year; he added the caveat that such an arrangement would require the sanction of the Senate of the University of New Zealand.

He resented the Committee's conclusion that graduates received insufficient training in either mechanical or operative dentistry, especially as he had not been questioned on this subject. He also resented the insinuations about the quality of the staff. He rejected criticisms of his own performance, noting that he did not have the power to limit the number of students entering his department, and that all graduates had no difficulty in finding highly paid employment after graduation – hardly likely to occur if they had received inadequate training – and other graduates had no difficulty in obtaining their DDS degrees in America. He concluded:

> there is not a single valid reason for the suggestion contained in the majority addendum that the School should be transferred to Auckland. There would be no more clinical material – no facilities for the medical portion of the course, no compensating advantages whatever. On the other hand, there would be loss of recognition of our degree by the [British] General Medical Council, and we should lose the proud distinction that a New Zealand graduate can practise anywhere in the Empire.[21]

The University of Otago Council, also highly offended, endorsed Pickerill's contention that the Committee grossly exceeded its terms of reference; it understood the inquiry was only to report to the Minister on the suitability of that part of the Medical School, currently occupied by the anatomy department and part of the physiological department, being converted for Dental School purposes. If the Committee had been authorised to report on other matters, the Council felt it should have been informed of this and given the opportunity to tender evidence and to cross-examine witnesses. The Council could only respond in a general way to the claim that 'conclusive evidence' had been presented on the inadequacy of training. Rather than accepting vague evidence of inadequacy, the Council presented complimentary testimonials from practitioners employing recent graduates; it also hoped that if any evidence of insufficient training were submitted it would need to be specific and allow thorough investigation. The Council also regretted that newspapers had been permitted to publish statements reflecting on the professional ability of its graduates before the Council had an opportunity to refute the charges.[22]

The newspapers had indeed made the most of the revelations in the report. The *ODT* published full details of the report in an article headed

'Graduates not sufficiently trained' and 'A startling recommendation',[23] the latter referring to the proposal to transfer the School to Auckland. The same issue contained statements from Cabinet Minister and former Dunedin mayor the Honourable Downie Stewart, and from Sir Henry Ferguson, Dean of the Medical School. Stewart confirmed the Committee had been set up to inquire into how best to enlarge the School in Dunedin; it had no Cabinet authority to explore options in any other centre. Ferguson had no knowledge of any evidence placed before the Committee, but commented it would be a 'grave mistake' to duplicate departments of physiology and anatomy anywhere else. The editorial in the following day's *ODT* sprang to the defence of the School and harshly criticised the extension of the mandate to consider a school elsewhere than in Dunedin.[24]

Auckland's *New Zealand Herald* pompously supported the removal of the School to Auckland on the grounds of the national interest: any satisfaction engendered by recommendation of removal of the School to Auckland would be trivial in comparison to the revelation of 'the appalling condition into which education has been permitted to fall at Otago University … Behind all the past prating of efficiency there was … a state of inefficiency which is a grave menace to the whole Dominion'.[25] The matter was so serious, the writer contended, that it could not be permitted to rest where it is: a sentiment echoed by Pickerill and the Council, which pointed out firmly that the fault lay with Government inaction, not with the University.[26]

The alleged 'evidence' of inadequate clinical training was eventually received and was answered in detail;[27] Pickerill concluded the reason Fowlds gave for the establishment of a new school in Auckland was little more than a protest about the cost to students travelling between Auckland and Dunedin. Fowlds had referred questions about facilities Auckland could provide and associated costs to a Dr Mackenzie who, according to Pickerill, had shown 'a lamentable lack of knowledge of the required dental curriculum. He is obviously utterly at sea as to the standard of training required in the "Medical" side of the course … He practically states that if a few Medical men can be got together to give honorarily [*sic*] a few demonstrations in Anatomy and a few dentists to visit the Dental Hospital and a Director of the Dental School is appointed, that is all that is required for a modern Dental school!' The Hospital Board, he went on, seemed to have the idea that students, for whom no salary would be needed, could cope with demands for dental treatment by patients unable to afford the fees of private dentists. The Auckland University College came under fire for 'two fundamental errors': that the provision of a dental school would be an inexpensive matter, and that the College could establish a course without reference to the Senate or the British General

Medical Council. Criticisms of Otago's course made by the dentist in charge of Auckland Hospital's Dental Department were dismissed as 'so puerile as not to merit notice', but the Otago University Council asked Pickerill to provide more information on several dental procedures, including methods of root-canal treatment and local analgesia, and on supervision in operative dentistry. In his response, Pickerill rather gleefully pointed out that Moses, who had given evidence for the Auckland Branch, had displayed a 'fundamental lack of knowledge of the Dental Curriculum'.[28]

Meanwhile, the Editor of the *Journal* (A.M. Carter of Auckland) was being very cautious. He acknowledged the importance of the School and the support it had received from the Association, but foresaw the possibility that 'new dental schools will in the course of time automatically arise in the main centres …'. Continued recognition of the BDS by the British General Medical Council was essential, and the facilities in any new school in any other centre would have to meet its requirements. But the Editor could see no reason why students for the COP, ' a mere licence to practise', could not 'take advantage of the large amount of clinical material at present going to waste, and receive a thorough and effective training in their own home centres'. The Committee's report, including Hunter's dissenting memorandum, was published in the March issue of the *Journal*.[30] Pickerill then pointed out to the Registrar that his rebuttal had not been included, although this may have simply been due to the Registrar not sending it to the Editor. He sarcastically added, 'Is it necessary for me to say that the journal is published in Auckland?'[31] Pickerill's rebuttal was published in the May issue.[32] An editorial note suggested, somewhat apologetically, that the report to the Council 'should be read by all those interested in dental education … and who are anxious to look at the question from an unbiased standpoint'. Another note reported that the contract for the new Dental School building had been let for over £23,000: progress was promising but by no means certain.

Prime Minister Massey met with the University Council in Dunedin in February 1924. Denis Ivory, a Tauranga graduate of the School and a Vice-president of the Dental Students' Association, heard about this and offered to come to Dunedin, at his own expense, to give evidence against shifting the School to Auckland. Pickerill asked the Registrar to accept the offer of 'a sensible and forceful speaker … graduates should have the opportunity of refuting insinuations against their ability'. The Council was grateful that Ivory made the long journey down, and the consensus was that he made a very able speech 'calculated to impress the Prime Minister'.[33]

Throughout all the controversy, the School struggled on as best it could; student numbers continued to climb. An exasperated Pickerill informed the

Registrar that he had to put men into the women's room, the result being that 'female staff, students, and patients had no access to lavatory accommodation … a condition of affairs no decent community should tolerate'.[34] He followed this up by regretting that 29 new students had been admitted, bringing the total to 123 and making the School 'an intolerably overcrowded department'. He questioned whether these students should have been admitted while their proper training could not be assured. He then vented his complete frustration in a tirade against the continued delay. This was triggered by the Director of Education asking whether Pickerill had discussed with the Senate the suggestion that students should undertake some of their clinical practice in other centres. Once this had been decided, according to the Director, it would no doubt be found that the amount of room required for clinical dentistry would not be as great as estimated. The Minister of Education had decided that no further action concerning the grant for the new building could be taken at that time.[35]

The Dean was furious at this new 'pretext' to delay authorisation. The continued postponement was 'clearly subterfuge and prevarication'. It was 'callous and unwarrantable that careers of 123 young people are being hazarded and juggled with'. He had no doubt that still further delays would be discovered; nothing had been done to relieve the congestion, and it was essential that the building, as planned, be provided as the 'bedrock minimum … I can no longer retain both my present appointment and my self-respect and unless something concrete is done at once to ensure faith being kept with our students I propose with great regret to ask the Council to relieve me of my position as Director of the Dental School at the earliest possible moment'.[36] His frustration with the Department of Education was now at bursting point. This episode followed another eruption three months earlier, when Marsden, the Assistant Director of Education and Chairman of the Committee of Enquiry, wanted details of equipment required by the School. Marsden thought it probable that the Government could obtain a better price than could the University, and that preferably the Education Department should arrange for its supply. Pickerill claimed his own prices were much lower than any the Government could obtain, and wanted the offer 'resisted to the utmost … It is an attempt to usurp the authority and functions of this University and to dictate to myself and the staff of the school here what apparatus, instruments etc we should or should not require'. He regarded the offer as 'the thin end of the wedge for more direct control over University Schools'.[37]

The Executive Council of the Association debated at length the report of the Committee of Enquiry at a meeting in April 1924; Bell and Marsden were present by invitation. The first motion proposed by the Chairman and seconded *pro forma* by Moses, the Secretary, was 'That the New Zealand Dental Association gives its support to the Otago Dental School'. This motion was quickly substituted, on the suggestion of Sherriff, a strong supporter of the School, by 'the Executive … is against the establishment of a second Dental School …'. This provided a much sharper focus, and allowed all issues to be addressed. Rishworth maintained his support for change, and once again was scathing in his views of the School in Dunedin. His amendment, agreeing that Otago should receive adequate support but that other centres 'should not be hampered from taking any course which they deem desirable', was eventually defeated. Pickerill informed the meeting by letter that Auckland students at the School all expressed 'freely and unanimously their preference for studying in Dunedin with its obvious advantages'; that he hoped to have scholarships for such students; that he hoped a fund would be established to be used toward purchase of gold and other precious metals for needy patients; and that it was his intention to establish a Dean's Prize to encourage students to do some, at least, of their mechanical work before coming to the School. Bell and Marsden addressed the meeting, but in committee, and no record of their contributions exists. Moses assured the meeting that although the Auckland Branch of the Association had not supported the proposed Auckland school, individual members promoted the move. He believed a school in Auckland was inevitable, and that the question really was whether it should be established without the Association's support. After further debate, Sherriff's motion was passed. His subsequent motion 'That this meeting … gives to the Otago Dental School its unqualified support. That it beseeches the Government to complete the grant of £38,000, as asked for by the Otago School, so that the building may be erected on the Beverly [King Street] site and suitably equipped' was withdrawn pending discussion at the conference in May: Rishworth, playing for time, had protested such a motion would have forced 'members to go further than they might intend'. Earlier in the proceedings he had acknowledged that the mood of the meeting was clearly to ensure the Otago School was brought up to a high standard; nevertheless he wanted 'the Executive to leave Auckland its freedom to go on with its desires'.[38]

This debate was a landmark in the history of the Association and the School; its outcome was renewed loyalty to the School. By the time of the conference, just a month later, the movement for a new school had died, and the only mention of it occurred when Sherriff, harking back to the very public controversy over school dental nurses, pointed out that 'some members of the Auckland Branch had taken part in the agitation for a dental school there, and it was a question of whether they should not be called upon to express contrition'. By now the Otago School was safe and, sensibly, the matter was dropped.[39]

As preparation for building progressed, the Chancellor sought Pickerill's advice on what might be required as the School developed over the next twenty years. The Dean produced a very thoughtful document, which proved prophetic in many ways. He predicted, on the basis of an increasing population and no change in the level of disease, an eventual need to train fifty students a year; that additions to the new building would become necessary; that a student to staff ratio of 8:1 was desirable for clinical training and 12:1 for mechanical work; that visiting staff, who must be paid for their specialised services, would continue to be needed; that research must be enhanced, necessitating more laboratories and equipment; that increasing numbers of postgraduate students would need increased facilities, but they would enhance the School's reputation; that there was great need for the care of adolescents after they left primary school; that if students, under supervision, were able to examine groups of workers in the city, they would provide a valuable public service by promoting oral health and thus enhance efficiency in the workplace; and that training dental mechanics would supply the profession with well-qualified assistants (he considered girls were most suited to this occupation, presumably because they might be less likely to extend their work into clinical fields than would males). And finally he made a plea for more 'benefaction' for the School, noting that it had no endowments for research or the library. He concluded:

> When the new School is built, fully equipped and staffed according to our recommendations, it will be without doubt the best Dental School in the Southern Hemisphere … With an efficient building and sufficient accommodation, equipment for research, and an enthusiastic staff, it is hoped to make the Dental school of the Otago University … the Mecca of Dentistry in the South.[40]

Building soon commenced, and the departing Governor-General, Lord Jellicoe, laid the foundation stone on 18 October 1924. It was a grand occasion, Jellicoe in his uniform of Admiral of the Fleet, and a Boy Scout guard of honour. Dental and medical students were present in force and enlivened proceedings with interjections. A casket containing historical Dental School items was laid beneath the foundation stone, and the Chancellor, the Governor-General, and Pickerill addressed the gathering. In his positive and distinguished speech, Pickerill mentioned that, despite visions of laying a foundation stone being so ephemeral that they thought it may never come, they were now 'reasonably certain' they would have a new school:

> Any school must, if it is to reach its fullest usefulness and success, have both traditions and ideals. We are young yet to have traditions, but during the last few years the dental faculty has been laying down … satisfactory traditions which will become more fixed and venerated with the passing years. We have three ideals of service. The first and most obvious is: we wish to serve New Zealand by providing courses and training for students which they in after years can look back upon and say 'It was second to none.' Secondly, we wish to serve Dunedin by providing a dental service within the reach of the poorest, and our ambition is to make Dunedin the most dentally fit city in the Dominion … Our third ideal is to carry on, extend, and develop the research work we have already done in the old building.

After suggesting that the design of the building might have been copied from the new School of Biochemistry at Cambridge University, he quoted from the Earl of Balfour's speech at that building's opening:

> How many are there who realise that the best way to serve mankind is so to master the secrets of Nature, that Nature turns her forces to our benefit instead of, as too often happens, turning them to our destruction?' It is along such lines as these that we hope to develop the school and make it worthy of our University and worthy of New Zealand.[41]

Wisely, he ignored all the rancour and bitterness that had marked events to this stage, and concentrated on what the future would bring.

The *Journal* enthusiastically greeted the event by reviewing the Association's role in founding the school. It praised the great organising ability of its 'young, charming, and enthusiastic' Director, the generous help of the ten honorary dental surgeons who supported him, and the crucial role of Sidey.[42] The Executive of the Association was now based in Wellington, away from the Auckland influence, and Richmond Dunn had taken over as Editor. Criticism of the School and of its Director seemed now to be in the past.

But the School still had to be completed, and frustration continued in Dunedin. The students vented their concerns over progress in a deputation to the Council in November 1925.[43] They wanted the School ready for the opening session the following year, and Pickerill was asked to report on the students' complaints that some equipment was obsolete and worn out. This was a classic buck-passing and delaying move; he had been making the same complaint to the Council for years.

The building was not ready until June 1926; the *Journal* gave a glowing description of it and its many amenities,[44] and Sidey, now Chancellor, presided at the official opening on 11 June. At what must have been for him personally a very moving occasion, he traced the development of dental education in New

Zealand, acknowledging generously the contributions of the Association and individual members, and the politicians who had played important roles. He was generous in praise of Pickerill: 'It was not too much to say that through the work of Professor Pickerill the Dental School of the University of Otago was known all over the world'. He urged the Government to increase funding for research. The recently appointed Minister of Education, the Honourable R.A. Wright, opened the building and described it as the 'finest and best equipped in the Southern Hemisphere'. He too acknowledged the contributions of the Association, including its support of the School Dental Service.

K.C. Morpeth, Chairman of the Association's Executive Council, took the opportunity to criticise the previous Minister of Public Health and 'those associated with him in their efforts to bastardize our profession and jeopardise the Public Health by the passage of a bill through Parliament to place on the Dental Register of N.Z. those who have not been efficiently trained, as we understand the word "trained" in the dental profession'.[45] Here he was referring to the failed 1924 Bill aimed at yet again prolonging 'back-door' entry into the profession, and yet another current and this time successful effort to amend the Dentists Act.[46] Having got that out of the way, he went on to proclaim the need to keep equipment up to date, to promise the students the support of the Association, to praise Sidey as the 'Father of Dentistry in New Zealand', and to assure the Minister of the Association's cooperation.

Pickerill prefaced his fine address by saying that his feelings were 'chiefly of praise and thankfulness that they at last found themselves in "the Promised Land". They really ought to have begun by singing the "Te Deum Laudamus" or the "Jubilate" or the "Hallelujah Chorus" or the "Old Hundred"'. He expressed deep gratitude to Sidey for his personal gift of £1,000 for research and for the purchase of gold and precious metals for the treatment of the indigent; he also thanked supply companies for their donations. He stressed that the School was a national institution. He believed it was not too big, as some had apparently claimed, and that its sixty-chair clinic was essential. He then stressed prevention as the only solution to the country's dental problems, pointing to indifference and expense as the reasons why simple preventive measures were not universally introduced. The day concluded with the Dental Students' Association hosting an 'elaborate' dinner.[47]

The victory had been won. Auckland's attempted coup had been repelled; somehow, despite the appalling conditions in the old building, dental education had survived and prospered in Dunedin; the Government's indifference and even opposition had been overcome. Pickerill now had a modern, spacious school. With one major extension and minor alterations, it was to service the profession for the next thirty-five years until it, too, was grossly overcrowded and inefficient. Then John Patrick (later Sir John) Walsh, another young, brash, and energetic Dean, also appointed from overseas, had the task of battling many of the same odds to achieve the University's third Dental School, next door on Great King Street.

16

Resignation

On 11 February 1927, just seven months after the new School opened, Pickerill informed the Chancellor that he was considering resignation in order 'to seek new challenges'.[1] The reasons he gave included a need for additional income: the children were growing up, as John Percival (Val) was now aged nineteen, Thomas Peverel Tuakana (Kana), was seventeen, Kathleen Marguerite (Kay), was sixteen, and Ethelbert Paul, fourteen; in addition, his position within the University would have brought social obligations and entertainment in the family's substantial home in Ravensbourne.

It seems that Pickerill was not offered any incentive to stay, for on 4 March he informed the Chancellor that, with great regret, he did intend to resign. For twenty years, he said, the progress and the welfare of the School had 'occupied first place'. He had found the work intensely interesting 'largely, perhaps, because it has been so much uphill …'. But now he believed a plateau had been reached, and everything should now be easier – there was a fine new building, sufficient students, excellent equipment, and the course continued to be recognised in Britain. He had great affection for the School and would be sad to leave it. In the past, he told the Chancellor, he had declined appointments in London and Sydney, but now he felt that family demands meant he should move to private practice.[2] The formal resignation, to take effect on 31 July 1927, was received with regret at the meeting of the Council on 15 March, at which appreciation of his services and recognition of his work as a facial surgeon were recorded, along with 'the outstanding success which he has attained in the ordinary work of the Dental School, as Professor and Director'.[3]

The Association was soon to be involved in the appointment of his successor. It still, with some justification given its crucial role in the School's foundation, regarded the School as its own, despite some influential members wanting to move it to Auckland. It watched the School with intense parental interest, as illustrated in August 1926 when it protested to the Registrar on two matters. It had previously been upset that Bell had been appointed without what the Association considered adequate advertisement. Now three associate professors had been appointed 'in direct contravention of the proper precedent of publicly advertising any vacancy, established when the late Professor Bell was appointed'. The second matter was directed at Pickerill's right of limited private consulting. The Executive resolved: 'That this Executive, representing the whole of the New Zealand Dental Association, is strongly of opinion that the size of importance of the Dental School necessitates the undivided attention of all Professors, and urges that it is not only against the interests of the School, but inimical to the interests of the Students, that Professors should be allowed to undertake part time outside work'.[4] This very public criticism would have hurt Pickerill deeply, perhaps even sown the seeds of his decision to resign.

It has not been unusual for the Council to consult the Association on the important matter of a new Dean; indeed, Dr Steven Simmons, when President of the Association in 2005, was involved in the appointment process for the current Dean, Professor Gregory Seymour. But it seems remarkably hasty for the Council, on 3 March 1927, to seek the Association's advice just two days after the formal resignation was received, and before it had even been placed before the Council.[5] The Executive was naturally pleased to inform the Registrar it had discussed the position fully, and 'appreciated the opportunity of assisting in the further advancement of the School'.

The Executive wrote to all the branch representatives on the Executive Council requesting their reaction to forming an investigative committee to make suggestions for reorganising the staffing of the school. This idea was dropped; as Davies pointed out, although the Association carried considerable weight with the University, a formal 'inquiry' would have gone too far. The Executive confirmed its belief that running the school had to be a full-time position. It also initially believed a 'good man' could not be attracted by a salary less than £1,100, and discussed the possibility of contributing £25 or £50 that would attract a government subsidy. Finally, however, the Executive recommended the salary be set at £1,000 as 'times had changed since last year [a major drop in farm export prices had occurred the previous year, and the economy was entering a period of deterioration[6]] and it might be quite possible to get a good man at £1,000, with the prospect of an increase later.[7]

The Editor of the *Journal* was also quick to have his say about the forthcoming appointment. He expressed surprise and regret at the resignation, and thought that:

> after the struggling years … the Professor would have settled down contentedly to put into practice many of the dreams of his enthusiastic years. But things often happen otherwise after strenuous times, and we find our Professor softly sighing his *Nunc Dimitis*, and leaving the new work to others with keen energy and fresh enthusiasm undamped by the difficult years.

The implication, even if unintended, that Pickerill was lacking energy, was a gross insult to a man who had shown incredible industry and vigour throughout his term as Dean. The Editor advised caution in appointing a successor, and called for an adequate salary that would 'be sufficient to tempt a first-class man to relinquish the emoluments of private practice in order to devote his whole energy and attention to the welfare of the school'. The Editor saw it as an indignity that the professor should have to supplement his salary in this way, and it must not be allowed to continue. He then went on to advocate that the appointee should not be both dentally and medically qualified, on the grounds that too much 'theoretical training' meant that:

> at present, a man entering the profession 'by the back door', passing a minimum examination in theory, but well up in practical dental mechanics and metallurgy, stands a much better chance of, say, obtaining a partnership than does a mere graduate of a dental school. This is not as things should be, but the graduate … should leave his university so well equipped that the older established practitioners of the Dominion should be tumbling over one another in their anxiety to compete for his services. We feel that an experienced dentist at the head of the Dental School would do very much towards the consummation of this ideal … No doubt other points will arise, mistakes of the past can be remedied in the light of new experience, and we hope that, even if the professorship has to remain in abeyance for some time, until a fixed policy has been well matured, the Council will duly consider the two points we have made it our business to emphasise … We have no doubt they will be well advised, and that they will not allow high academical qualifications to obscure their view of practical worth and personality.[8]

These condescending words betrayed the efforts made over the life of the School to raise dentistry above the status of being simply a mechanical exercise. It was also a further insult to Pickerill, which did not pass unnoticed by readers. H.E. Suckling chastised the Editor in a letter that was not published, on the feeble grounds that it had arrived too late for the May issue (no mention of the July issue in which it could have appeared) and that, by the September issue, sufficient time had elapsed for the healing of any 'lacerated feelings, and that no useful purpose could be served by reopening the subject'. Nevertheless the Editor acknowledged that no slur was intended, and that the remarks were 'a genuine attempt by the writer to help … by calling attention to a possible weakness in the present educational system that, as he had gathered from many sources, tended to put the newly graduated student at a disadvantage in competing with those whom legislation in recent years has enabled to enter, by a short cut, the ranks of commercial dentistry'.[9] One doubts that the feelings of either Suckling or Pickerill were mollified by this defensive response.

A month before his resignation took effect, Pickerill wrote to the Registrar in terms suggesting he was dismayed at the salary being offered to attract a suitable successor. He thought his advice would have been helpful in drawing up the new conditions of appointment, especially as 'I have given the best part of my life to the development of our Dental School and … it is now favourably known throughout the world …'. He believed an 'adequate man' could be obtained for much less than the starting level of £1,000 being offered. 'My successor is not likely to have anything like the hard work I have had and the Council has had these services for the past 20 years for an average of less than £700 p.a.'[10] Although this reaction is far from uncommon – many people retiring or resigning have felt they have been short-changed when they learn of the salary and conditions being offered to their replacements – Pickerill obviously took the matter very personally.

He introduced in that letter two other matters that had troubled him for some time. The first was the right of limited private consulting practice. He believed it important for teachers of clinical subjects to be 'kept keen' and up to date, and this could only be done by 'competitive association' with the outside world. He felt, appropriately so, that the exclusion of this right from the conditions of employment was 'a sad blow for the prestige and future of the Dental School'. He had received many referrals from medical and dental practitioners and he had been forced to defend himself in 1915 and again in 1922 against serious accusations that he was engaged in extensive private work.[11] He wanted his successor to enjoy the privilege he had been granted and to be free to accept referrals without having to face the suspicions he himself had endured.

The second matter was a warning against the influence of the Association on the policies and activities of the School. His warning was ill tempered but, in his defence, he had endured much innuendo and insult that provoked a series of real and imagined complaints. He felt it was his duty to inform the Council that the influence of the Association, though outwardly favourable, 'has always been secretly antagonistic to the best interests of the Dental School'. He went on: 'It was not until I decided to cut myself completely adrift from this body that the School became really successful numerically, and it will be found, I suggest, that in proportion as this Association gains any control, so will the number of students drop'. In this he ignored the success of Davies in increasing the number of students, and he had no grounds for the latter prophecy. He concluded by stating that it had been said at a meeting of the Association that: 'The aims and objects of the Dental School are so diametrically opposed to those of the Association that the head of the one can never be the head of the other'. On the face of it, this signifies a deep antagonism between the School and the Association, but in practice, and even if relations were entirely amicable, serious conflicts of interest would arise if one person had both responsibilities; the situation would be most unlikely ever to be considered. Members of the staff of the School have been presidents of the Association, but the presidency remained, until 1989, a non-executive position, and the real power rested in the office of Chairman of the Executive Council. Staff members have edited the *Journal*, but occasions when they diverged from the policies of the Association have been rare. Pickerill's advice to the University Council, although understandable, was exaggerated.

Pickerill received numerous compliments as the date of leaving approached. The Professorial Board expressed its appreciation of his work, noted his international record that had brought distinction to the School and University, and acknowledged his endurance of the 'serious disability of inadequate accommodation'. The Board felt he had the gratification of having procured a new building, but 'By his going the University is deprived of an able organiser and administrator'.[12] The students received the news of the resignation of 'the father of the Faculty' with great regret: 'We students will always remember his optimism and ready encouragement; the loss is not ours alone but that of the whole of New Zealand'.[13] J.L. Saunders described him as 'a first-class teacher and a fluent lecturer. He had a natural gift for reducing problems to their simplest forms and elucidating them in an interesting way that could be readily understood'. The distinguished graduate Dr Basil Bibby recalled:

> I remember Doctor Pickerill as a well groomed alert individual, with a quiet military type of carriage. He was easily approachable and friendly, but undoubtedly a disciplinarian although this was seldom shown … There is no question that his example had a good influence upon many of us, and he has made a lasting contribution in setting the tone of dental education in New Zealand.[14]

The Faculty recorded its appreciation 'of the valuable services Dr. Pickerill has rendered the University and the community as Professor, as Dean of the Faculty and as Director of the Dental School – and expresses its hope that he will meet with great success in his new sphere of work'.[15] In his response, Pickerill explained the history of a picture in the library, described as 'possibly a Hogarth', and the chair he had presented to the School as the Dean's Chair, a replica of that used by the Venerable Bede. (It is currently in the School's Staff Common Room.) His colleagues at the Medical School presented him with a superb silver tray.

Pickerill's resignation as Surgeon in Charge of the Facial and Jaw Department was accepted at a meeting of the Hospital Board on 29 July. The Chairman commented that Dr Pickerill:

> had continued a valued member of the honorary medical staff for 19 years without break as honorary dental surgeon, honorary stomatologist and honorary surgeon in charge of the facial and jaw department. The brilliant plastic surgery work carried out by Dr Pickerill during the Great War, and continued since in Dunedin, would be gratefully remembered by those who had been assisted, and the new Dental School recently erected and opened stood for all time as a monument to Dr Pickerill's energy … Dr Pickerill would be missed sadly not only in Dunedin, but throughout New Zealand …[16]

In a sad commentary on the state of plastic surgery at that time, yet a compliment to Pickerill's pioneering but lonely status, the Medical Superintendent added that as no surgeon had taken up this department of surgery, he did not consider there was any necessity to appoint anyone to fill the vacancy. New Zealand had, for the time being, lost its only plastic surgeon.

That same evening Pickerill was guest of honour at a meeting of the Officers' Club, where once again many fine tributes were made, and he lectured on 'Work in a Facial and Jaw Hospital During the War'. He hoped he would 'be fortunate to find as staunch fellows in Sydney'. He was presented with an inscribed silver cigarette case.

The University Council presented him with an illuminated address at a farewell function on 9 August. The Vice-Chancellor, W.J. Morrell, praised Pickerill's contributions:

> it was a great wrench to lose services which had extended over a period of over 20 years. No one could feel more deeply than the council the debt that the University owed to Dr Pickerill, and he [Morrell] knew that opinion was shared by every dental student … he had brought a great deal of lustre to the school, as he was known not only all over the Dominion, but throughout the world … His ability as a surgeon in peace and war was well known … the school would scarcely seem itself without the doctor, and the council regretted very much that he had found it in his own interests to remove his sphere of activities to the other side of the Tasman.[17]

In his reply Pickerill expressed his regret that such an occasion was necessary, and that his long association with the University 'made him feel that it was part of his being'. He concluded his acknowledgement with the wistful comment that entry to the profession still had not been restricted to a 'single portal'.

He lectured to senior students and the whole Faculty on 'Plastic surgery in peace and war' at a function hosted by the students on 9 August. 'All felt privileged that they were able to catch a glimpse of what our Dean had done during the war and in civilian practice'. The staff and other members of the Faculty met the following day, when Associate Professor Dodds, now the Acting Dean, presented Dr and Mrs Pickerill each with a silver-mounted dressing case. That evening the dental and medical students combined to give Dr Pickerill a farewell dinner.[18]

The date Pickerill left Dunedin for Sydney is uncertain, but he was there in November 1927. The University council would have been surprised to receive at its meeting on 29 November a message from him stating that Sydney was not suiting him, and that, if it were not too late to apply for his old position, he would reimburse the expenses of his resignation and abide by the new conditions. The Council resolved not to make an appointment from the present applicants in the meantime, and to ask the University of New Zealand to approve Pickerill as an applicant. It also asked him to cable a formal application immediately, and said he would probably be required to contribute to the Superannuation Fund.[19] His immediate response was to enquire how much that would cost for a man of forty-six years – in view of his previous financial concerns, he would want to ensure he would not be further disadvantaged by a net reduction in salary. The University of New Zealand agreed his application could be considered, but in his telegram to the Registrar on 5 December he thanked the Council 'sincerely for [its] very kind consideration but have regretfully decided not to apply'.[20]

He now established himself in Sydney in private and hospital practice as a plastic surgeon. He had gone to Sydney without Mrs Pickerill and the children, the intention being for them to join him at a later date. One who did travel to Sydney was, however, Cecily Mary Wise Clarkson, who had graduated MB, ChB just the previous year.

The selection process went ahead without the complication of having the former Dean as a candidate. The outcome, to the delight of the Association,[21] was that Robert Bevan Dodds, BDS (1916), DDS (1924) was appointed to the position. The Pickerill era at the School had now ended.

17

Plastic surgeon in Sydney

Pickerill's move to Sydney in 1927 resulted in two life-changing events. Firstly, after abandoning his academic connections, he became a full-time specialist in plastic surgery. Although he was acknowledged nationally in New Zealand for his expertise in the discipline, and also in maxillofacial surgery, surgery had formed a relatively small part of his duties in Dunedin. In Sydney, however, the distractions of heading a dental school and the turmoil he faced in the post-war years were behind him; he could now devote his energies and skills to the challenge of building his reputation as a surgeon in a much larger environment. He became the pioneer in Australia, as well as in New Zealand, in what was to become a major surgical specialty. (His former colleague at Sidcup, Sir Henry Newland, had returned to Adelaide after the war, but did not confine his work to plastic surgery.[1])

The second life-changing event in Sydney was the arrival of his former Dunedin house surgeon, Cecily Clarkson. Born in Taihape on 9 February 1903, she was the daughter of the town's first Anglican vicar. Educated at the Taihape Public School and the Diocesan School for Girls in Auckland, she graduated MB, ChB from Otago in 1925. The following year she was Pickerill's house surgeon, and early in 1927 she sought a residency in Los Angeles: her father at that time was vicar of an Episcopal church in Laguna Beach,[2] but he then established a congregation of the obscure American Catholic Church in the same community. Pickerill wrote in a reference for her: 'I have been impressed with her keenness, ability and efficiency. She is the best house surgeon I have had for many years'.[3] She also had glowing references from Hercus, then Sub-dean of the Faculty of Medicine, and from the Medical Superintendent of Dunedin Hospital.[4] Whether she went to California for a period is not known, but she did move to Sydney to study plastic surgery under its leading exponent. She in effect became Pickerill's apprentice, learning all her surgical skills as his assistant, and later his associate. She was to become widely recognised as a skilled surgeon in her own right, but her lack of higher surgical qualifications was probably a barrier to full acceptance in the medical profession. She was, however, to be acknowledged publicly by becoming New Zealand's first medical Dame – she became a Dame of the British Empire in 1977. Daughter Margaret Frazer believes Cecily initially acted as secretary and nurse to Pickerill, but an undated card shows both Dr H.P. Pickerill and Dr C.M. Clarkson as 'Plastic Surgeons'. They eventually purchased and developed a property at Narabeen, which they named Caradoc.

Her move to Sydney to be the associate of Pickerill no doubt raised questioning eyebrows amongst his colleagues and friends back in Dunedin; family sources confirm it caused great anguish for Mabel Pickerill and the children. No correspondence between Pickerill and Mabel has been traced, but it would have been surprising if Mabel and the children had not anticipated joining him after he was settled in Sydney. Pickerill's former students certainly expected this to happen, for they presented Mabel with a handsome engraved leather suitcase on his retirement. Whatever were the reasons, the family stayed in Dunedin, and it was Pickerill who petitioned for divorce in 1931, on the grounds of having been 'wilfully deserted' for 'three years and upwards'. This was a cruel denunciation of Mabel who, family sources suggest, was a loyal and devoted wife and mother. Grandchildren still express deep resentment against Cecily for her perceived role in the break-up, although Pickerill himself could hardly have been blameless. *Decree nisi* was granted on 4 May 1934, and made absolute on 20 November 1934. Cecily and Percy were married at Enfield, New South Wales, on 17 December 1934. The witnesses were Constance Ross and Gertie Killworth, the latter was presumably the wife or relative of the officiating minister, Arthur Killworth, suggesting this was a small and private ceremony. He was fifty-five, Cecily thirty-one.

What preparations Pickerill made for his arrival in Sydney is unclear, but his brief flirtation with returning to Dunedin suggests he faced some initial problems. Various notes, including reminiscences by Cecily,[5] state that he went directly to an appointment at the Royal North Shore Hospital, but this could not be confirmed. It is likely, however, that he had operating privileges before a formal position was established at that hospital in 1934.[6] He is also believed to have operated during his early years in Sydney at the St Luke's Hospital,[7] a private hospital established by the Anglican Church in

1919,[8] but this also could not be confirmed from hospital archives. He did, however, obtain consulting rooms at 193 Macquarie Street, and from there he announced his arrival to the medical and dental professions.

He was fully aware of the importance of establishing contacts with future colleagues on arriving in this new location, particularly with those likely to initiate referrals. Early in October 1927, just a few weeks after his arrival in Sydney, Pickerill presented a paper to the Dental Association of New South Wales on the subject 'The complications and sequelae [*sic*] of the extraction of teeth and their treatment'.[9] Although he spoke ably on the topic, unfortunately, or perhaps fortunately, his slides were back in Dunedin; but he did have slides on other topics: 'illustrating the surgical work in which he had been engaged during the late war and afterwards. These showed what was possible in the way of restorative surgery'. The published photographs showed dramatically a sample of the scope of his practice: reconstruction of upper and lower lips following war injury; restoration of the noses of a man and a woman, one following trauma, the other following infection; treatment of ankylosis (fusion) of the mandibular joint; treatment of an infant with cleft lip and palate; and grafting of muscles to alleviate the effects of facial paralysis. It was a lecture that must have engrossed his audience by vividly illustrating the skills of this new arrival in the city.

Another step he took to publicise his arrival was to send a note, probably to a range of medical and dental professionals, saying 'how pleased I should be if I can be of any assistance to you in the treatment of any of your cases in which my experience may be of value? As my specialty is not a usual one I should like to indicate the kind of case in which I may be of service …'.[10] Then followed a list of oral and facial conditions that would undoubtedly attract attention, including 'All tumours, ulcers, cysts, deformities and disfigurement of the face, mouth, jaws and nose (external) – treatment by endothermy and plastic reconstruction'. He thus announced his arrival in a very professional manner. Possibly the outcome of this announcement confirmed that he did indeed have a future in Sydney.

A wide-ranging article written in emotional language, which was published in the *Sydney Guardian* in 1930, gave him a great deal of publicity.[11] Although his name was only mentioned in a quote from a New Zealand newspaper, Pickerill was undoubtedly one of the two Sydney surgeons praised. (The other was a Dr Max Herz.) Although somewhat light-hearted in considering the possibilities of plastic surgeons changing the faces of 'crooks' and other 'wanted underworlders', it outlined some of the ways people's appearance, and lives, can be transformed by plastic surgery. It quoted a New Zealand newspaper as stating: 'His loss to surgery, medicine, and the whole of New

Zealand is irreparable, for Sydney will now claim probably the greatest plastic surgeon in the world'. His reputation in Sydney would appear to be firmly established, although the tone of the article may well have caused concern to him, and to the medical establishment, in view of its advertising potential.

The position of honorary plastic surgeon at the Royal North Shore Hospital was established in 1934, the first such post in Australasia. Pickerill was appointed to this position later in the year. He resigned it in 1936, but by then he had returned to New Zealand. B.K. Rank, a prominent Australian plastic surgeon, later wrote: 'The restricted opportunities then presenting among the small population in New Zealand he [Pickerill] augmented by periodic visits to Sydney, where he had a regular clientele'.[12] It therefore appears he commuted several times a year from Wellington to Sydney during 1935 and until his retirement from the Royal North Shore Hospital.

In contrast to his extensive correspondence and other writings, and the copious other material documenting his career up to this point, information on the Sydney period is sparse. He appears to have held no positions of responsibility in professional organisations. This was a time of consolidation of his skills and his reputation, but not a time marked by spectacular achievements or controversy. He was, however, productive in writing, and he had a number of articles published in journals in Australia and overseas, as listed by Schmid,[13] the Swiss doctoral candidate, who focused chiefly on Pickerill's caries research. These publications included reports on the repair of facial lesions, the treatment of tic douloureux (trigeminal neuralgia, a very painful disorder of the fifth cranial nerve) by injection of alcohol, treatment of deformities of the genitalia, repair of clefts of the lip and palate, grafting of muscle to overcome facial paralysis, management of impacted wisdom teeth, repair to defects of the skull, restoration of the buccal sulcus by skin grafting and the preparation of the mouth for dentures, and repair of defects of the larynx. No doubt also he was in demand for the treatment of victims of trauma to the face and jaws, restoration following the excision of tumours, and general maxillofacial surgery. Presumably Cecily became increasingly involved as his surgical assistant and associate plastic surgeon.

What brought him to return to New Zealand is not known, but a need for more involvement with his children may have been a major factor. Accompanied by his new wife, he returned shortly after their marriage.

18

Wellington, Bassam, and Middlemore

The Pickerills settled in Wellington in 1938, and set up as specialist plastic surgeons, with consulting rooms in Kelvin Chambers on The Terrace. They treated their private patients at the Lewisham Hospital in Newtown, which later became the Calvary Hospital and is now Wakefield Hospital. They also operated, between 1941 and 1951, on a small number of patients, mostly with cleft lips and palates, at the Home of Compassion, Island Bay.[1]

Wellington Hospital

Both Pickerills held appointments at Wellington Hospital, but the exact dates of these appointments could not be determined from hospital archives. Pickerill held the position of Senior Plastic Surgeon, probably until 1945, but the date when this position was created could not be found. The Photographic Negative Register records that Pickerill operated there between 1942 and 1946.[2] A 1948 publication shows him as 'Consulting Plastic Surgeon' at the Hospital, and it is likely that, although no longer operating, he retained that title after his resignation as Senior Plastic Surgeon.[3] Cecily also held positions at Wellington Hospital. She had a part-time appointment between 1940 and 1942, and in 1943 had the title of Part-time Assistant Plastic Surgeon. She was appointed Senior Plastic Surgeon for a period in 1946, after a year as Acting Senior Plastic Surgeon.[4] Mr Frank Hutter became Senior Plastic Surgeon in 1947. In one of those regrettable failures to acknowledge Pickerill, Hutter has been credited with founding the Plastic Surgical Unit at Wellington Hospital,[5] overlooking the fact that Pickerill had been Senior Plastic Surgeon for some years previously.

The operations recorded in the Photographic Register cover a range of conditions, including skin grafts for burns and trauma, cleft lip, various tumours, jaw abnormalities, excision of scar tissue, and syndactyly (fusion of digits). His publications following his return from Sydney include articles published in overseas journals such as *The Lancet*, *The British Journal of Surgery*, *British Medical Journal*, and *British Journal of Plastic Surgery*. He also published in the *New Zealand Dental Journal*, the *New Zealand Medical Journal*, and *The Australian and New Zealand Journal of Surgery*.[6] Themes included plastic surgery following burns and malignancy, the importance of early treatment of cleft lip and palate, repair of defects of the skull by means of autogenous bone grafts, and surgery to improve appearance in children with congenital facial defects. The Pickerills also jointly produced several issues of the *Bulletin of Plastic Surgery.*

Pickerill's Wellington period is now best remembered for his work at Bassam, the private hospital he founded with Cecily specifically for plastic surgery for infants.

Bassam

Pickerill's belief that successful plastic surgery depended on the prevention of infection in the surgical area grew out of his wartime experiences. Cross infection – the spread of infection between patients and staff – remains a major concern in hospitals. In plastic surgery, especially in highly vulnerable infants with cleft lips and palates, it had to be avoided at all costs: results could be disastrous if the repair failed. Pickerill first described how cross infection might be prevented in one of his earliest papers on the repair of clefts: the infant given over to him many years earlier by Batchelor, the Dunedin surgeon who thought the child had no hope of survival.[7] Pickerill wanted the baby to be gaining weight before surgery, but the intensive care necessary for this to be achieved could not be provided in a busy hospital ward, where cross infection was endemic. The solution was obvious to Pickerill: the mother was the only person who could devote the time and loving care necessary to reverse the decline. Years later, he recalled this experience in a pamphlet on mothers nursing their babies in hospital. He arranged accommodation for the mother and baby in a 'nice, clean, sunny room, with fortunately a kind landlady who did everything possible for her, and there she nursed her baby so well that each operation went smoothly without setback or infection, and the baby continued to gain weight throughout'.[8] Keeping children out of the usual hospital environment became an overriding principle of his work.

The Pickerills' ambition was to have their own small, private hospital where mothers would do all the nursing. Pickerill discussed the establishment of such a clinic with the then Minister of Health, the Honourable Arnold Nordmeyer, early in 1941. The Minister was interested, and wanted information on how many babies they could take at a time, and how many they could treat in a year.[9] He also asked if the Pickerills would consider full-time salaried appointments, and what salaries they would expect. The Pickerills would be under no obligation, but this would be an option he could take to Cabinet. Full-time appointments would have meant no right of private practice.

This must have brought a testy response, for the Minister regretted that, although he saw nothing in his letter that justified the Pickerills' fears, the terms of his letter 'have apparently been so misunderstood'; he simply needed something in writing to take to the Cabinet, but he also wanted them to consider working on a wider basis than confining their work to infants. He told them that, even if they rejected the salaried suggestion, he still wanted details on the clinic proposal.

Their suggestions received support, and they achieved their goal. Bassam (named after Bassam Common, near Hereford) was a spacious bungalow situated in the pleasant Bloomfield Terrace in Lower Hutt, near Wellington. Initially it acted as a hostel for babies and their mothers, and operations took place at the Lewisham or Wellington Hospitals. The building was subsequently modified to include operating facilities, a new bedroom wing was added, and it became a self-contained hospital. By 1947, the Bassam building had eight bedrooms, and a further four bedrooms were at Audley Lodge, nearby at 183 Waterloo Road. Each infant and mother had a private room where the mother looked after her baby just as she would at home: preparing the baby's food, bathing, changing napkins, and feeding, which could be a long and tedious process for the infant with cleft lip and palate. Mothers carried out these essential duties in a much more relaxed and efficient way than could nurses in busy wards and, most importantly, without risk of infection being spread between patients via nursing staff.

The other major advantage of mother-nursing was maintenance and enhancement of the mother-child bond, frequently mentioned in the publications arising from the Bassam experience, and a topic of international interest in the early 1950s.[10] During the day, weather permitting, mothers could take their babies into the attractive gardens, and at night attend immediately to any need arising, be it feeding, changing, comforting, or adjusting dressings. Except when the infant was undergoing surgery, no person other than the mother had physical contact with the child. Dressings were changed under light general anaesthesia. The aim was to 'insulate' the mother and child from infection by foreign or other people's bacteria.

Staff at Bassam consisted of a full-time theatre sister, two live-in part-time registered nurses, two non-live-in part-time nurses, a manageress, and two domestics, one being full-time. Although a private hospital, it was sanctioned and supported by the Department of Health. Hospital benefits of nine shillings a day were available, but operating costs in private hospitals could not be met at this time from the Social Security Fund. In 1944, the Hospital Benefits for Out-patients Regulations were amended, with specific provision for children with cleft lip and palate. The amended regulations allowed such children to be operated on by specialists 'in specially-equipped private hospitals and under conditions which could not be readily duplicated in many public hospitals'.[11] The Minister of Health was thus convinced of the value of the Pickerills' methods. Subsidies from the Crippled Children's Society were also available for some children.

Bassam functioned during the 1940s virtually as the national centre for babies with clefts and other serious congenital conditions requiring plastic surgery.[12] The Pickerills held contracts with most of the hospital boards in the country; Canterbury, Otago, and Southland were the only regions with boards that did not have contracts. The standard contract covered 'all cases referred by the board where the age of the child is such that it needs to be accompanied by its mother, and where treatment at the hostel is desirable'. Each board's medical superintendent was required to assess the severity of the deformity before referral. The contracts stated that all such cases in the boards' areas were to be referred; they could not be admitted to other institutions. In 1946, the Pickerills were paid twelve and a half guineas per operation, and the boards were responsible also for anaesthetic, theatre, and 'chemists' accounts where necessary'. The Pickerills had to submit to the referring board the number of operations required for each child, and could not charge for any operations that exceeded this estimate. After completion of treatment, patients were referred back to the referring hospitals. Financial records show that in the two years from 1 March 1948, hospital boards or the Crippled Children's Society were billed for 208 patients, and accounts were sent to the parents or guardians of 112 children treated privately.

A brief report of the results at Bassam after eight years showed a 0.3 per cent post-operative mortality for all infants having plastic surgery, much lower than that reported overseas (1.4–3.4 per cent).[13] No instances of cross infection, failures of surgery, or post-operative shock had occurred. Children with the full range of disabilities were treated, and no patients needing surgery had been turned away; the Pickerills accepted any child in need. The system was highly successful. But the Pickerills also had great success at Wellington, operating at either the Wellington or Lewisham Hospitals before Bassam was fully established. Commenting on Cecily's report of seventy consecutive cleft-palete patients, Pickerill noted:

> all have been completely successful – no mortality, no sloughing, no non-union, and no operation has had to be 'repeated'. This is a unique record and thus I hope will be opened up a new era in cleft palate surgery by the hostel system of nursing.[14]

This was in stark, but unverifiable contrast with the situation before they, as specialists in the field, were appointed to Wellington Hospital; his handwritten footnote on a copy of the above-quoted paper stated: 'In 3 years prior to our taking over, 92% of cleft palate cases failed in Wellington Hospital, and this was regarded as inevitable!'

Their claim of success is well justified. Photographs taken before and after surgery reveal remarkable transformations,[15] although more modern methods, as were developed in units such as Middlemore, improved even further on their results. Testimonies to their skills can be seen in the many letters of gratitude from their patients' parents, and reports in newspapers and magazines.

After mother and child were discharged and before the next pair were admitted, the room they had occupied was thoroughly aired and spring-cleaned. Annually the hospital was cleared of all patients, staff had their holidays, and opportunity taken for repainting, ventilating, and repairs, and the interior was sprayed with DDT, all with the aim of breaking up any chain of infection. After eleven years' experience at Bassam, there was still not a single instance of cross infection:

> Because we have no cross-infection and because of the general buoyancy of our infants, our over-all mortality-rate for the past eleven years averages 0.3% (including 1 anaesthetic death only). Because operation wounds remain uninfected (though we use a minimum of antiseptics and antibiotics) primary union is the rule. This means a great saving of time, work, and *number of nurses*, as well as vastly less worry for the surgeon. Infants remain in hospital for a shorter time per operation ...[16]

'These babies want mothering more than expert nursing', wrote Pickerill in 1947.[17] 'With their mothers, they are happier, more contented, and are able to have more constant attention day and night, and an operation for a contented baby is much more likely to be successful'. Although not the only advocates of mother-nursing at the time, their approach attracted international attention; a leading article in *The Lancet* praised the Bassam procedures, noting that the Pickerills rarely needed to use pre- or postoperative sedation – 'the best sedative for any baby is the mother'.[18] The birth of a baby with severe facial deformity comes as a great shock to its parents. Involvement of the mother in every step of rehabilitation, seeing the improvement occurring at each surgical stage, and contributing vitally to the whole procedure through day-to-day nursing and care, provided mothers with a priceless investment in their infants' well being, and gave them hope for the future: a mother's child was not to be maimed for life. This was reinforced through socialising with other mothers facing similar difficulties; the mutual support gave the mothers encouragement and comfort, not least by seeing progress in other babies. Although mainly children with cleft lips and palates were treated at Bassam, children with other problems – for example, burns, syndactyly, and children with abnormal genitalia – were also treated.

Initially the surgery was shared between the Pickerills, but Percy developed sensitivity to ether, and Cecily became primarily responsible. He continued overall supervision until shortly before his death in 1956. Bassam continued for a further eleven years under Cecily's full control. For her distinguished services, she was awarded the Order of the British Empire in 1958, and in 1977 was created Dame of the British Empire. In addition to this public recognition, she received many grateful acknowledgements from former patients and their parents. Although these were well deserved, Pickerill family members have reminded the writer that primary recognition must go to Percy; she herself acknowledged that she learnt everything from him: he was her teacher and guide until his death. It is not possible to say whether the surgical outcomes achieved by one were better than those achieved by the other. Cecily attended some conferences in the United States and Europe,[19] did a modest amount of lecturing at professional gatherings, and was in demand as a speaker at meetings of organisations such as the Crippled Children's Society. Her publications are sparse, and in only one was she the first author in a joint paper with her husband. Family bitterness continues over her being made a Dame, whereas Percy was not knighted. Although it cannot be formally documented, their daughter, Margaret Frazer, has informed the writer that, according to one of the children of the first marriage, he declined such an honour in 1923, the year he received the CBE. A knighthood was, however, expected in the 1957 New Year's Honours, but his death precluded what would have been an appropriate tribute.

After indifferent health and partial blindness in her latter years, Cecily suffered a devastating stroke in 1986. Bassam is now the Bloomfield Medical Hospital and, perhaps fittingly, is where Dame Cecily died in 1988.

The Second World War

Pickerill quickly offered his services on the outbreak of the Second World War. He wrote to the Director of Medical Services at Defence Headquarters: 'If you can utilise my services as a plastic surgeon in the present emergency I beg to place them at your disposal',[20] but he was not required for active service. Repatriated servicemen with facial and jaw injuries were mostly sent to Burwood Hospital, Christchurch, but some would have been among his patients at Wellington Hospital. He also offered to assist wounded passengers from the refrigerated cargo ship *Rangitane*,[21] sunk by German raiders off the East Cape of New Zealand in November 1940.[22] The Prime Minister thanked him warmly:

> I sincerely thank you for your generous gesture of Saturday and on behalf of the Government desire to express deep appreciation of the very generous and highly valued offer of services which it conveys and which has brought to the notice of the unfortunate people referred to.[23]

It is not known if any passengers who returned to New Zealand accepted the offer.

Although his surgical expertise was not specifically called upon in the Second World War, his wartime experience was put to very good use in another sphere: the training of personnel of the Dental Corps. He lectured at courses for dental officers held at Trentham Military Camp, and his papers were included in manuals for ongoing training.[24] His services in the Second World War were thus modest compared with those of the First; he had by now given way to the next generation of maxillofacial and plastic surgeons, amongst whom his son Paul was a prominent member.

Surgery at Middlemore

Early in 1946, the Pickerills considered a move to Auckland. The Auckland Hospital Board had taken over the American military hospital at Middlemore, near Otahuhu, south of Auckland city, and the Board negotiated with the Pickerills, with a view to them moving north. In February 1946, they were informed that Cabinet had agreed to them being employed as full-time plastic surgeons at a combined remuneration of £4,000 per annum, contingent on satisfactory arrangements being made for the establishment of a plastic surgery unit at Middlemore 'in accordance with the proposals set out in correspondence from the Board and yourself'.[25] Nothing came of this development, but they did begin regular visits to Middlemore from Wellington.

Details of these visits are not clear, for once again Pickerill's pioneering work was not adequately recorded. *Middlemore Memories*, the publication to mark the first fifty years of Middlemore Hospital, fails to mention the Pickerills,[26] but they were acknowledged in a history of nursing in Auckland:

> The plastic surgery unit was part of Middlemore from the very beginning. Many of the patients with severe burns were nursed there and the Doctors Pickerill used to come up from Lower Hutt on a Friday and spend the weekend at Middlemore, operating on children who had a cleft palate and/or a cleft (hare) lip.[27]

The pattern between 1947 and 1950 seemed to be that they held a clinic on the Saturday morning, and Cecily, who did most of the surgery, operated that afternoon and on the Sunday. They were away from Wellington for one week each month, travelling by car, and they probably held clinics in various centres on the way to or from Auckland. Their work at Middlemore included general plastic surgery, facial and jaw surgery, and repairs of cleft lips and palates. A former staff member has suggested the system was not conducive either to successful surgery or to positive relationships; post-operative care was left to others, who were reported to be generally unhappy with the arrangement.[28]

Because of time constraints, the Pickerills were working under unfavourable conditions, but nevertheless they provided a vital service. This was recognised when they ceased work at Middlemore in November 1950.[29] The Superintendent-in-Chief of the Auckland Hospital Board, H. Selwyn Kendrick, acknowledged their fine work and the growth in the clinic since they began. They were by that time said to be handling up to fifty consultations and up to sixteen operations each weekend they were in Auckland, an enormous commitment. The clinic served an area that included practically the whole of the northern half of the North Island; by then, hospital boards in the area were no longer contracted to Bassam.

A different structure was needed at Middlemore. In an interview on the occasion of his Middlemore retirement in 1950, Pickerill reviewed their experiences at the hospital and noted: 'the clinic had grown to a very considerable extent, and the board has now appointed a resident plastic surgeon, Mr W. Manchester, formerly at Christchurch, and recently doing post-graduate work in England, to carry on the work'.[30] Manchester (later Sir William) was a New Zealand surgeon who served in England during the Second World War, and then specialised in plastic surgery. He was appointed second in command at the military plastic surgery unit at the

Burwood Hospital in 1944 and, after further training in England, was appointed to Middlemore in 1950.[31] An outcome of the First World War was that Pickerill brought back to New Zealand the most up-to-date plastic surgical techniques and concepts of the day. In turn, he was succeeded by the younger generation of plastic surgeons, whose experience and skills had also been nurtured in war, and refined afterwards under Gillies, Pickerill's former Sidcup colleague.

Reflections on Pickerill's management of cleft lip and palate

A marked difference between the published methods of the Pickerills in the repair of cleft lips and palates and those of later surgeons, particularly Manchester at Middlemore, was the Pickerills' apparent lack of any systematic follow-up care, particularly orthodontic treatment. Pickerill was undoubtedly a highly skilled surgeon, but operations on clefts in infants are just the beginning of a long rehabilitative process. Speech therapy was an important part of their on-going care,[32] but the Pickerills did not report any long-term outcomes of their surgery on appearance and function. An advantage enjoyed by Manchester at Middlemore was that he was able to establish a plastic surgical 'unit', in contrast to the Pickerills' 'clinic' of consultation and surgery. Manchester reported in *Middlemore Memories* that he received:

> the necessary leverage to convince the board that the unit needed a small dental department, not only to help in the treatment of jaw fractures but to provide orthodontic treatment for cleft lip and palate cases. You must realise that the specialty of cleft lip and palate orthodontics was then virtually non-existent in the world ...[32]

Manchester developed a team approach, a crucial member of the team being the orthodontist. At that time, understanding was growing that a frequent outcome of surgery, which immediately transformed appearance, was inhibition of facial growth: the 'dished-in faces' of many cleft patients. 'Orthodontics was able to bring to the treatment of cleft lip and palate not only the skills of straightening the teeth but also, and more basically, the knowledge and expertise of facial growth, the use of long-term studies and the discipline of accurate record taking'.[34] The concept of 'pre-surgical orthopaedics', whereby segments of the maxilla separated by the clefts are held in their 'normal' position for a period before surgery, was evolved at Middlemore.[35] Combined with advanced surgical techniques, the management of cleft lips and palates made huge progress under Manchester's leadership. These advances received international acclaim, as had Pickerill's methods after the First World War and in the early Bassam period.

These new developments occurred after Pickerill retired. Cecily continued at Bassam until 1967, and her patients, and those of Hutter (until the Plastic Surgical Unit at Hutt Hospital was established), received orthodontic treatment only on an 'ad hoc basis' on referral.[36] Her writings and newspaper interviews suggest she had no formal team association with the orthodontists at that time; apparently, according to an orthodontist of the day, to the disadvantage of her patients. But this should not detract from Pickerill's long and distinguished contribution to the care of these children – in his later years, his pioneering methods were simply overtaken by a new and more holistic approach.

Retirement in Wellington

In December 1950 Pickerill wrote that his work at the Lewisham Hospital was 'tailing off rapidly' and that 1951 would probably be his final year practising surgery;[37] he was not now taking any fresh big operations, and Cecily was responsible for the surgery at Bassam. Nevertheless, he retained his enthusiasm for the advancement of plastic surgery into the final years of his life but, as his health became a burden, sometimes his enthusiasm was misplaced. In 1951, before he 'completely gave up work', he sought approval of the Medical Superintendent of Wellington Hospital to initiate a programme of clinical research into how sufferers of varicose ulcers could be aided by skin grafts. He wanted to hand on his experience 'before it was too late' (he had only recently recovered from a coronary thrombosis). At this time he proposed the establishment of skin banks that would ensure a source of suitable tissue to cover large areas where skin had been lost through burns.[38] He believed skin grafting would effectively treat varicose ulcers once all the pathological tissue had been excised. He presented this method of treatment as an original idea, and wanted to demonstrate the method to Hutter. But, unknown to him, the method was already widely accepted, and indeed was being practised at Wellington Hospital; Hutter had presented a paper on the subject at a recent meeting of the Royal Australasian College of Surgeons. This was an embarrassing episode, but Pickerill was driven by the highest of motives. He acknowledged he was falling behind modern developments, not least because his deafness meant sitting through lectures and not hearing anything was 'beyond human endurance'. He was delighted to know that patients were having ulcers grafted, but he would still like to have had the opportunity to pass on some of his methods to Hutter; he had found it rare that any doctors at Wellington or Middlemore hospitals had come to 'see how it was done'. These were the words of a true pioneer: for most of his career as a plastic surgeon he had followed a lonely road; now he was approaching its end.

But there was still work to do, and shots to be fired.

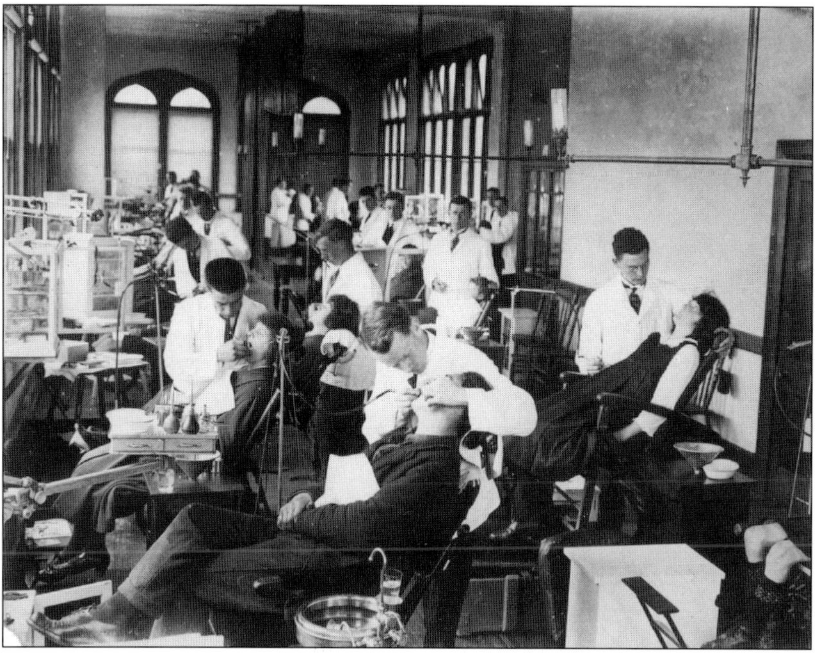

Top: *Serious overcrowding in the main clinic of the Dental School, c. 1924.*
Bell Collection, School of Dentistry.

Bottom: *Students posing in the mechanical laboratory of the School, c. 1924.*
Bell Collection, School of Dentistry.

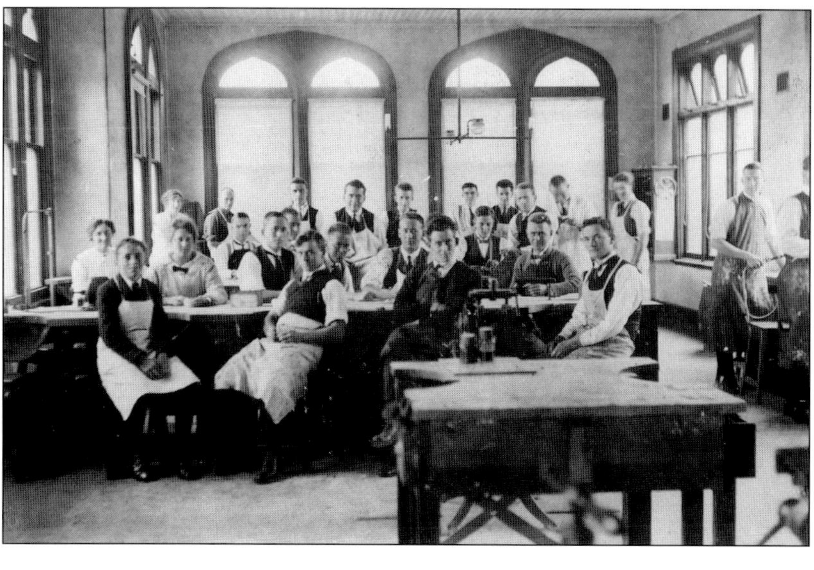

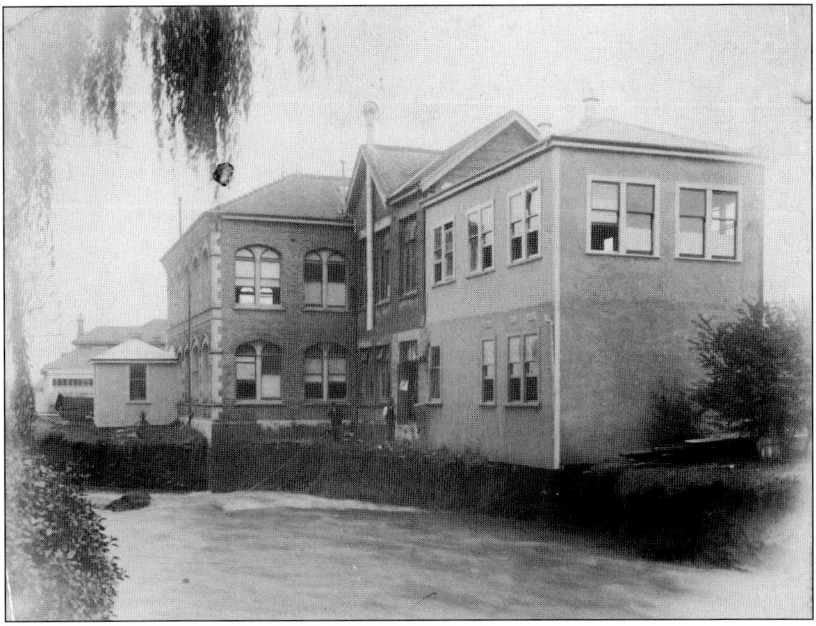

The great flood of 23 April 1924. ***Top****: the Leith Stream at its height, undermining the main building and the newly completed extension;* ***Bottom****: the aftermath, showing the seriously undermined extension and the main building in danger. Bell Collection, School of Dentistry.*

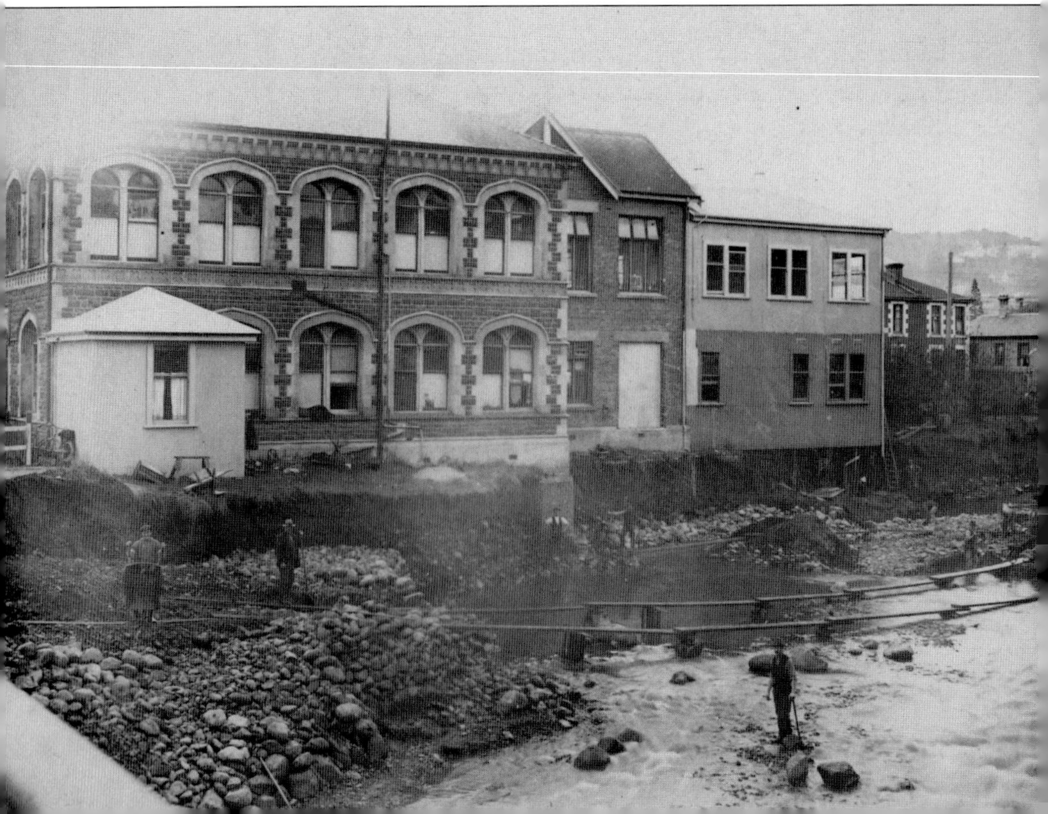

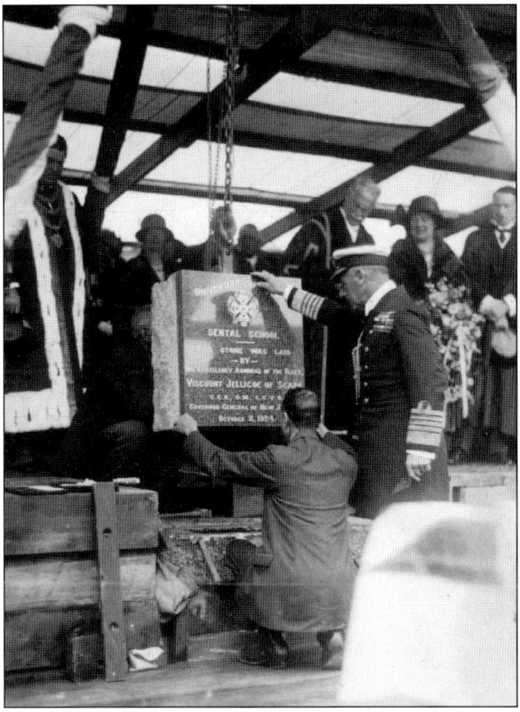

His Excellency Viscount Jellicoe laying the Foundation Stone of the new School in Great King Street, 18 October 1924. *Bell Collection, School of Dentistry.*

Bottom: *The new School, later to become part of the Department of Zoology.*

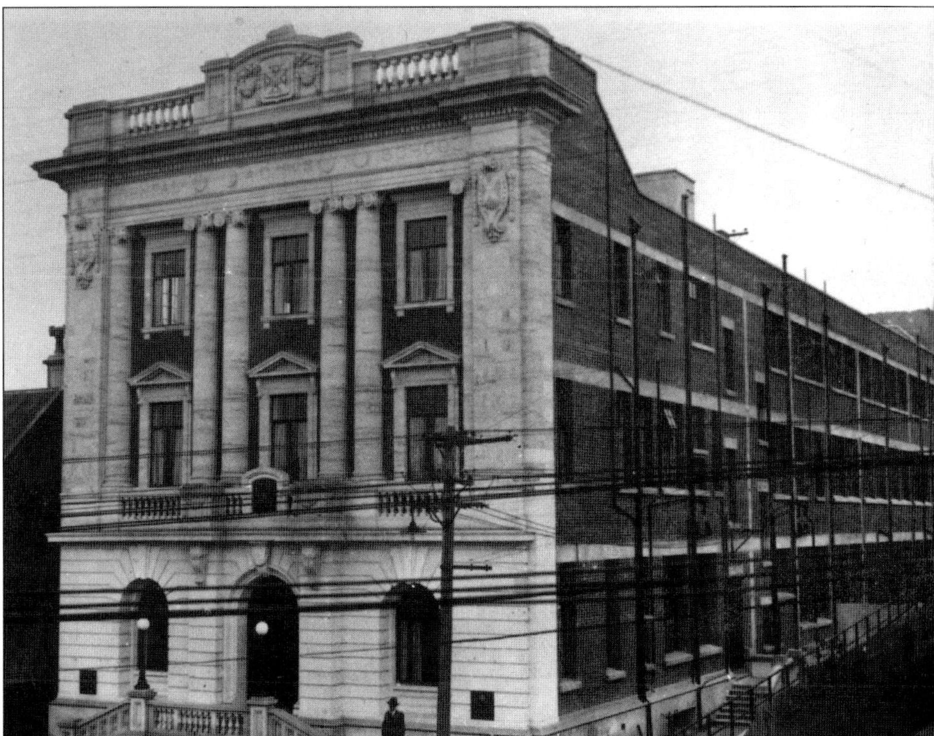

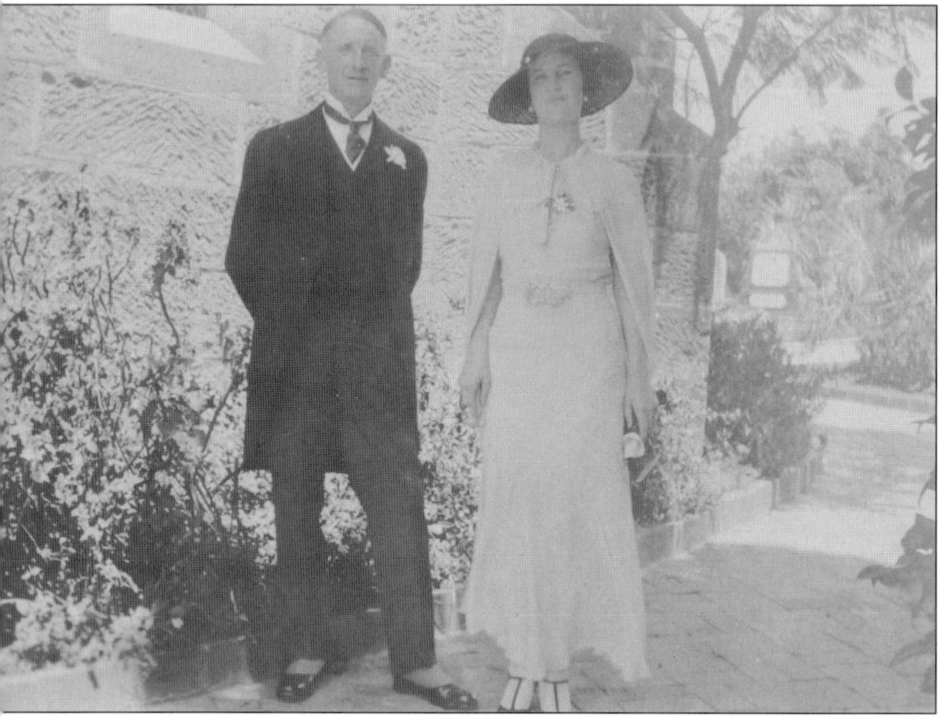

Pickerill and his new bride, Cecily (née Clarkson) on their wedding day, the Enfield Church, Sydney, 17 December 1934.

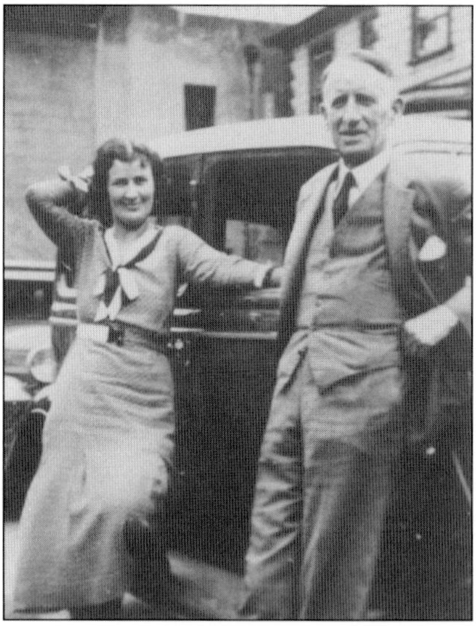

Pickerill and Cecily outside the Lewisham (now the Wakefield) Hospital, Wellington. Date unknown.

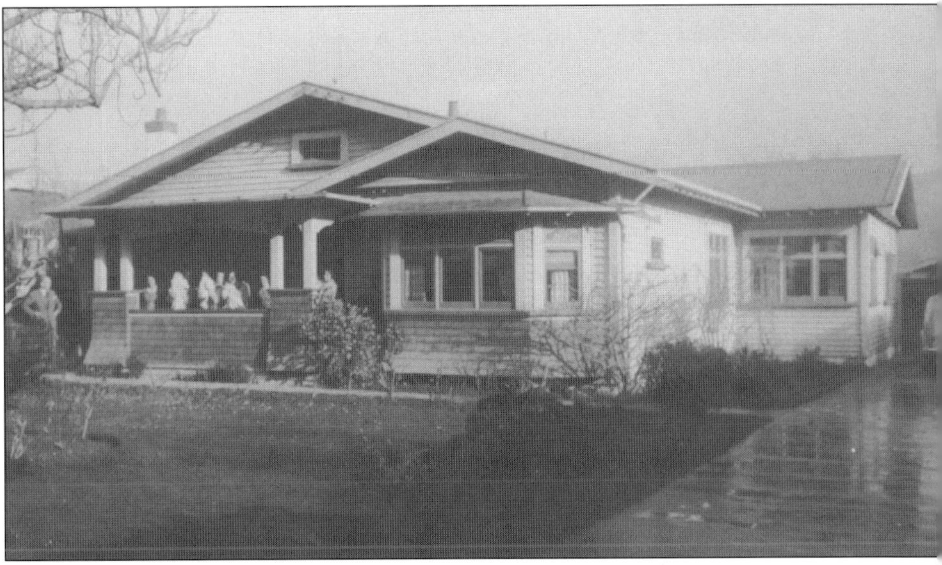

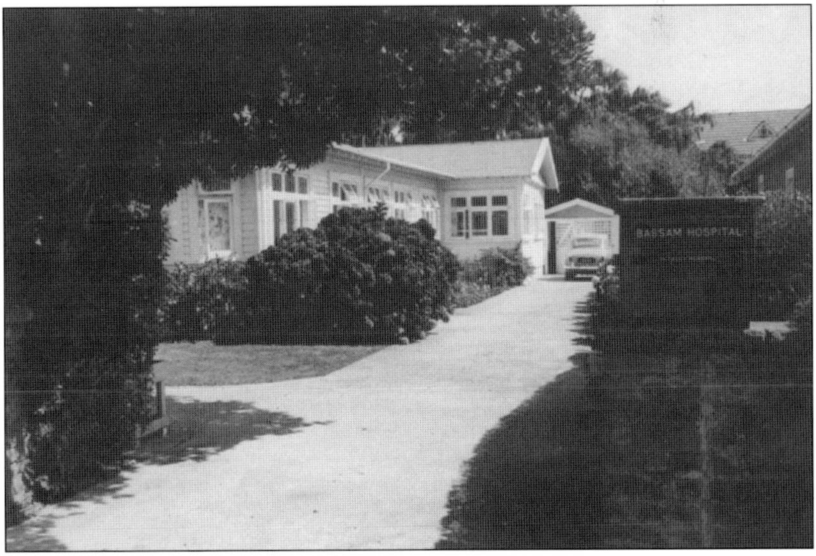

Top: *Bassam Hospital, Lower Hutt. Pickerill can be seen at the left of the porch, on which are standing mothers and their babies.*

Bottom: *Bassam Hospital after alterations increased the number of bedrooms.*

Following page: *Examples of the Pickerill's cleft-lip surgery at Bassam.* ***Left****, the babies on admission;* ***right****, approximately nine months after the first operations.* *Pickerill Papers, Hocken Collections.*

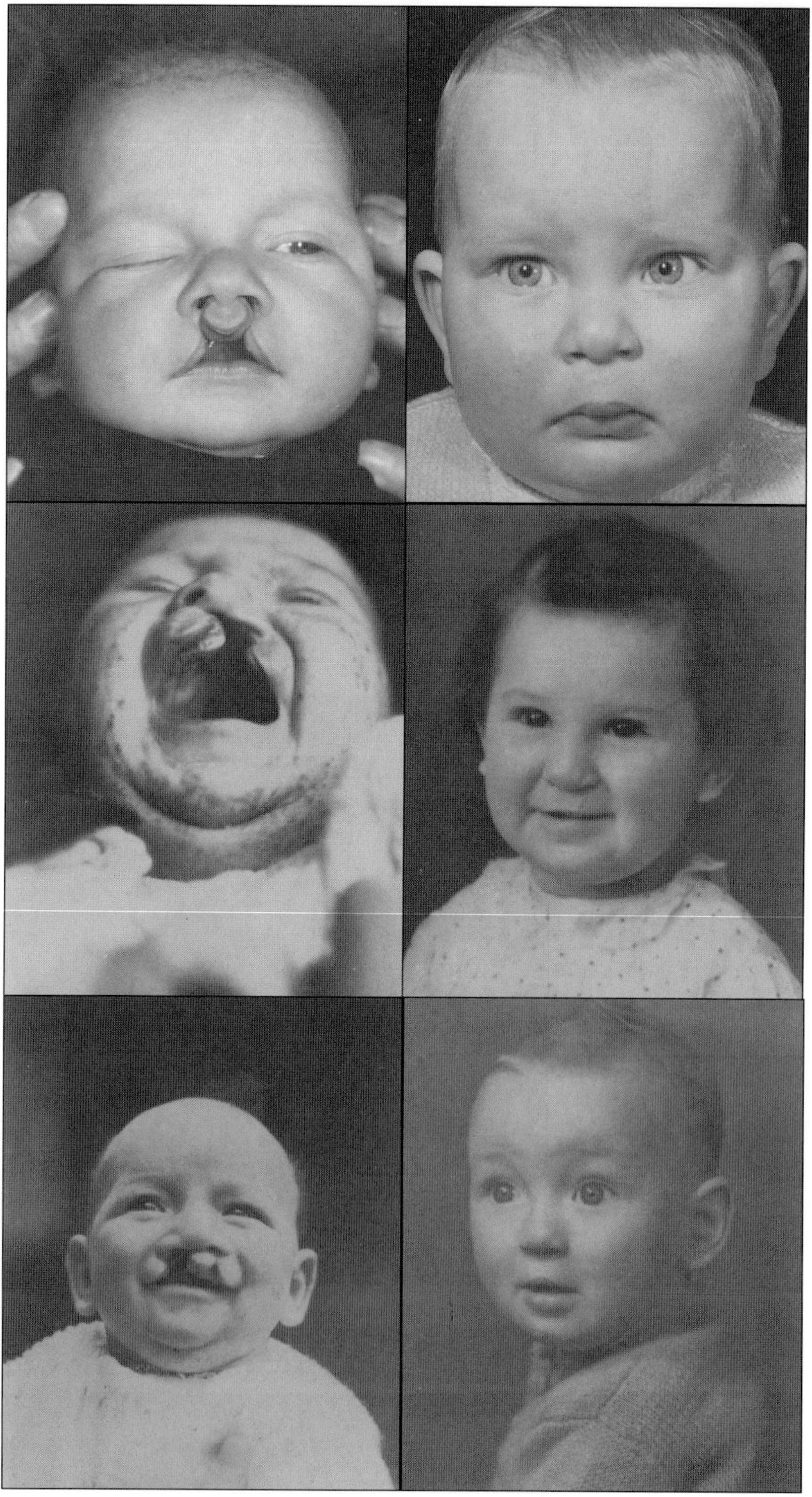

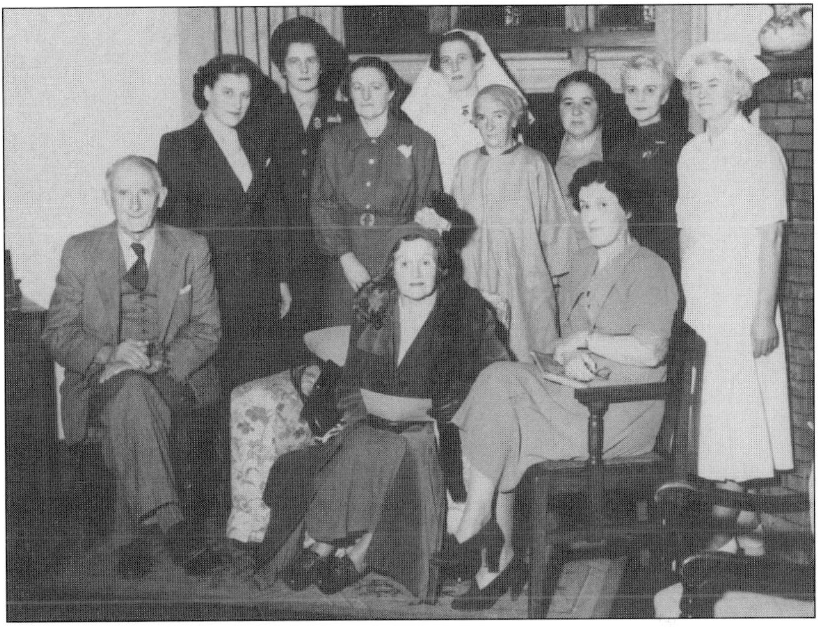

The Pickerills (seated left and right) and staff of Bassam on the occasion of the visit of Lady Freyberg, wife of the Governor-General Sir Bernard Freyberg, 31 May 1951. Photograph by Laurence A. Hoare, Lower Hutt.

Lois White's 1956 portrait of H.P. Pickerill in the first-floor foyer of the present School of Dentistry, completed in the final months of his life and presented by the New Zealand Dental Association to the Faculty of Dentistry at the fiftieth Jubilee Celebrations of the School on 21 August 1956, just eleven days after he died.

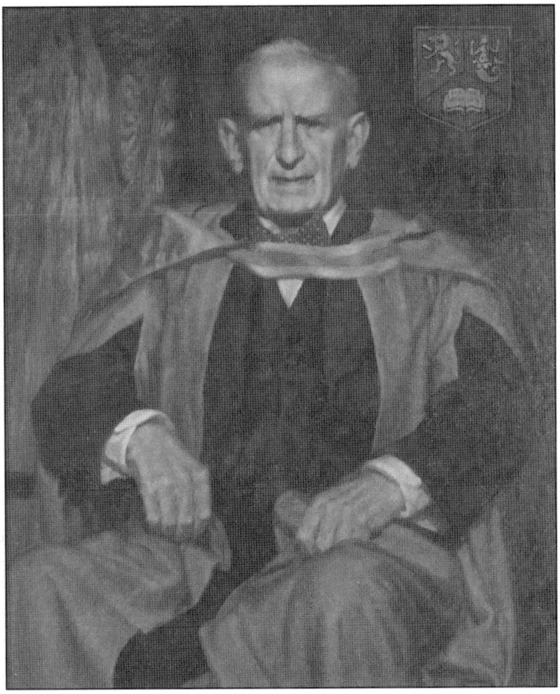

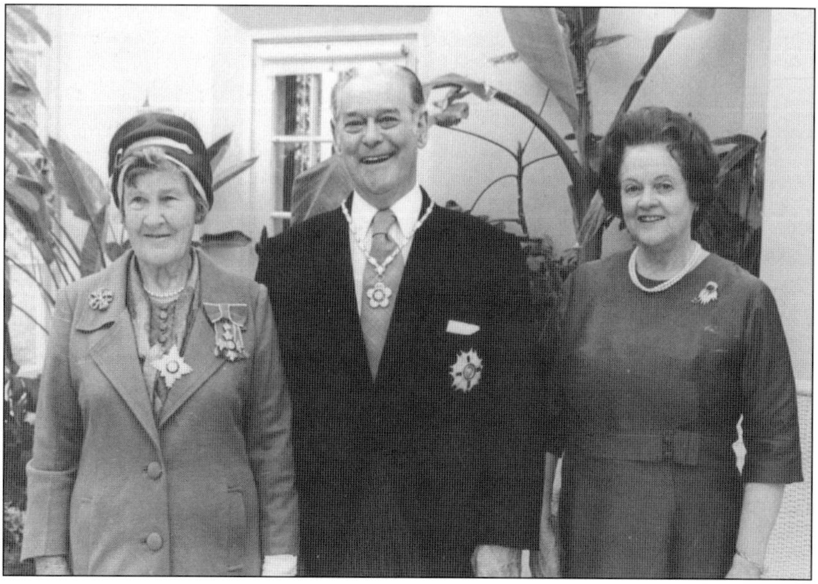

Pickerill never received a knighthood, but his second wife and surgical colleague, Cecily, became Dame Commander of the British Empire. Dame Cecily is pictured on the day of her investiture, 2 December 1977, with Their Excellencies Sir Keith and Lady Holyoake.
Photograph courtesy of The Weekly News.

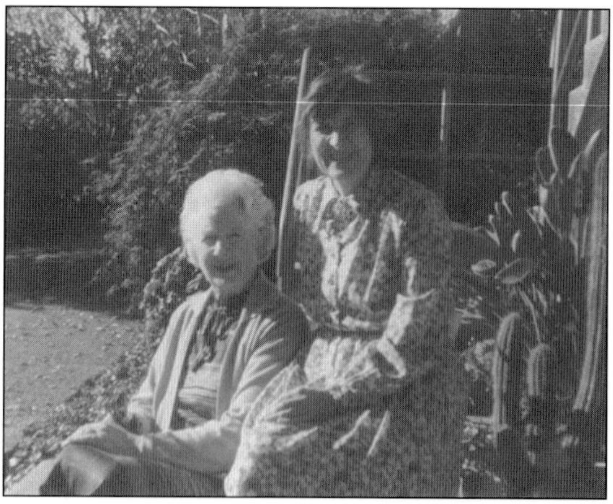

The two Pickerill daughters. On the left is Kathleen (Kay) Fogg, daughter of Percy and Mabel Pickerill, and on the right is her half-sister Margaret Frazer, daughter of Percy and Cecily Pickerill.

19

The final months

Pickerill's final months were far from restful. His last paper appeared just a month before he died,[1] and he had the energy to protest about an inverted figure in the paper a fortnight before the end.[2] He was also tested on three separate fronts. Each caused him much anguish that would not have helped him in this time of failing health: he had suffered a coronary thrombosis, and periodic episodes of angina were limiting his activities; his increasing deafness made telephoning and taking part in meetings very difficult. His correspondence related to the three events suggests growing frustration and impatience with those who sought to honour him in his declining years, but he persisted with typical vigour.

The Royal Australasian College of Surgeons

Pickerill's final contribution to surgery was his role in the formation of the Plastic Surgery Section (now the Section of Plastic and Reconstructive Surgery) of the Royal Australasian College of Surgeons. He and others saw the annual scientific meeting of the College, to be held in Christchurch in April 1956, as the golden opportunity to promote the section, especially as Gillies was to be present. Sir Archibald McIndoe, the distinguished New Zealand plastic surgeon of the Second World War, had also been invited. Despite Pickerill's increasing deafness and occasional attacks of angina, he felt it was vital to promote the specialty of plastic surgery within the College. As the 'senior plastic surgeon in this part of the world', he wrote to Gillies, he wanted to be present to welcome his old colleague from Sidcup days and, although 'not in very good form now', he hoped to be there 'to help give the wandering son of N.Z. a famous welcome'. He described his hearing as 'completely negative' but, if Cecily were permitted to attend (she was not a Fellow of the College), she could take notes for him. He was expecting to get 'some real good oil straight from the horse's mouth', but felt that, as his hearing was then so bad, he would profit the least from the lectures.

Writing to McIndoe, he commented that he and Cecily were not very 'persona grata' with some Fellows of the College, owing probably to 'our heresy over mother-nursing of babies'. He added that few hospitals could claim to have had no single case of cross-infections in thirteen years, and no sign of resistant staphylococci. The College granted Cecily permission to attend, but he was disappointed to learn that McIndoe was unable to come.

Pickerill suggested he should open the discussion of Gillies' paper on cleft palate, hoping that the lecture and his angina 'would not clash'. He also questioned the topic: if Gillies were to speak at length on cleft palate, he thought only about four people would be able to follow him. He suggested an alternative: an oration on the 'Past, Present, and Future of Plastic Surgery' as being of much more general interest. Such a topic would also have been a powerful tool to advance the cause of the specialty within the College.[3]

His request to open the discussion of Gillies' paper on cleft palate was not only declined, but also his presence was not even acknowledged, for he was incorrectly reported by the President to have been absent. Complaining about this slight, he told the Secretary that, although he did not mind not making a speech, he would like to have had the opportunity to comment that, almost twenty years previously, he had read a paper on the use of tubed-pedicle grafts in cleft-palate surgery, which, he claimed, Gillies opposed at the time but now advocated:[4] the old rivalry still thrived!

The minutes of the meeting of plastic surgeons record contributions from Gillies, B.K. Rank (a leading Melbourne plastic surgeon and a member of the College's Council), J.J. Brownlee (Melbourne), Manchester, Cecily Pickerill, Frank Hutter, and David Poswillo, prominent New Zealand maxillofacial surgeon practising in London, who spoke on behalf of dentally qualified members of the British Association of Plastic Surgeons.[5] The outcome was support for the formation of a plastic surgery section within the College, rather than the formation of a New Zealand group within the British Association of Plastic Surgeons. Rank proposed that a provisional committee of Pickerill, A.R. Wakefield (Melbourne), and D.O. Brown (Sydney) be formed.

Pickerill anticipated the formation of the section would be his 'last effort' on behalf of the specialty,[6] and so it was to prove. The plastic surgeons present at the meeting developed draft objects and regulations, but Pickerill was pessimistic about their acceptance. In June 1956 he said to Rank: 'You will have gathered that our proposals will be opposed by the President and possibly by the S.A. [South Australian] councillors. The proposal will be made, I think, that there should be instead a group in the B.M.A. or that consideration should be postponed until there is a larger number of plastic surgeons'. He argued that a section on plastic surgery would be an inducement for surgeons to enter the specialty and would encourage attendance at meetings of the College; a section would also remind general surgeons of the possibilities presented by plastic surgery, rather than adopting the still common recommendation made to patients to 'leave well alone'.[7]

But lobbying by Rank, Brown, and Wakefield proved successful in gaining support for the section; on 6 July the Secretary of the Royal Australasian College of Surgeons told Pickerill that his preliminary proposals had been welcomed by the College's Council at its meeting on 23–24 June, and were approved in principle. The Council looked forward to receiving further details. Encouraged, Pickerill sent the latest draft objects and rules for comment to Rank and Wakefield on 31 July. To the latter, he expressed surprise that the thoracic section of the College had no such documentation: although simplicity was desirable, he thought this was going too far.[8]

His final action in the formation of the section, also on 31 July, was to request photographs from those attending that first meeting of the plastic surgeons of Australasia so that he could make a composite record of the occasion. Completion of this task fell to Cecily, for Percy Pickerill died just ten days later.

The formation of the Plastic Surgery Section of the Royal Australasian College of Surgeons was a major achievement, and in many ways a fitting epitaph to a long and distinguished career. He had carried the torch for plastic surgery virtually alone in Australasia for many years. Now it was recognised as a legitimate specialty within the mainstream of surgery, and its status thus greatly enhanced.

The portrait saga

To mark its Fiftieth Jubilee in 1955, the New Zealand Dental Association decided to present a portrait of Pickerill to the Dental School,[9] the presentation to take place the following year at the Association's conference in Dunedin. The artist chosen was A.J.C. Fisher, Director of Auckland's Elam School of Fine Arts. Thanking the Association for this honour, Pickerill could not help reminding the Association, whose headquarters were by then back in Auckland, of 'the great battle which raged 30 years ago over the site of the "new" Dental School'.[10] Then followed a flurry of correspondence between Fisher, Pickerill, Maurice Priestley (acting on behalf of the Association), and

Ronald Tonkin, the Association's President. Tonkin was especially apologetic over the failure to reach agreement with Fisher about where the portrait would be painted: Fisher was unable to spare the time to be away from Auckland, and also had health problems, and Pickerill's own state of health prevented him from travelling to Auckland. Tonkin assured Pickerill that the Association was 'firmly of the opinion that no more suitable presentation could be made to the Dental School than a portrait of yourself as first Dean … and we are highly honoured that you have given your consent …'.[11]

The outcome was that a new artist, Lois White, was commissioned, but problems soon arose, with the portrait itself and with relations between artist and subject. Pickerill did not like the result. He complained to Priestly about its scowling look, but her response had been that that was how she saw him at the time. He thought she was 'Too much the art school mistress repeating what she has so industriously instilled into her pupils and mechanical transference to the canvas, not a study of the victim's average or usual disposition'. He had stipulated 'that the portrait should not in any way resemble Southerland's [*sic*] of Churchill', which he detested, but that was how the first attempt appeared to him. He added: 'I take it you and N.Z.D.A. want a record of H.P.P. not just a "a study of an old man's head by Miss. Lois White" tho' doubtless the latter might have greater artistic merit, but it is not to go into an art gallery but to a University department as a record of service, and the 2 things may be miles apart'. She also upset him with her language. He further commented to Priestley:

> You are doubtless more than a little upset at the outcome of our initial attempt at the portrait, for which I am truly sorry. It is possibly much my fault for being a perfectionist and not being familiar with the argot of the art school, but the great Australian adjective … coming from a woman's lips is more than I can stand, it defiles her, and puts her on a level with half drunken sailors or soldiers in camps. I think Miss White really wants to please you (but not *me* she as good as told me, but quite nicely). But if you want my portrait I must have some little say in it – it would be something totally contrary to my nature otherwise, as you possibly realise.[12]

Hers was not an easy task, especially as his health interfered with sittings. He apologised to her for what proved to be an unfortunately timed last visit she made to his Beechdale home to collect her equipment, and she wrote a gracious reply, including warm thanks for the hospitality and kindness shown to her.[13] Priestley then suggested that a new painting be made from coloured slides, a proposal gladly accepted by Pickerill, albeit with instructions on how the slides should be stored and viewed. 'If she … will cooperate, I am sure a successful method will be found'.[14] He instructed that the shield of the

University of Birmingham be included in the background, and that he would commission a smaller version if the shield came out well.

Apparently the revision was still not satisfactory, for the eyes were almost invisible. Priestley, probably by now very tired of the whole business, assured Pickerill that:

> Every possible effort has been made to ensure that the portrait is the best we can procure, both in the very careful selection of the artist on the recommendation of our highest authorities, and in the ample time for its execution.
>
> The fact that the sitter is looking downward rather than directly forward does not appear to me to matter in the least and I cannot agree that it will be an insult to you or a disgrace to any one of us, but re-iterate that it is an honourable, fitting and permanent expression of your service to the School and the profession, and of the esteem with which you are held by your old students and the N.Z. Dental Association.

The portrait by then was packed and ready to be shipped south, but it was retrieved, and the artist tried to make the necessary alterations. She was, however, doubtful of the outcome if the eyes were given greater prominence. Four days later, Priestley triumphantly cabled Pickerill: 'Optoplasty completed and entirely successful'.[15]

Pickerill was glad that the artist had 'been able to rectify the mistake and had the missing optics restored'. He would hate to think that past and present students would think he was blind, for he claimed he could still thread a quarter-inch needle 'with the finest silk, and give the patient an incision line which is almost invisible'. He was cheered, too, that he had just received word that, from a list of British paediatric surgeons, he was one of eight who had 'rendered outstanding service to paediatric surgery'.[16]

The saga was now almost over, for the portrait duly arrived at the School. It now hangs, with portraits of later deans, in the foyer on the first floor. It appears to this writer that it is a finely executed work, but one that bears little resemblance to photographs of Pickerill taken in those final months of his life. Nevertheless it is a distinguished work that is exhibited with pride, and is a fitting expression of the Association's appreciation, despite periods of bitterness, of his contribution to New Zealand dentistry.

The Dental School Jubilee

The Association planned to present the portrait at the Dental School's Fiftieth Jubilee. Although the School had opened its doors in June 1907, the celebrations took place in 1956. The role of the Association in the founding of the School was so crucial that the University Council felt honour-bound to accede to requests to mark the occasion during the Association's conference, held that year in Dunedin; it justified its decision on the grounds that building actually commenced in 1906.

Pickerill had hoped to be able to attend this important occasion. The Secretary of the conference, Associate Professor Frank Shroff, reserved suitable accommodation for the Pickerills at the Grand Hotel, and invited the former Dean to attend official conference functions. Shroff, the Head of the Department of Basic Dental Science at the School, also wanted Pickerill to visit his department: 'It would also make me very happy if you could spare the time and the effort to make a short visit to your old Dental School and see what we have done, particularly in the way of scientific dentistry and research …', adding in his next letter: 'Many of your former graduates will be looking forward to meeting you again and even those who were not privileged to be your students I am sure will be grateful for the opportunity of meeting one who did so much to put the Dental School on a firm foundation and achieve its place among other schools of the world'. Shroff informed Pickerill that the 'Jubilee ceremony was to be held in the Town Hall Concert Chamber, with 'only a short flight of steps to the stage'. Paul Pickerill was to bring his father and presumably also his stepmother down from Timaru.[17]

The Dean of the Faculty at this time was John (later Sir John) Walsh, with whom Pickerill had previously had amiable correspondence, as Dean and as Editor of the *Journal*. Pickerill had previously informed Walsh that he planned to attend, health permitting, and, as the foundation Dean, expected to have the opportunity to speak. If he were not able to attend, he hoped that Walsh or his son Paul Pickerill could read the message.[18] On receiving Walsh's reply, he wrote to Stanley Wilson, presumably a member of the Jubilee committee: 'I have just had a most astonishing slap in the face from Walsh'. In what Pickerill described as a 'very formal letter', Walsh said he could be 'given' a seat on the platform, but would not have the opportunity to speak:

> I think that some of you fellows should tell him where he gets off. Such rudeness is the more astonishing as he and I have always been quite friendly. I certainly don't feel inclined to go if I am denied ordinary courtesies. Besides it is a Jubilee and I should be exhibit 'A' as being the only one alive now who can say anything from the inside University aspect of 50 or 60 years ago. I applied for the job and was appointed in 1906 [*sic*] and I did a bit to put it on the map.

He felt Davies and others could speak on behalf of the Association, but pointed out that Walsh had no knowledge of events in those early days. He wondered if Walsh thought he, Pickerill, wanted to 'steal his thunder'. He added that he would certainly not be touching on anything controversial, and that it 'Seems to me Walsh is saying "I'm the boss now! You shan't play in my backyard" – childish!'[19]

The storm soon settled after he took his concerns to the Chancellor;[20] the Registrar replied that there had never been 'any objection to your speaking at all',[21] although the official programme and invitations had been printed before Pickerill's letter of 29 June had been received: it seems Pickerill had indeed been thoughtlessly overlooked when the programme and invitations were prepared. The Registrar added that he was sure there would be no objection to Pickerill acknowledging the honour to be paid to him and giving a brief message of 'hail and farewell' to former students, but this would be after the formal speeches. His son could read the message if he could not make the trip to Dunedin.

Sadly, Pickerill did not make it to the Jubilee held on 21 August. In a letter dated 10 August, the day he died, he told the Registrar: 'Things have taken a turn for the worse with me and it is more doubtful than ever if I can make the journey … with apologies for all the trouble I have caused you.' He asked the Registrar to write and ask Paul to read the message if he could not make it. He thought Paul was 'a little diffident', but was sure he would do it well.[22]

The following day Dunedin newspapers announced his passing and noted that the portrait was to be presented at the celebrations; a statement from Walsh read: 'It is a matter of deep regret to the staff that Dr Pickerill will not hear the tributes which will be paid to him as the founder of formal dental education in New Zealand'.[23] The present writer, one of Walsh's final-year students in 1956, believes nothing personal was involved in the initial failure to invite Pickerill; it was simply an oversight, but it was an unfortunate blunder that caused a great deal of distress.

The Registrar sent the Council's sympathy to Paul, formally inviting him to read the message his father had already sent to Dunedin.[24] The celebrations and the conference duly took place. Walsh spoke generously about him in his Jubilee address. After listing the names of some of Pickerill's internationally distinguished graduates, he added: 'It is fitting on this occasion of the Jubilee of the School that his portrait should be presented to the School as a reminder of the early traditions of dental education and research so ably laid down by him at the very beginning of formal dental education in New Zealand. We honour his memory.'[25]

The Association's President, A.D. Brice, reminded the conference that Pickerill would have been attending as 'a guest of honour'; the audience stood in silence as a mark of respect.[26] Walsh informed Cecily that the celebrations were very successful, that Paul 'read his father's speech very well',[27] and that it and a photograph of the portrait would be published in the next issue of the *Journal*.[28]

At its November meeting, the Faculty placed on record 'its deep feeling of regret at the death of its first Dean and Director of the School …', and acknowledged his distinguished career as 'teacher, administrator, research worker, scholar, dentist, surgeon …' in each of which his fame was international. It also recorded that the University of Otago was the first university in the Empire to establish a Faculty of Dentistry. 'That the Faculty not only prospered but provided an example which other and older universities copied was due to Pickerill's genius, courage, and devotion. It is with respect and gratitude that the Faculty pays this tribute to his memory'.[29]

The Pickerill era at the Faculty of Dentistry was indeed now ended.

20

Hail and farewell

'Hail and Farewell' was the theme Pickerill hoped to present personally to the Jubilee Celebrations of the School of Dentistry, when his portrait was to be gifted to the School by the New Zealand Dental Association. The words are also appropriate in concluding this story of an exceptional life.

His death on 10 August 1956 produced many fine tributes touching all aspects of his career. Obituaries were published in newspapers throughout the country and in medical and dental journals in New Zealand and overseas.

Fellow plastic surgeon, Frank Hutter, Pickerill's successor at Wellington Hospital, acknowledged him as the 'founder of maxillo-facial surgery in New Zealand and in the world-wide renaissance of plastic surgery during and after the first world war … He had many critics, but the name of H.P. Pickerill will be remembered long after most of his critics are forgotten'.[1]

By coincidence, the obituary of Sydney Devenish (Tommy) Rhind, his surgical associate at Sidcup and a highly respected surgeon in Wellington and Lower Hutt, also appeared in the same issue of the *New Zealand Medical Journal*. Auckland surgeon Douglas Robb added a further obituary of Pickerill in the next issue of the same journal:

> The account of the late Dr. Pickerill … records the facts of the life of this remarkable man. May I be allowed to add the impressions he made on me as a student and at intervals up to the end?
>
> He brought a fresh and inquiring mind to everything he took up, and was affected and deterred very little by what others thought. He might have been difficult at times as a colleague, and it was not hard to quarrel with him. But he was always stimulating and often right – going to basic principles for his working ideas.
>
> When one considers the range of his interests – dental science, dental caries,

> the teaching of odontology to both dental and medical students, maxillo-facial surgery, infant nursing and management in hospital – and the influence made on each, his total performance was amazing. Many consider that his most outstanding contribution was his pioneering with Dr. Cecily Pickerill of the Bassam Hospital, and the management of infants with their mothers.
>
> His knowledge of fundamentals allowed him to make interesting and useful suggestions to persons working in quite different fields, and demonstrated the basic unity of all medical and biological approaches.[2]

The obituary in the *New Zealand Dental Journal*, unsigned but presumably by the Editor, F.W. Craddock, recorded that Pickerill's work at Sidcup

> firmly established him as a plastic surgeon of exceptional ability; and it is in this field that he will be remembered for his outstanding and original work. It is no exaggeration to say that his scalpel has given new hope and encouragement to countless people otherwise doomed to a life of misery and isolation.

It then quoted the words of the President of the Dental Association when the portrait was presented to the School during the Jubilee celebrations:

> No reproduction on canvas can do him justice. Pickerill the surgeon … the scientist, the teacher and disciplinarian, the idealist and humanitarian; all were parts of the man we knew, facets of a brilliant personality. He taught us to 'Follow the gleam'. He impressed on us a concept of dentistry far beyond the confines of a tooth …[3]

The writer of the obituary in *The Lancet* considered that 'many doctors in this country and in this decade will remember him best for the enterprise of his old age, when he successfully eliminated cross-infection from a children's hospital by bringing the mother to the bedside'. A colleague of that writer described him as 'a man of great and original intelligence and insight … He was always stimulating to talk to, provocative, and almost quarrelsome at times … Pick will be remembered affectionately and with admiration by many medical and dental colleagues throughout the Commonwealth'.[4]

Writers of these obituaries, unanimous in praise of his achievements, saw fit to comment on relations with colleagues. The stormy problems with the New Zealand Dental Association and with staff at the School of Dentistry are well documented, but the reasons for problems with medical colleagues are unclear. In the lead-up to the formation of the Plastic Surgery Section of the Royal Australasian College of Surgeons, Pickerill himself implied that he was out of favour with many colleagues. The late Brigadier J. Ferris Fuller, a former Director of Defence Dental Services and a great admirer of Pickerill, told the present writer of his sadness that, when he returned from service overseas, he found Pickerill was 'for some reason on the outer … When I mentioned the name of the Pickerills among the medical establishment I found they were dismissed curtly'.

There are several possible reasons for this, in addition to the obvious one that Pickerill could be prickly, outspoken, and had definite opinions that he defended vigorously. He acknowledged that the revolutionary mother-nursing system introduced at Bassam was not widely approved, despite its success preventing the serious complications of cross infection. He wrote to niece Vivien Jones after her graduation at the University of Birmingham:

> But I am & always have been a heretic & that's why many people don't like me. The surgeons here for instance are out after our blood because of the success of our baby hospital which is now quite contrary to accepted lines, rules and regulations but results are miraculous & that's an unforgivable sin. If you depart from the hunting pack you are liable to become the hunted … Take my advice stick to the pack & keep your opinions to yourself![5]

Today, with mothers increasingly being expected to be involved in the nursing of their infants in many hospitals, the Pickerills' pioneering approach has been more than vindicated. Another problem may have been resentment and even jealousy that Cecily, without any post-graduate qualifications, achieved eminence in plastic surgery – even to the extent of being awarded the equivalent of a knighthood – and that the stature of her husband, her mentor and guide, suffered by comparison. 'Her hands transformed the lives of thousands' was a typical newspaper headline announcing her retirement and the closing of Bassam in 1967;[6] high praise indeed. Or it may be that their actual union was still considered offensive even long after this second marriage had taken place: Pickerill's retiring from a prominent position in the University, being joined in Sydney by a young graduate many years his junior, and leaving behind his four children and wife of twenty years, may have remained imprinted in the minds of a conservative medical establishment and been held against them both.

Whatever the reasons, the apparent souring of relations with the medical profession does not detract from what was undoubtedly a brilliant career. He left a rich legacy, not just in one field, but in many. It was Pickerill who brought the School of Dentistry in the University of Otago to the forefront of dental education in the world. It was Pickerill who brought similar world notice for New Zealand dental research through his groundbreaking studies and writings on dental caries. It was Pickerill who, despite the most unfortunate break with the New Zealand Dental Association, remains as one of its most distinguished servants through his roles as Secretary and Editor of the *Journal.* It was Pickerill who, as one of the dynamic leaders of the Association, brought into being what is now the Royal New Zealand Dental Corps, the clear leader in dentistry for the armed forces in the First World War. It was Pickerill who, alongside Sir Harold Gillies and other pioneers in plastic surgery, alleviated great suffering and mutilation experienced by servicemen in the war, and established the foundations of modern plastic surgery. It was Pickerill who twice led the defence of Otago's Dental School against the forces wanting to move dental education to Auckland. It was Pickerill who endured, with his staff, the dreadful trials of providing education in a grossly deficient environment, and who led the campaign to build a new school. It was Pickerill who established plastic surgery services in Sydney: he was a pioneer of the specialty in that country, indeed in Australasia. He, an Englishman, was New Zealand's first plastic surgeon, despite that title commonly but incorrectly being assigned to Gillies, who never practised in his native country. It was Pickerill who trained Cecily; they received the everlasting gratitude of hundreds of patients and parents for their skills, especially in restoring infants afflicted with cleft lip and palate to normality and acceptance within their families and communities. It was Pickerill who contributed to the scientific and clinical literature well over 100 articles, three major textbooks, and several treatises and pamphlets for the education of professionals, parents, and the public.

A person associated with any one of such achievements deserves to be honoured: there have been few men or women in medicine or dentistry with such a diversity and number of notable achievements. His was an exceptional career.

But what of the man himself and his family? Pickerill's incredibly busy life while Dean, and his absence overseas during the war, meant that Mabel Pickerill bore a heavy load managing the household and bringing up the children. But worse was to follow when her husband left for Sydney. The relationship of Percy and Cecily, at least on a professional level, had begun before the departure for Sydney. Being left alone in Dunedin, and then facing the scandal of separation and divorce, must have been devastating and humiliating for Mabel and the children. She was now a single parent with four children, a dramatic change for the wife of one of the University's most prominent professors, Dean of a faculty, and a national and international leader in his professional fields. After the divorce she changed her style of address from 'Mrs H.P. Pickerill' to 'Mrs M.L. Pickerill', a very public and no doubt daring public acknowledgement of her changed status. Her endurance in adversity showed she was indeed a remarkable woman.

The family continued to occupy the house at Ravensbourne after Pickerill left. Until her marriage in 1934 to dental surgeon Stanley Fogg, daughter Kathleen (Kay) stayed there with her mother. The house was sold shortly afterward and Mabel moved to Timaru to be near Kathleen and Stanley. Later, Stanley sold his practice to brother-in-law Paul Pickerill who, like Kathleen, was close to his mother. Kathleen and Stanley then moved to Christchurch, where Stanley limited his practice to oral surgery. Mabel died in Timaru in 1953. All her children are now deceased.

Grandson Gerald Fogg, son of Kathleen, describes his 'Granma' as 'a lovely lady. Very strong, compassionate, fun loving and good looking … a firm believer in God … had good health and was a great walker'. Gerald used to spend school holidays with her in her flat at Timaru. There she lived frugally, in totally different surroundings from the spacious home she and Percy had built in the open spaces of Ravensbourne. Gerald and his grandmother enjoyed many outings together, long and vigorous walks, picnics by the river or at Caroline Bay, and evensong at the Anglican church. Gerald records that, at the end of his stays with her, his mother would drive down from Christchurch to collect him and stay overnight. He remembers many private and tearful discussions between the two women of an evening; there was no doubt what the subject was, although details were not shared with him. Nor were they shared widely with the Pickerill family back in England; indeed niece Vivien Jones informed the writer that her generation believed Mabel had died. Although Vivien and her sister, Sylvia Lamb, were always aware of some mystery about what happened to Mabel, divorce was never mentioned.

Pickerill's move to Australia in 1927 and their parents' divorce in 1934 must have been devastating for Mabel's children. It was particularly so for Kathleen; she was always reluctant to talk about it and, to the best of son Gerald's knowledge, saw her father only once after his remarriage. In her latter years she warmed to her half-sister Margaret Frazer.

Gerald Fogg believes that Val, the oldest, fell out with his father, who wanted him to study medicine. Val also suffered from the after-effects of the Second World War. Gerald speaks warmly of his Uncle Val, who built him a radio; he worked in broadcasting and, with wife Ailsa, lived in Abbotsford, a suburb of Dunedin.

Kana, as described by Gerald, was the child who most resembled his father, and was probably the closest to him, certainly in distance terms. He was a wool-buyer and, with his wife Eila and their two daughters, lived at Eastbourne, a suburb on the east side of Wellington Harbour.

Paul Pickerill had a distinguished career in dentistry, of which his father was probably very proud. Paul's wartime skills in maxillofacial surgery were mentioned prominently in the history of New Zealand Dental Services,[7] and were highly praised by Ferris Fuller, his commanding officer in the Second World War, who described him to this writer as a 'chip off the old block, totally dedicated to the care and treatment of his patients, a touch of genius in his clinical work, and just different from anyone else'. Paul was President of the New Zealand Dental Association in 1968–9, and died in Timaru in 1974; he is buried next to his mother.

Although older first-marriage descendants appear not to have developed easy relationships with Cecily, relations were warmer with the only child of the second marriage, Mary Margaret Ann (Frazer), who was born in July 1936. Margaret became a registered nurse, specialising in theatre work, and was at Lower Hutt Hospital at the time of her father's death.

The home of Percy and Cecily was Beechdale, a beautiful house in Silverstream in the Upper Hutt Valley north of Wellington. Margaret describes many happy gatherings there for her birthdays and at Christmas, often attended by members of the Clarkson family and by her half-brother Kana Pickerill and his wife, Eila. Extended caravan holidays were a feature of family life, as were outings over the Rimutaka Ranges for picnics in the Wairarapa district. Margaret described her father as not having many friends, and at times she thought he felt very isolated: perhaps an indication that all was not well in his relations with medical colleagues. Despite this he had many personal interests. They purchased the Beechdale property of four acres in 1935, and their English-style garden became one of Wellington's most acclaimed;[8] Margaret recalls many happy childhood days in the beautiful surroundings. Their dogs were a source of joy. Pickerill was a great outdoor person, and in his younger days mountaineering, tramping, and flyfishing were favourite recreations. Farming, too, was a major interest, and while he was still in Dunedin he owned a property at Heriot in West Otago where his Jersey cows were highly regarded; indeed, the clearance sale of his 'Meadows' Jersey stud in October 1926 attracted buyers from all over the country, and top prices were paid for the best of his pedigree stock.[9]

In his latter retirement years he kept up a vigorous flow of correspondence on various subjects to newspapers under the pseudonym 'Viator' (a 'traveller' or 'messenger'). He was an accomplished silversmith and a very keen photographer, the latter interest having existed from his early days in New Zealand, in his Urewera expeditions, his mountaineering, and his meticulous recording of his clinical work.

Henry Percy Pickerill died at Beechdale at 4 p.m. on 10 August 1956, just a week after his seventy-seventh birthday, and not long after his second coronary thrombosis. Apart from his deafness, he retained his faculties to the end. His loving daughter Margaret recalls that, as he lay back on his pillow, he said: 'I think I'll go to sleep now'. And so he did. His funeral took place at his parish church, St John's, Trentham, where he is remembered by an elegant memorial window. Cecily and Margaret took his ashes back to Hereford, where they were cast into the River Wye at Holme Lacy.

Sir Douglas Robb provides a fitting farewell:

> *Like other prophets he was known and admired beyond his own country and immediate sphere of his work. It will be a long time before we have another 'Pick'.*

References

1

1 Information on the Gurney family, the residences in Harold Street, and the Hereford Census provided by the Hereford Record Office, through J. Harnden.
2 Hereford Registration District. *Register of Births and Deaths.*
3 M.S.V. Gill to D. Bullar, grandson of Thomas Pickerill, 28 August 2004.
4 *Directory* for Herefordshire, 1891.
5 'Responsions' was previously a name describing the first of the three examinations once required for an academic degree at the University of Oxford.
6 Pickerill to F.W. Craddock, 3 November 1955. Pickerill Papers, Hocken Collections.

2

1 *University of Birmingham. Faculty of Medicine and Dentistry* (Booklet). University of Birmingham, 1982. This brief (18pp) publication is an excellent overview of the development of the Faculty and lists dates of significant events.
2 *Ibid.* (p. 4.)
3 R.A. Cohen. *The History of The Birmingham Dental Hospital and Dental School 1858–1958.* Birmingham: Board of Governors of the United Birmingham Hospitals, 1958. (p. 27)
4 University of Birmingham. *Proceedings at a Congregation of the University of Birmingham, holden on July sixth, MDCCCCI.*
5 University of Birmingham. *Proceedings at a Congregation of the University of Birmingham, holden on July fourth, MDCCCCIII.*
6 *University of Birmingham Calendar, 1899–1900.*
7 *University of Birmingham Calendar, 1901–1902.*
8 University of Birmingham. *Proceedings at a Congregation of the University of Birmingham, holden on July ninth, MDCCCCIV.*
9 University of Birmingham. *Proceedings at a Congregation of the University of Birmingham, holden on July eighth, MDCCCCV.*
10 Aesculapius [H.P. Pickerill]. *The Treatment of Caries in the Temporary Teeth Both with Regard to Their Own Well Being and the Influence Exerted by Their Condition Upon the Teeth of the Permanent Series.* Unpublished manuscript, 1902. Pickerill Papers, Hocken Collections.
11 Queen's College Medical Society. *Minute Book.*
12 *University of Birmingham Magazine* 1 No. 2, December 1900.
13 *University of Birmingham Magazine* 2 No. 4, March 1902.
14 *University of Birmingham Magazine* 3 [incorrectly titled Vol. 1] No. 3, November 1902.
15 *The Mermaid (University of Birmingham)* 1: 49, December 1904.
16 Guild of Undergraduates, University of Birmingham. *Minutes.*

17 *The Mermaid (University of Birmingham)* 2 No.1: 7–9, December 1905.
18 G.H. Duckworth to Pickerill, 15 April 1905. Pickerill Papers, Hocken Collections.
19 Minutes of the Meeting of the Students' Representative Council, 17 February 1903.
20 *The Mermaid* 1 No. 1: 1–2, October 1903.
21 O. Lodge. Testament supporting the application of H.P. Pickerill for the post of Director of the Dental School, University of Otago. Copy undated. Hocken Collectons AG180/33.
22 R.A. Cohen. *Sixty Years Being a History of the Birmingham Dental Students' Society 1886–1946, Together with a Short Account of Early Dentistry in Birmingham*. (Reprinted with additions from the *Birmingham Medical Review*, December 1946.
23 N.G. Bennett. The University of London and dental education. *British Dental Journal* 24: 781–96, December 1903. Following issues of the *BDJ* contained letters on the topic and a report of an Extraordinary General Meeting of the British Dental Association (*BDJ* 25: 91–131, February 1904), which concluded that the granting of degrees 'is undesirable'.
24 H.P. Pickerill. (Correspondence). *Evening Post* (Wellington), 29 July 1948.
25 *The Mermaid* 1 No. 1: 28–30, October 1904.
26 University of Birmingham. Report of the Senate. For Presentation to the Council on 4th April, 1906.

3

1 W.P. Morrell. *The University of Otago. A Centennial History*. Dunedin: University of Otago Press, 1969.
2 R.F. Stockwell. *The Origins of the Dental Profession in New Zealand.* Dunedin: New Zealand Dental Association, 1976. Collected reprints from the *NZDJ* 71, July 1975 to 72, July 1976.
3 Stockwell (p. 7–8).
4 J.H. Scott to the Dunedin Dental Examining Board. Quoted by Stockwell (p. 9).
5 Stockwell (p. 9).
6 Aspirations of 1890 (Correspondence). *NZDJ* 3: 104, April 1907.
7 T.W.H. Brooking. *A History of Dentistry in New Zealand*. Dunedin: New Zealand Dental Association, 1980 (p. 41).
8 Brooking (p. 42).
9 Scott to Edwin Cox. Quoted by Stockwell (p. 13).
10 Scott to Edwin Cox. Quoted by Stockwell (p. 13).
11 Brooking (p. 50).
12 Carter A.M. Dental legislation. *NZDJ* 1: 25–32, July 1905.
13 First Day's Proceedings of the New Zealand Dental Association at their Conference, held in Wellington, June, 1905. *NZDJ* 1: 9–24, July 1905.
14 Dental Conference at Wellington. *NZDJ* 1: 16–33, October 1905.
15 A call to action (Editorial). *NZDJ* 1: 3–4, October 1905.
16 Editorial. *NZDJ* 1: 3–4, January 1906.
17 *University of Otago Calendar*, 1906.
18 Discussion on the Dental Curriculum drawn up by the University N.Z. *NZDJ* 1: 16–27, 1905.
19 Council Minutes Vol. 3, 8 January 1906. Hocken Collections AG–180–1/03.
20 Report of the N.Z.D.A. Syllabus Committee. *NZDJ* 3: 112. April 1907.
21 Council Minutes Vol. 4, 14 January 1907. Hocken Collections AG–180–1/04.
22 Report of the Executive Committee, New Zealand Dental Association. *NZDJ* 1: 3–4, January 1905.

23 New Zealand Dental Conference *NZDJ* 2: 11, April 1907.

24 F.W. Thompson. Presidential Address. *NZDJ* 2: 112–20, April 1907.

4

1 A message from the late Dr. H.P. Pickerill. *NZDJ* 52: 193–4, October 1956.

2 James Belich, in *Paradise Reforged. A History of the New Zealanders*, Auckland: Penguin, 2001, p. 76–86, describes New Zealand as 'the Better Britain' and New Zealanders as 'Better Britons', terms that would have appealed to an ambitious young professional wanting to make his mark in the world.

3 M. King. *The Penguin History of New Zealand*. Auckland: Penguin Books, 2003 (p. 272).

4 W.P. Reeves. *The Long White Cloud*. Quoted by King (p. 269).

5 Pickerill application and testimonials. Staff Appointment Files. Hocken Collections AG–180/33/A.

6 Kennaway to the Registrar, 4 January 1907. Inward Letters No.12. Hocken Collections AG–180–28/12.

7 Council Minutes, 18 February 1907. Hocken Collections AG–180–1/04.

8 Council Minutes, adjourned meeting 19 February 1907. Hocken Collections AG–180–1/04.

9 High Commissioner to Pickerill. Inward Letters. Hocken Collections AG–180–28/12.

10 Registrar to Pickerill, 27 February 1907. Letterbook No. 7. Hocken Collections AG–180–30/8.

11 *ODT*, 20 February 1907.

12 Pickerill to Kennaway; Kennaway to Pickerill, 20 February 1907. Inward Letters No. 12. Hocken Collections AG–180–28/12.

13 High Commissioner to the Registrar, 22 February 1907. Inward Letters No. 12. Hocken Collections AG–180–28/12.

14 Registrar to the High Commissioner, 5 March 1907. Letterbook No. 7. Hocken Collections AG–180–30/8.

15 H.P. Pickerill. Salivary calculus in the submaxillary gland. *British Dental Journal* 27: 18–20, 1906.

16 Morrell (p. 90).

17 Kennaway to the Registrar, 31 August 1907. Council Minutes, 2 September 1907. Hocken Collections AG–180–1/03.

5

1 Council Minutes, Vol. 4, 7 October 1907. Hocken Collection AG–180/1/04.

2 H.P. Pickerill. Impressions on first arrival in New Zealand. *NZDJ* 3: 47–8, October 1907.

3 A message from the late Dr. H.P. Pickerill. *NZDJ* 52: 193–4, October 1956.

4 Taste of Tudor. *The New Zealand Woman's Weekly*, 6 November 1995 (p. 85).

5 Council Minutes Vol. 4, 11 December 1907. Hocken Collections AG–180–1/04.

6 A Chair of Dentistry established. *NZDJ* 5: 74–5, January 1908.

7 Pickerill to F.W. Craddock, 3 November 1955. Pickerill Papers, Hocken Collections.

6

1 School of Dental Science (1904–). The University of Melbourne. http://chs.unimelb.edu.au.programs

2 History of Dentistry at the University of Sydney. http://www.dentistry.usyd.edu.au
3 Owen Vivian Davies (Obituary). *NZDJ* 66: 364–7, October 1970.
4 R.F. Stockwell. Owen Vivian Davies (Obituary). *NZDJ* 66: 364–7, 1970.
5 H.P. Pickerill. Impressions on first arrival in New Zealand. *NZDJ* 3: 47–8, October 1907.
6 The Dental School. Opening Ceremony. *NZDJ* 3: 123–8, April 1908.
7 The Dental School, University of Otago (Editorial). *NZDJ* 4: 3–4, July 1908.
8 The Dental School (News item). *NZDJ* 4: 124, May 1909
9 The Dental School (News item). *NZDJ* 4: 36–7, December 1908.
10 University of Otago. *Syllabus of the Dental School 1908*. Pickerill Papers, Hocken Collections.
11 Minutes of the Faculty of Dentistry, University of Otago, 17 April 1918. Faculty Minutes of that period are included with the records of the NZDA, Otago Branch. Hocken Collections MS 0689/M.
12 H.P. Pickerill. Matters affecting dental education in New Zealand. *NZDJ* 4: 103–6, May 1909.
13 Advertisement. *NZDJ* 5: 37, July 1909.
14 The 'L.D.S.' of New South Wales (Editorial). *NZDJ* 5: 96–7, January 1910.
15 R. Cape-Williamson. The Dental Boards (Correspondence). *NZDJ* 5: 99–100, January 1910.
16 Association Intelligence. The Executive Council. *NZDJ* 5: 100–1, January 1910.
17 The Dental Curriculum in New Zealand (News and Comment). *NZDJ* 4: 15–16, July 1909.
18 The equipment of the Dental School (News item). *NZDJ* 5: 138–9, March 1910.
19 [Notes by] C.E. Hercus. Case of fracture of the upper and lower jaws. *NZDJ* 6: 62–3, October 1910.
20 *Syllabus of the Dental School. Loc cit.*
21 H.P. Pickerill *Prevention of Dental Caries and Oral Sepsis*. London: Ballière, Tindall and Cox, 1912.
22 H.P. Pickerill. *Physiological Secretion of the Salivary Glands in the Human Subject*. London: Ballière, Tindall and Cox, 1914.
23 These two theses, MD and MDS, are in the Library of the University of Birmingham.
24 H.P. Pickerill. *Stomatology in General Practice.* London: Oxford Medical Publications, 1912.
25 H.P. Pickerill. The medical aspects of dentistry and the necessity of dental instruction for medical students. (Paper read before the Otago Section of the British Medical Association). *NZDJ* 5: 125–32, March 1910. (Reprinted from the *British Medical Journal*, 15 February 1909.)
26 Falconer and Pickerill. *Otago Medical and Dental Schools' Pharmacopoeia*. Dunedin: John McIndoe, 1909.
27 O.V. Davies. *Otago Medical and Dental Schools' Pharmacopoeia*. (Book review). *NZDJ Journal* 5: 32–3, July 1909.
28 Pickerill to Council, 31 March 1909; Registrar to Pickerill, 1 April 1909. Letterbook No. 8. Hocken Collections AG–180–30/9.
29 Pickerill to Council, 2 July 1909. Inwards Letters No.15. Hocken Collections AG–180–28/15.
30 Pickerill to Council, 3 July 1910. Inwards Letters No. 18. Hocken Collections AG–180–28/18.
31 Copy of Agreement Sent to the High Commissioner for New Zealand, 24/11/06. Attachment to the Minutes of the Council of the University of Otago, August 1906 –

June 1910, adjourned meeting 19 February 1907. Hocken Collections AG–180–1/04.
32 Pickerill to the Registrar, 8 July 1910. Inwards Letters No.18. Hocken Collections AG–180–28/18.
33 Pickerill to Council, 4 November 1911. Inwards Letters No. 20. Hocken Collections AG–180–28/20.
34 Council Minutes, Vol. 5. Meeting of 6 November 1911. Hocken Collections AG–180–1/05.
35 Pickerill to Council, 16 September 1912. Inwards Letters No. 22. Hocken Collections AG–180–28/22.
36 Registrar to Pickerill, 19 September 1912. Letterbook Vol. 11. Hocken Collections AG–180–30/12.
37 Pickerill to the Chancellor, 4 May 1915. Inwards Letters No. 28. Hocken Collections AG–180–28/28.
38 Registrar to Pickerill, 21 July 1915. Letterbook No. 14. Hocken Collections AG–180–30/15.
39 The shortage of dental students – recent suggestions (News item). *NZDJ* 10: 165–7, March 1915.
40 Minutes of the Faculty of Dentistry, University of Otago. Report of the Director of the Dental School for the Year Ending 31 March 1915. Hocken Collections MS 0689/M.
41 Minutes of the Faculty of Dentistry, University of Otago, 14 October 1915. Hocken Collections MS 0689/M.
42 Minutes of the Faculty of Dentistry, University of Otago, 8 August 1916. Hocken Collections MS 0689/M.
43 Minutes of the Faculty of Dentistry, University of Otago. Report of the Director for the Year Ended 31 March 1916. Hocken Collections MS 0689/M.
44 Minutes of the Faculty of Dentistry, University of Otago. Report of the Acting Dean for the Year Ended 31 March 1917. Hocken Collections MS 0689/M.
45 Minutes of the Faculty of Dentistry, University of Otago, 8 December 1916. Hocken Collections MS 0689/M.
46 Minutes of the Council of the University of Otago, Volume 6, 1914–1919, Meeting of 19 December 1916. Hocken Collections AG-180–1/06.
47 Minutes of the Council of the University of Otago, Volume 6, 1914–1919, Meeting of 16 October 1916. Hocken Collections AG–180–1/05.
48 University of Otago General File No. 3. Hocken Collections AG–180–31/003.
49 Minutes of Meetings of the Council of the University of Otago, Vol. 6, 1914–1919. Special Meeting of 8 December 1916. Hocken Collections AG–180–1/06.
50 University of Otago General File No. 3. Hocken Collections AG–180–31/003.
51 University of Otago Inward Letters No. 29. Hocken Collections AG–180–28/29.
52 Minutes of Meetings of the Council of the University of Otago, Vol. 6, 1914–1919. Meeting of 21 December 1916. Hocken Collections AG–180–1/06.
53 University of Otago General File No. 25. Hocken Collections AG–180–31/0025.

7

1 'Aesculapius' [H.P. Pickerill]. The Treatment of Caries in the Temporary Teeth Both with Regard to Their Own Well Being and the Influence Exerted by Their Condition Upon the Teeth of the Permanent Series. Unpublished manuscript, 1902. Pickerill Papers, Hocken Collections.
2 Some technical details are included in this chapter to illustrate the nature and scope of his findings.

3 *Prevention of Dental Caries and Oral Sepsis* (Review). *NZDJ* 7:161–2, January 1912.
4 Quoted by J.R. Tagg. Studies of BLIS-ful oral bacteria. *NZDJ* 87: 14–16, 1991.
5 H. Cox. Auckland Branch. Presidential Address. *NZDJ* 9: 22–5, May 1913.
6 Auckland Branch. [Report of address by Professor H.P. Pickerill] *NZDJ* 9: 924, September 1913.
7 C.F. Bödecker to Pickerill, 21 November 1913. Pickerill Papers, Hocken Collections.
8 C.F. Bödecker. Enamel caries and immunity. *Review* 29: 338–44; 612–19, 1915
9 Tomes to Pickerill, 6 February 1912. Pickerill Papers, Hocken Collections.
10 H.P. Pickerill, Dr. Med. *Verhutung von Zahnkaries und Mundsepsis*. Berlin: Hermann Reusser, 1913.
11 *Verhutung von Zahnkaries und Mundsepsis* [Book review] *NZDJ* 9: 158, March 1913.
12 T. von Beust to Pickerill. Pickerill Papers, Hocken Collections.
13 H.P. Pickerill. Inspection of school children: method of charting the teeth. *NZDJ* 8: 133–40, September 1912.
14 *Prevention of Dental Caries and Oral Sepsis*. (Book review) *NZDJ* 11: 30–2, May 1915.
15 Interview with the Minister for Public Health (News item). *NZDJ* 8: 38–40, September 1912.
16 J. Binney, G. Chaplin, and C. Wallace *Mihaia. The Prophet Rua Kenana and His Community at Maungapohatu*. Auckland: Auckland University Press, 1979 (p. 109).
17 H.P. Pickerill and S.T. Champtaloup. An investigation into the causes of immunity to dental disease in the Maori of the Urewera. *NZDJ* 9: 169–82, March 1914.
18 Etiology of dental caries (Editorial). *NZDJ* 9: 187–9, March 1914.
19 This is a further quotation from Pickerill to Champtaloup. An investigation into the causes of immunity to dental disease in the Maori of the Urewera. *NZDJ* 9: 169–82.
20 H.P. Pickerill. The etiology of dental caries. *British Dental Journal* 36: 314–3, 1 April 1915; 36: 361–85, 15 April 1915. Reprinted in *NZDJ* 10: 129–38, January 1915; 11: 7–10, May 1915; and 11: 35–51, July 1915.
21 H.P. Pickerill. Recognition of research work prior to the War, 2/2689. Attachment to the military records of Henry Percy Pickerill. Wellington: New Zealand Defence Forces, 1920.
22 H.P. Pickerill. *Prevention of Dental Caries and Oral Sepsis*. London: Ballière, Tindall and Cox, third edition, 1923.
23 H.P. Pickerill. Salivary secretions and acid dentifrices. *NZDJ* 20: 64–71, September 1924.
24 Included in the Pickerill Papers, Hocken Collections.

8

1 Notes and General News. *NZDJ* 4: 96, March 1909.
2 F. Armstrong. A paper on the workings of the New Zealand Dental Association. *NZDJ* 4: 67–70, March 1909.
3 Fifth Annual Conference held at Parliament House, Wellington, January 1909. *NZDJ* 4: 107–9, May 1909.
4 W.F. Goulstone. The work of dental societies. [Paper presented to the Auckland Branch]. *NZDJ* 5: 121–4, March 1910.
5 Proceedings of Annual meeting, 1912. *NZDJ* 8: 85–9, November 1912.
6 H.P. Pickerill. Matters affecting dental education in New Zealand. *NZDJ* 4: 103–6, 1909.
7 The Executive Council. *NZDJ* 5: 26–8, October 1909.

8 Report of the 1910 Conference. *NZDJ* 6: 11–17, July 1910.
9 Annual meeting of the New Zealand Dental Association. Toronto Degree. *NZDJ* 7: 60–83, October 1911.
10 The back door (Editorial). *NZDJ* 6: 64–5, October 1910.
11 The Amendment Act (News and Comment). *NZDJ* 6: 142–3, April 1911.
12 New Zealand Parliamentary Debates. Reprinted in *NZDJ* 6: 107–12, January 1911.
13 Dentists Amendment Act. Reprinted in *NZDJ* 7: 124–5, January 1912.
14 Dental politics (Editorial). *NZDJ* 7: 120–1, January 1912.
15 New Zealand Dental Association. Annual Report and Balance Sheet. *NZDJ* 8: 52, September 1912.
16 Annual meeting, Wellington, July, 1913. Foreign degrees. *NZDJ* 9: 117–21, November 1913.
17 Dental Conference Proceedings. Registered dentists. *NZDJ* 12: 46, May 1916.
18 Fifth Annual Conference held at Parliament House, Wellington, January 1909. *NZDJ* 4: 71–2, March 1909.
19 Editorial. *NZDJ* 5: 9–10, July 1909.
20 Organisation (Editorial). *NZDJ* 5: 21–2, October 1909.
21 The parting of the ways. (Editorial). *NZDJ* 5: 135–6, March 1910.
22 The 'L.D.S.' of New South Wales (Editorial) *NZDJ* 4: 96–7, January 1910.
23 The back door (Editorial). *NZDJ* 6: 65–6, October 1910.
24 Retrogression (Editorial). *NZDJ* 6: 103–4, January 1911.
25 The Debate in the House on the Dentists Amendment Bill. NZDJ 6: 107–12, January 1911.
26 Association Intelligence. Annual meeting. *NZDJ* 7: 53, October 1911.
27 *Sine curriculo* degrees (Editorial). *NZDJ* 7: 51–2, October 1911.
28 The recent Conference (Editorial). *NZDJ* 7: 22–3, July 1911.
29 Annual meeting. *NZDJ* 7: 54–7, October 1911.
30 New Zealand Dental Association. Discussion on the 1912 Annual Report and Balance Sheet. *NZDJ* 8: 51–4, September 1912.

9

1 Belich, *loc. cit.* (p. 81).
2 Annual Meeting of the New Zealand Dental Association, 11–14 July 1911. *NZDJ* 7: 85–6, October 1911.
3 H.P. Pickerill. Recognition of research work prior to the War, 2/2689. Attachment to the military records of Henry Percy Pickerill. Wellington: New Zealand Defence Forces, 1920.
4 Dentistry and the War (Editorial) *NZDJ* 10: 85–6, September 1914.
5 Report from the Auckland Branch. *NZDJ* 10: 89–90, September 1914.
6 Dentistry with the Expeditionary Force (News item). *NZDJ* 10: 117, November 1914.
7 Dentists with Expeditionary Force. *NZDJ* 10: 117, November 1914.
8 Dental examiners to the forces (Editorial). *NZDJ* 10: 150–1, January 1915.
9 The War and the dental profession (Editorial). *NZDJ* 11: 25–6, May 1915.
10 *Ibid.*
11 University of Otago Inward Letters No. 28. 31 May 1915. Hocken Collections AG-180-28/28.
12 University of Otago Inward Letters No. 28, 14 June 1915. Hocken Collections AG-180-28/28.
13 University of Otago Inward Letters No. 28, 29 June 1915. Hocken Collections AG-28-28/28.

14 University of Otago Inward Letters No. 29, 25 August 1915. Hocken Collections AG-28-28/29
15 Minutes of the Faculty of Dentistry, University of Otago. Report of the Director for the Year Ended 31 March 1915. Hocken Collections MS 0689/N.
16 J.H. Don. Making history. Dentistry in the trenches at Gallipoli. *NZDJ* 11: 70, September 1915.
17 An official dental service (Editorial). *NZDJ* 11: 87–9, September 1915.
18 *Ibid.*
19 Military records, Department of Defence, Wellington.
20 *New Zealand Gazette* No. 143, 16 December 1915.
21 The N.Z. Dental Corps (Editorial). *NZDJ* 129–30, November 1915.
22 Progress of the New Zealand Dental Corps (Editorial). *NZDJ* 160–1, January 1916.
23 Council Minutes Vol. 6, 21 December 1915. Hocken Collections AG-180-1/06.
24 Dental treatment of returned soldiers (News item). *NZDJ* 11: 162, January 1916.
25 Davies to Secretary, Otago Branch, 4 August 1916. NZDA Otago Branch, Correspondence, 1912–18. Hocken Collections MS-0689/A
26 Treatment of recruits and returned soldiers. Debate at Annual Meeting, May 1916. *NZDJ* 12: 7–30, May 1916.
27 Otago University Officer Training Corps. Military Committee Minute Book and Correspondence, Hocken Collections 95–157. Box 26.
28 Minutes of the Meetings of the Council of the University of Otago, Vol. 6, 1914–1919. Meeting of 21 December 1916. Hocken Collections AG-180-31/0025.
29 The departure of Dr. Pickerill ('Passing notes'). *NZDJ* 12: 180–1, March 1917.
30 *Ibid.*
31 B.S. Finn. The Dental Unit on active service. *British Dental Journal* 38: 33–40, January 1917. Reprinted in *NZDJ* 12: 204–8, May 1917.

10

1 The departure of Dr. Pickerill ('Passing notes'). *NZDJ* 12: 180–1, March 1917.
2 Minutes of the Faculty of Dentistry, University of Otago, 3 April 1911. Hocken Collections MS 0689/M.
3 H.P. Pickerill. Double resection of the mandible. *Dental Cosmos* 54: 114–19, 1912.
4 Christchurch Branch (News item). *NZDJ* 8: 91, November 1912.
5 Southland Branch (News item). *NZDJ* 8: 91–2, November 1912.
6 Reported from a meeting of the Professorial Board, *ODT*, 17 November 1913.
7 H.P. Pickerill. Cleft palate. *Dental Cosmos* 57: 1304–5, 1915.
8 H.P. Pickerill. Treatment of fractured mandible accompanying gunshot wounds. *NZDJ* 12: 75–80, July 1916.
9 War Supplement. *British Dental Journal* 37: 1– 232, 1916.

11

1 H.P. Pickerill. New Zealand Expeditionary Force, Jaw Department. *NZDJ* 13: 35–8, September 1917.
2 A.D. Macalister. The Queen's Hospital, Sidcup: the Foundation of British Oral Surgery. The Menzies Campbell Lecture, The Royal College of Surgeons of England, 1987. (Unpublished). Pickerill Papers, Hocken Collections.
3 H.P. Pickerill. *NZDJ* September 1917. *Op. cit.*
4 *NZDJ* 13: facing page 96, January 1918.

5 HM Queen Mary. *Requiescat in Pace et Honore.* Unpublished and undated manuscript. Pickerill Papers, Hocken Collections.

6 H.P. Pickerill. *War Diary: New Zealand Section of the Queen's Hospital, Sidcup, England.* 14 July 1918. Archives New Zealand (Wellington) War Archives Series 143, Item 1.

7 R. Pound. *Gillies. Surgeon Extraordinary.* London: Michael Joseph, 1964 (p. 15).

8 A. Bamji. Gillies: an historical vignette. *Trauma* 1: 267–9, 1999.

9 Brochure. *The Queen's Hospital Sidcup Kent, 1917–1929* Undated. Publisher not stated.

10 H.P. Pickerill. Untitled and undated manuscript, Pickerill Papers, Hocken Collections.

11 *The Queen's Hospital Sidcup Kent, 1917–1929. Op. cit.* (p. 4).

12 A.N. Bamji The Macalister Archive: records from The Queen's Hospital, Sidcup, 1917–21. *Journal of Audiovisual Media in Medicine* 16: 76–84, 1913.

13 *The London Times*, 22 January 1918.

14 Pound (p. 14).

15 Pickerill. *Op. cit.*

16 Macalister. *Op. cit.*

17 A. Bamji. Personal communication.

18 S.J. Callister *War, Seen Through Photographs, Darkly; the Photographic Representation of World War One from a New Zealand Perspective.* A thesis submitted in partial fulfilment of the requirements for a Doctorate of Philosophy, The University of Auckland, November 2005. In the chapter 'Broken gargoyles. The photographic representation of severely wounded New Zealand soldiers' (p. 168–215), Dr Callister very movingly describes the archive more fully, and examines what the injuries might have meant to the men concerned. The water-colours are of particular interest. The senior artist at Sidcup was Henry Tonks, Professor of Fine Arts at the Slade School of Fine Arts, and other artists included Daryl Lindsay and Herbert R. Cole.

19 New Zealand Section *War Diary. Op. cit.*

20 Macalister. *Op. cit.*

21 A.D. Carbery. *The New Zealand Medical Services in the Great War 1914–1918.* Auckland: Whitcombe and Tombes, 1924 (p. 488).

22 Pickerill to the Chancellor, 11 January 1918. University of Otago General File No. 9 Hocken Collections AG–180–31/0009.

23 Registrar to Pickerill, 6 April 1918. University of Otago General File No. 9. Hocken Collections AG–180–31/0009.

24 Pickerill to the Chancellor, 7 April 1918. University of Otago General File No. 9. Hocken Collections AG–180–31/009.

25 G. Harper. *Spring Offensive. New Zealand and the Second Battle of the Somme.* Chapter 9: Weathering the Storm: 5 April 1918. Auckland: Harper Collins, 2003 (p. 140–50). On a personal note, the present writer's uncle, Private Reginald Herbert Belliss, NZRB, was killed in this battle on 6 April 1918.

26 Richardson to Pickerill, 2 June 1918. Pickerill Papers. Hocken Collections.

27 Allen to Pickerill, 4 September 1918. Pickerill Papers. Hocken Collections.

28 New Zealand Section *War Diary. Op. cit.*

29 H.D. Gillies. *Plastic Surgery of the Face. Based on Selected Cases of War Injuries of the Face Including Burns*. London: Hodder and Stoughton, 1920 (Fig. 363, p. 195).

30 Pound (p. 54).

31 H.P. Pickerill. Intra-oral skin-grafting: the establishment of the buccal sulcus. *Proceedings of the Royal Society of Medicine* 12: 17–22, 1919.

32 Gillies (p. 9).

33 H.P. Pickerill. *Facial Surgery*. Edinburgh: Livingstone, 1924 (p. 10).

34 H.L. Hunt. *Plastic Surgery of the Head, Face, and Neck*. Philadelphia: Lea and Febiger, 1926 (p. 97).
35 Pound (p. 62).
36 H.P. Pickerill. *Facial Surgery (*p. 24),
37 Amy Gambier to Margaret Frazer, 4 January 1969. Pickerill Papers, Hocken Collections.
38 H.D. Gillies and D.R. Millard *The Principles and Art of Plastic Surgery*. Boston: Little Brown, 1957.
39 Gillies to Pickerill, 5 February 1955. Pickerill Papers, Hocken Collections.
40 Photographic group (News item). *NZDJ* 14: 13; photograph p. 14, July 1918.
41 King (p. 301–3).
42 Photographic group. *Op. cit.*
43 H.P. Pickerill. Methods of control of fragments in gunshot wounds of the jaws. *The Lancet* 1: 313–16, 7 September 1918. Reprinted in *NZDJ* 14: 109–18, January 1919.
44 H.P. Pickerill. Orthodontics in war surgery. *NZDJ* 14: 140–1, March 1919.
45 H.P. Pickerill. *Facial Surgery*. Thesis for the Master of Surgery (ChM) of the University of Birmingham, Faculty of Medicine, 1923.

12

1 Richardson to Pickerill, 22 December 1918. Pickerill Papers, Hocken Collections.
2 W. Wright to Pickerill, 13 January 1919. Pickerill Papers. Hocken Collections.
3 *Evening Star*, 6 March 1919. Otago Hospital Board Cuttings Book 1918-1919. Archives New Zealand (Dunedin) DAHI D292/5c.
4 Otago Hospital Board (OHB) Minutes 1915-1921. Ordinary Meeting, 20 March 1919. Archives New Zealand (Dunedin) DAHI D270/3.
5 J. Angus. *A History of the Otago Hospital Board and Its Predecessors*. Dunedin: OHB, 1984 (p.153).
6 *Evening Star*, 26 March and 21 May 1919. OHB Cuttings Book 1918-1919. Archives New Zealand (Dunedin) DAHI/D292/6a.
7 Jaw Hospital. *The New Zealand Red Cross Record* April-May 1919 (p.12). New Zealand Red Cross, Dunedin Branch 96-113/92.
8 *Evening Star*, 21 May 1919.
9 OHB Minutes 1915-1921. Ordinary Meetings 26 June and 24 July 1919. Archives New Zealand (Dunedin) DAHI D270/3.
10 Pickerill to the Chancellor, 21 June 1919. University of Otago General File No. 17. Hocken Collections AG-180-31/0017.
11 *Otago Daily Times* (*ODT*), 19 May 1919 ('Facial Disfigurment'); *Evening Star*, 6 November 1919 ('Salvage').
12 *Otago Witness*, 28 May 1919.
13 *Otago Witness*, 9 July 1919.
14 Pickerill to the Director General of Medical Services, 14 June 1919; A. Gray to Pickerill, 9 June 1919. Archives New Zealand (Wellington) AD 1, Box 1224, 49/229/1. Dental Hospital – Dunedin, 1916-26.
15 Jaw Section, Otago. *NZDJ* 15: 74-6, September 1919.
16 F. Armstrong (Correspondence and circular to Executive). *NZDJ* 15: 103-4, January 1920.
17 Otago Hospital Board (OHB) Minutes 1915-1921. Ordinary Meeting 22 October 1919. Archives New Zealand (Dunedin) DAHI D270/3.
18 Pickerill to Ferguson, 17 April 1920; Ferguson to Pickerill, 20 April 1920. Medical School Correspondence 1920, Hocken Collections 94-121-4.

19 OHB Minutes 1915-1921. Ordinary Meeting, 22 April 1920. Archives New Zealand (Dunedin) DAHI D270/3.
20 Secretary, Otago Hospital and Charitable Aid Board (OHCAB) to the Registrar, University of Otago General File No. 39. Hocken Collections AG-180-31/0039.
21 Secretary, OHCAB to the Registrar, 25 June 1920. University of Otago General File No. 39. Hocken Collections AG-180-31/0039.
22 OHB Minutes 1915-1921. Ordinary Meeting, 22 July 1920. Archives New Zealand (Dunedin) DAHI D270/3.
23 University of Otago General File No. 25. Hocken Collections AG-180-31/0025.
24 Registrar to Officer in Charge, War Expenses Office, NZ Military Forces, 8 April 1920. University of Otago General File No. 25. Hocken Collections AG-180-31/0025.
25 Council Minutes Vol. 7. Meeting of 20 April 1920. Hocken Collections AG-189-1/07.
26 Report of meeting of the Medical Committee 29 June 1920. University of Otago Committee Reports, Vol. 3A, December 1919 – March 1924. Hocken Collections AG-180-2-03A.
27 OHB Minutes 1915-1921. Ordinary Meeting, 28 October 1920. Archives New Zealand (Dunedin) DAHI D270/3.
28 OHB Minutes 1915-1921. Ordinary Meeting, 16 December 1920. Archives New Zealand (Dunedin) DAHI D270/3.
29 Proceedings of a Court of Inquiry (Defence Headquarters) in the 1st day of December, 1920. Archives New Zealand (Wellington) AD1, Box 1250, 49/755, Hospital Military – Dunedin.
30 S. Marshall, Assistant Director of Medical Services (Southern), to Director General of Medical Services, 14 December 1921. Dental Hospital – Dunedin, 1916-1926. Archives New Zealand (Wellington) AD 1, Box 1224, 49/229/1.
31 The extensive correspondence on the fate of the records is held in Archives New Zealand (Wellington) AD 1, Box 1224, 49/229/1, Dental Hospital – Dunedin, 1916-1926. A further record source is a file prepared by Captain Turner, NZDC, one of Pickerill's assistants at Sidcup. This is a collection of radiographs of patients with gunshot wounds to the mandible, accompanied by Turner's own superb line drawings from the radiographs and details of the splints for which he was responsible; case notes are included. This file is currently held in Defence Dental Headquarters, Wellington.
32 One gain from the War … *ODT*, 19 September 1923.

13

1 The shortage in dental students (Editorial). *NZDJ* 10: 178–80, March 1915.
2 The shortage of dental students – recent suggestions (News item). *NZDJ* 10: 165–7, March 1915.
3 Minutes of the Faculty of Dentistry, University of Otago, 30 May 1917. Hocken Collections MS 0689/M.
4 C. Hay to C.H. Moses, 7 August 1917. Davies Papers, Box 4, File 1. Hocken Collections MS 1146.
5 Minutes of the Faculty of Dentistry, University of Otago. Report of the Acting Director for the Year Ended 31 March 1917. Hocken Collections MS 0689/M.
6 Minutes of the Faculty of Dentistry, University of Otago, 17 April 1918. Hocken Collections MS 0689/M.
7 O.V. Davies Papers, Box 4, File 1. Hocken Collections MS 1146.
8 Minutes of the Faculty of Dentistry, University of Otago. Report of the Acting Director for the Year Ended 31 March 1918. Hocken Collections MS 0689/M.

9 Pickerill to the Council, 3 July 1910. Inwards Letter No. 18. Hocken Collections AG–180–28–18.

10 Pickerill to the Registrar, 21 September 1910. Inward Letters No.18. Hocken Collections AG–180–28–18.

11 Davies Papers, Box 8. Hocken Collections MS 1146.

12 O.V. Davies, G.V. Black. Club methods. *NZDJ* 7: 106–10; Discussion, 110–14, Jan. 1912.

13 Pickerill to Davies, 21 March 1912 (supplied to the Chancellor); Davies to the Chancellor, 22 March 1912; Pickerill to the Chancellor, 29 May 1912; Allen to Davies, 2 June 1912. Letterbook No. 21. Hocken Collections AG–180–28/21.

14 O.V. Davies. A short history of the founding of the New Zealand Dental Association *NZDJ* 51: 94–101, July 1955.

15 Pickerill to M. Priestley, 27 July 1955. Pickerill Papers, Hocken Collections.

16 Priestley to Pickerill, 1 August 1955. Pickerill Papers, Hocken Collections.

17 Davies to the Registrar, 20 March 1917. General File No. 3. Hocken Collections AG–180–31/003.

18 Davies to the Registrar, 31 August 1917. General File No. 9. Hocken Collections AG–180–31/009.

19 Pickerill to the Public Service Commissioner, 5 September 1919. University of Otago General File No. 34. Hocken Collections AG–180–31/0034.

20 University of Otago Council. General File No. 9. Hocken Collections AG–180–31/0009.

21 Pickerill to the Chancellor, 12 July 1919. General File No. 25. Hocken Collections AG–180–31/0025.

22 Minister of Defence to the Chancellor, 2 March 1920. General File No. 25. Hocken Collections AG–180–31/0025.

23 Registrar to Pickerill, 3 July 1919. University of Otago General File No. 17. Hocken Collections AG–180–31/0017.

24 Davies to the Vice Chancellor, 9 July 1920. Davies Papers, Box 8. Hocken Collections MS 1146.

25 Owen Vivian Davies (Obituary). *NZDJ* 66: 364–7. October 1970.

26 Dr. Raynor Colin Bell (Obituary). *NZDJ* 21: 227–8, May 1926.

27 Scott and Pickerill to the Otago Hospital Board, 5 September 1915. Otago Hospital Board Minutes. National Archives (Dunedin) HDAHI D289/17.

28 Otago Hospital and Charitable Aid Board Special Committee Report to the Resgistrar, 17 October 1912. Inward Letters No. 22. Hocken Collections AG–180–28/22.

29 Sixth Annual Dental School report, 1913. Inwards Letters No. 23. Hocken Collections AG–180–28/23.

30 Pickerill to Registrar, 1 April 1914. Inwards Letters No. 25. Hocken Collections AG–180–28/25.

31 Secretary of the Board to the Registrar 20 October 1917. General File No. 13. Hocken Collections AG–180–31/0013.

32 Pickerill to the Registrar, 4 August 1921. General File No. 43. Hocken Collections AG–180–31/43.

33 *Evening Star*, 28 October 1921.

34 Secretary of the Board to the Registrar, 29 November 1921. General File No. 47. Hocken Collections AG–180–31–0047.

35 Pickerill to the Registrar, 15 September 1922. General File No. 31. Hocken Collections AG–180–31/00.

36 Cuddie (Otago Branch Secretary) to Registrar, 30 April 1923; Registrar to Cuddie 11 May 1923; Cuddie to Registrar, 16 May 1923. General File No. 58. Hocken Collections AG–180–31/0058.

37 Pickerill to the registrar, 10 May 1923. General file No. 58. Hocken Collections AG–180–31/0058.
38 Board Secretary to the Registrar, 29 November 1921. General File No. 39. Hocken Collections AG–180–31/0039.
39 Pickerill to the Registrar, 5 April 1922; Registrar to Pickerill 17 May 1922. General File No. 51. Hocken Collections AG–180–31/0051.
40 Registrar to Bell 29 November 1922; Pickerill to Registrar, 13 December 1922; Bell to the Registrar, 14 December 1922. General File No. 58. Hocken Collections AG–180–31/0058.
41 Otago Hospital Board Minutes, 1921–25, Ordinary Meeting 22 March 1923. National Archives (Dunedin) DAHI D270/4; Secretary, Hospital Board to Registrar 15 June 1923 and 1 October 1923. General File No. 67. Hocken Collections AG–180–31/0067; Registrar to Pickerill 4 July 1923. General File No. 65. Hocken Collections AG–180–31/065; Secretary, Hospital Board to Registrar 9 April 1924. General File No. 83. Hocken Collections AG–180–31/0083.
42 Pickerill to Registrar 20 May 1927. General File No.108. Hocken Collections AG–180–31–/108; and Registrar to Pickerill, 20 July 1927. General File No. 115. Hocken Collections AG–180–31/115.
43 Pickerill to the Council, 1 February 1911. Inwards Letter No. 18. Hocken Collections AG–180–28/18.
44 Minutes of the Faculty of Dentistry, University of Otago, 3 April 1911. Hocken Collections MS 0689/M.
45 Pickerill to the Chancellor, 29 June 1915. Inwards Letters No. 28. Hocken Collections AG–180–28/18.
46 Pickerill to the Registrar, 17 May 1921. General File No. 43. Hocken Collections AG–180–31/0043.
47 Meeting of the Medical Committee, 27 March 1922. Committee Reports, Vol. 3. Hocken Collections AG–180–2/03A.
48 *ODT*, 24 April 1923; 26 April 1923.
49 Report on Dental School. General File No. 58. Hocken Collections AG–180–31/0058.
50 Report of the Dental Conference, 21 May 1920. *NZDJ* 15: 69–70, July 1920.
51 NZDA, Minutes of the Executive Council, 17 November 1920 and 1 December 1920. *NZDJ* 16: 169–71, January 1921.
52 NZDA, Minutes of the Executive Council, 1 February 1921. *NZDJ* 16: 205, March 1921.
53 Report of the 1921 NZDA Conference. *NZDJ* 16: 49–52, July 1921.
54 *Ibid.*
55 Registrar to the Secretary NZDA, 20 July 1921. *NZDJ* 17: 96, September 1921.
56 NZDA, Minutes of the Executive Council, 13 October 1921. *NZDJ* 16: 126–7, September 1921.
57 NZDA, Minutes of the Executive Council, 13 November 1921. *NZDJ* 17: 175–85, March 1922.
58 Dentists' Act Amendment Bill (Editorial). *NZDJ* 17: 163–4, March 1922.
59 Syllabus for Special Examination to be held in December, 1922, in accordance with Section 7 (1) (C) of the Dentists Amendment Act, 1921. *NZDJ* 18: 6–9, July 1922.
60 University of New Zealand. Examinations in Dentistry. *NZDJ* 18: 142–4, March 1923.
61 Annual Dinner of the Association. *NZDJ* 20: 34, July 1924.
62 NZDA, Minutes of the Executive Council, 7 February 1923. *NZDJ* 18: 156, March 1923.
63 Passing Notes. *NZDJ* 18: 141, May 1923.
64 NZDA, Minutes of the Executive Council, 11 November 1924. *NZDJ* 19: 104–6, November 1924.

65 Editorial. *NZDJ* 22: 1–4, September 1926.
66 H.P. Pickerill. *Prevention of Dental Caries and Oral Sepsis*. London: Ballière Tindall & Cox, third edition, 1923.
67 *Prevention of Dental Caries and Oral Sepsis* (Review). *Dental Record* 45: 27–8, 1925.
68 H.P. Pickerill. Surgical conditions of the jaws in relation to mastication and development. *NZDJ* 20: 23–31, July 1924.
69 Pickerill to Hercus 6 August 1954 (enclosure). Pickerill Letters *in* Hercus Papers. Hocken Collections MS–1533/35.
70 H.P. Pickerill. *Facial Surgery*. Edinburgh: Livingstone, 1924.
71 H.D. Gillies, *Plastic Surgery of the Face. Based on Selected Cases of War Injuries of the Face Including Burns*. London: Oxford University Press and Hodder and Stoughton, 1919.
72 Facial surgery (Book reviews). *The Lancet* 241–2, 31 January 1925.
73 H.P. Pickerill. *Stomatology*. Dunedin: McIndoe, second edition,1925.
74 *Stomatology* (Review). *NZDJ* 21: 180–1, March 1926.
75 *Stomatology in General Practice* (Book review). *British Dental Journal* 47: 844–5, 1926.
76 H.P. Pickerill (Correspondence) *British Dental Journal* 47: 1257–8, 1927
77 H. Allaeys to Pickerill, 7 July 1921. Pickerill Papers, Hocken Collections.
78 J. de Arkovy to Pickerill, undated. Pickerill Papers, Hocken Collections.

14

1 'Aesculapius' [H.P. Pickerill]. *The Treatment of Caries in the Temporary Teeth Both with Regard to Their Own Well Being and the Influence Exerted by Their Condition Upon the Teeth of the Permanent Series*. Unpublished manuscript, 1902. Pickerill Papers, Hocken Collections.
2 F.W. Thomson. The teeth of our children. *NZDJ* 1: 11–20, January 1906.
3 Editorial. *NZDJ* 2: 71, January 1907.
4 Correspondence. *NZDJ* 4: 129–30, May 1909.
5 Society for the Health of Women and Children. Fifth Annual Report. Annual Reports of Council, 1908–1923. Hocken Collections AG–007–001–003/001.
6 Editorial. *NZDJ* 6: 9–10, July 1909.
7 T.A. Hunter. On the duty of the State and the public towards the prevention of dental diseases. *NZDJ* 6: 2–7, July 1910.
8 A. Paterson. Presidential Address to Seventh Annual General Meeting, Wellington, 1911. *NZDJ* 7: 1–9; 30–1, July 1911.
9 H.P. Pickerill. Inspection of school children: method of charting the teeth. *NZDJ* 8: 33–8, September 1912.
10 Interview with the Minister of Public Health. *NZDJ* 8: 38–43, September 1912.
11 *Ibid*.
12 After many years (Editorial). *NZDJ* 8: 26–8, July 1912.
13 Medical inspectors of schools and the examination of the teeth. *NZDJ* 8: 41–3 September 1912.
14 School dentistry (Editorial). *NZDJ* 8: 84–5, November 1912.
15 Annual Meeting of the New Zealand Dental Association, 1912. *NZDJ* 8: 149–52, March 1913.
16 N.K. Cox. Presidential Address to the Ninth Annual Meeting of the New Zealand Dental Association. *NZDJ* 9: 33–7, July 1913.

17 Discussion, *NZDJ* 9: 38–47, July 1913.
18 A School Dental Service (Editorial). *NZDJ* 9: 56–8, July 1913.
19 State Dentistry. Deputation to the Minister. *NZDJ* 9: 48–50, July 1913.
20 Editorial, *NZDJ*, July 1913, *Loc. cit.*
21 News and Comments. *NZDJ* 10: 19, May 1914.
22 R. Dunn The prevention of dental disease and the adequacy of dental service. *NZDJ* 12: 198–203, May 1917.
23 N. Cox. State dentistry. *NZDJ* 12: 276–84, May 1917.
24 Dental education. Extending the facilities. Important debate. *NZDJ* 12: 269–76, May 1917.
25 Report of State School Committee set up by the New Zealand Dental Association, April 25th, 1917. *NZDJ* 13: 70–1, November 1917.
26 State School Committee. N.Z. Dental Association's Deputation to Hon. G.W. Russell and Hon. J.A. Hanan. *NZDJ* 13: 73–8, November 1913.
27 Editorial. *NZDJ* 13: 65–6, November 1917.
28 Dr. H.B. Macdonald's letter on the dental problem [to the Auckland Hospital and Charitable Aid Board]. *NZDJ* 13: 49–50, September 1917.
29 Dental service to schools (Editorial). *NZDJ* 14: 137–8, March 1919.
30 Minutes of a Special Meeting of the Executive Council, 6 March 1920. The position of Chief Dental Officer (Association News). *NZDJ* 15: 157–8, March 1920.
31 Thirteenth Annual Conference. Cheif Dental Officer. *NZDJ* 16: 28–30, July 1920.
32 Minutes of the Faculty of Dentistry, University of Otago. Special Meeting, 12 July 1920. Hocken Collections MS 0689/M.
33 Pickerill to the Registrar, 13 July 1920. General File No. 34. Hocken Collections AG–180–31/0034.
34 Minutes of the Executive Council, 26 July 1920. *NZDJ* 16: 111, September 1920.
35 State dental scheme. Serious complications. Important legal opinion. *ODT*, 17 November 1920.
36 Dental treatment of school children. Statement by Dr Pickerill. *ODT*, 20 November 1920.
37 The methods of Mr Parr (Editorial). *ODT*, 20 November 1920.
38 State Dental Scheme, *ODT*, 22 November 1922. (The Minister's response to Pickerill's rejoiner; Armstrong's letter.)
39 *ODT*, 23 November 1920 (Editorial); 25 November (opposition by Otago and Canterbury dentists); 27 November ('A woman's point of view'); 29 November (Wanganui and Auckland opinions); 30 November (further rejoiner by Pickerill); 9 December (reply by Hunter to Pickerill, Pickerill's response; opposition from Wanganui dentists, Dunedin Women Citizens' Association, and Dunedin branch of the New Zealand Education Institute); 10 December (editorial opposing the scheme); 15 December (statement by Hunter and reply by Pickerill).
40 Report of a Special Meeting of the NZDA Executive, 5 September 1920. *NZDJ* 15: 140, November 1920.
41 An Auckland opinion. *ODT*, 29 Novenber 1920.
42 Moses to Davies, 2 December 1920. Davies Papers, Box 3. Hocken Collections MS–1146.
43 *ODT*, 23 November 1920.
44 School children's dental troubles. Government scheme condemned. *ODT*, 9 December 1920.
45 Major Gray to the Chancellor, 11 December 1920: the Registrar to Gray. University of Otago General File No. 34. Hocken Collections AG–180–31–0034.

46 The State Dental Scheme and the New Zealand Dental Association (Editorial). *NZDJ* 16: 145–8, January 1921.
47 Minutes of the NZDA Executive Council, 1 December 1920. *NZDJ* 16: 171–5, January 1921.
48 The Government Scheme for the training of dental nurses. (Report by the Director of State School Dental Service.) *NZDJ* 16: 179–81, March 1921.
49 Dental service to the children (Editorial). *NZDJ* 16: 177–8, March 1921.
50 President's Address and discussion. *NZDJ* 17: 2–11, July 1921.
51 T.A. Hunter. Progress of School Service, Dental Hygiene. *NZDJ* 17: 216–9; Discussion, 219–20, May 1922.
52 H. Ziele. Correspondence. *NZDJ* 17: 96, 1923.
53 Dental nurses in New Zealand (News item). *NZDJ* 17: 127, November 1923.
54 Correspondence involving the NZDA Secretary and Treasurer, the Secretary of the Otago Branch NZDA, the NZDA's Solicitor and Pickerill to 19 March 1923 when Pickerill resigned. The resignation was accepted on 11 April 1923, and the Otago Branch informed. Records of the NZDA, Otago Branch. Hocken Collections, MS 0689/C and L.
51 'Dr. Pickerill's criticism'; Hunter's letter to the *Spectator*; extract from *New Zealand Herald*, 30 November 1927. *NZDJ* 23: 82–6, January 1928.

15

1 E. Siedeberg to Davies, 24 April 1918. General File No. 9. Hocken Collections AG–180–31/0009.
2 Davies to the Council, 25 March 1919; 4 February 1920; Pickerill to the Council, 16 July 1920. General File No. 17. Hocken Collections AG–180–31/0017.
3 Pickerill to the Registrar, 10 April 1922. General File No. 51. Hocken Collections AG–180–31/0051.
4 King (p.317).
5 Pickerill to the Registrar, 2 May 1922. General File No. 51. Hocken Collections AG–180–31/0051.
6 A boy's death. Succumbs under anaesthetic. *ODT*, 18 May 1922.
7 Dental School, Overcrowded building, Efficient teaching impossible, Patients put to discomfort (Article). A congested institution (Editorial). *ODT*, 19 May 1922.
8 Pickerill to the Registrar, 12 October 1922; Bell to Pickerill, 16 October 1922. General File No. 58. Hocken Collections AG–180–31/0058.
9 Pickerill to the Registrar, 17 February, 1923. General File No. 58. Hocken Collections AG–180–31/0058.
10 Council Meeting, 29 February 1923. Council Minutes Vol. 7 Hocken Collections AG–180–1/07.
11 The Dental School. 'Shocking conditions'. *ODT*, 18 April 1923.
12 The Dental School (Editorial). *ODT*, 19 April 1923.
13 Pickerill to the Registrar, 19 April 1923. General File No. 58. Hocken Collections AG–180–31/0058.
14 Report of a Special Committee set up to formulate a request to be placed before the Prime Minister setting out the necessities of the University in their order of urgency, 4 May 1923. Committee Reports Vol. 3A. Hocken Collections AG–180–2/03A.
15 Report signed by 89 students to the Registrar (undated). General File No. 58. Hocken Collections AG–180–31/0058.
16 Pickerill to the Registrar, 25 May 1923. General File No. 65. Hocken Collections AG–180–31/65.

17 Pickerill to the Registrar, 19 March 1924. General File No. 70. Hocken Collections AG–180–31/0070.
18 Morrell (p.134).
19 Otago University. Position of Special Schools. Mr Fowld's complaint. Reply by Dr Cameron. *ODT*, 20 June 1923. This is a full report of the Council meeting, 19 June 1923.
20 Report of the Dental Committee to the Minister of Education, 21 December 1923. Hocken Collections AG–180–31/70.
21 Report by the Dean of the Dental Faculty submitted to the Otago University Council on the Report of the Committee Set Up by the Minister of Education to Inquire into the 'Provision of Accommodation for the Training of Dental Students' (undated). General File No. 70. Hocken Collections AG–180–31/0070.
22 The Registrar to the Minister of Education, 26 February 1924. General File No. 70. Hocken Collections AG–180–31/70.
23 *ODT*, 25 January 1924.
24 Dental education (Editorial). *ODT*, 26 January 1924.
25 *New Zealand Herald*, 28 January 1924.
26 *ODT*, 30 January 1924.
27 Pickerill to the Registrar, 3 March 1924. General File No. 65. Hocken Collections AG–180–31/78.
28 Pickerill to the Registrar, 12 March 1924. General File No. 65. Hocken Collections AG–180–31/78.
29 One Dental School, or more? (Editorial). *NZDJ* 19: 153–4, January 1924.
30 Report of the Committee set up to Enquire into the Provision of Accommodation for the Training of Dental Students. *NZDJ* 19: 221–4, May 1924.
31 Pickerill to the Registrar, 20 March 1924. General File No.70. Hocken Collections AG–180–31/0070.
32 Report by the Dean of the Dental Faculty submitted to the Otago University Council on the report of the Committee set up by the Minister of Education to Enquire into 'The Provision of Accommodation for the Training of Dental Students.' *NZDJ* 19: 221–4, May 1924.
33 Ivory to Pickerill, 7 February 1924; Pickerill to the Registrar, 8 February 1924; Registrar to Ivory, 21 February 1924. General File No. 70. Hocken Collections AG–180–31/0070.
34 Pickerill to the Registrar, 14 March 1924. General File No. 70. Hocken Collections AG–180–31/0070.
35 Director of Education to the Registrar, 13 March 1924. General File No. 70. Hocken Collections AG–180–31/0070.
36 Pickerill to the Registrar, 17 March 1924. General File No. 70. Hocken Collections AG–180–31/0070.
37 Marsden to Pickerill, 21 November 1923; Pickerill to Registrar, 24 November 1923. General File No. 70. Hocken Collections AG–180–31/0070.
38 Minutes of the NZDA Executive Council, 13 April 1924. *NZDJ* 19: 238–44, May 1924.
39 Business Meeting [NZDA] *NZDJ* 19: 37, July 1924.
40 H.P. Pickerill. Report to the Chancellor on the future development and requirements of the Dental School during say the next twenty years. Hocken Collections MS 689/M.
41 New Dental School (reprinted from the *ODT*). *NZDJ* 19: 83–4, November 1924.
42 Editorial. *NZDJ* 20: 78, November 1924.
43 Minutes of the Council, January 1924 – December 1927. Meeting of 24 November 1925. Hocken Collections AG–180–1/08.

44 New Dental School. *NZDJ* 21:203–5, May 1924.
45 The new Dental School. The Official Opening. (Adapted from the *ODT*, 12 June 1926) *NZDJ* 21: 235–46, July 1926.
46 The September 1926 issue of *NZDJ* (22: 5–30) contained a full report of evidence placed before the Dental Commission established 'to Investigate and Report upon the Cases of Persons who should be enabled to Qualify for Registration as Dentists', the report itself, and the consequent Dentists Amendment Act, 1926.
47 The new Dental School. The Official Opening. *Loc. cit.*

16

1 Pickerill to the Chancellor, 11 February 1927. General File No. 108. Hocken Collections AG–180–0108.
2 Pickerill to the Chancellor, 4 March 1927. General File No. 108. Hocken Collections AG–180–0108.
3 Council Minutes, Vol. 8. Meeting of 15 March 1927. Hocken Collections AG–180–1/08.
4 NZDA Executive Meeting 24 August 1926. *NZDJ* 21: 31–4, September 1926.
5 Minutes of the Central Executive NZDA, 28 March 1927. *NZDJ* 23: 182, May 1927.
6 King (p.332–3).
7 Minutes of the NZDA Executive Council, 17 May 1927. *NZDJ* 23: 229–30, July 1927.
8 Editorial. *NZDJ* 23: 107–9, March 1927.
9 Correspondence. *NZDJ* 23: 35, September 1927.
10 Pickerill to the Registrar, 27 June 1927. General File No. 108. Hocken Collections AG–180–31/0108.
11 Meeting of the Medical Committee, 27 March 1922. Committee Reports Vol. 3 Hocken Collections AG–180–2/03.
12 Professorial Board Minutes 1912–1933. Meeting of 13 July 1927. Hocken Collections AG–180–15/05.
13 Otago University Dental Students' Association. Notes. *NZDJ* 23: 181, May 1927.
14 H. Schmid. *Henry Percy Pickerill (1879–1956): Inaugural-Dissertation zur Erlangung der Doktorwürde der Zahnheilkunde der medizinschen Fakultät der Unisität Zuürich.* Zürich, 1960 (p. 138–9).
15 Minutes of the Faculty of Dentistry. Meeting of 12 July 1927. Hocken Collections MS–0689/M.
16 Dr Pickerill's resignation. Tribute by the Otago Hospital Board. No fresh appointment to be made. Entertained by Officers' Club. *ODT*, 29 July 1927.
17 University's loss. Dr Pickerill's departure. *ODT*, 10 August 1927.
18 Farewell to Dr Pickerill. *NZDJ* 23: 3–4, September 1927.
19 Council Minutes Vol. 8. Meeting of 29 November 1927. Hocken Collections AG–180–1/08.
20 Pickerill to the Registrar, 1 December 1927; 5 December 1927. General File No. 115. Hocken Collections AG–180–31/0115.
21 Professor Robert Bevan Dodds, D.D.S. *NZDJ* 23: 112–13, March 1928.

17

1 B.W. Taylor. *Plastic Surgery Origins and Innovators*. Private publication, 2000.
2 Tiny Laguna Beach Church squeezes into history. *The Register* (Laguna Beach), 27 February 1977.

3 References for C.M.W. Clarkson by Pickerill (January 1927), Hercus (22 February 1927), and AR Falconer (24 February 1927). Pickerill Papers, Hocken Collections.
4 A.R. Falconer to T.B. Ponton (Los Angeles), 24 February 1927). Pickerill Papers, Hocken Collections.
5 Cecily Pickerill. An outline of the work of H.P. Pickerill. Undated and unpublished. Pickerill Papers, Hocken Collections.
6 R. Vanderfield (Archivist, Royal North Shore Hospital) to the author, 12 December 2005. Pickerill Papers, Hocken Collections.
7 B.W. Taylor. *Foundations of Australasian Plastic Surgery*. Melbourne: Division of Plastic and Reconstructive Surgery, Royal Australasian College of Surgeons, 1991.
8 *The Story of St. Luke's Hospital, Sydney, 1919–1927.* Sydney: St Luke's Hospital, 1929.
9 P. Pickerill. The complications and sequelae of the extraction of teeth and their treatment. *The Australian Dental Summary* 8: 277–91, November 1927.
10 Included in the Pickerill Papers, Hocken Collections.
11 M. Lawson. Facing the world as somebody else. *Sunday Guardian*, 28 September 1930.
12 B.K. Rank. *Heads and Hands. An Era of Plastic Surgery*. Sydney: Harper and Row, 1987 (p.173). Rank's autobiography, and Taylor's *Foundations of Australasian Plastic Surgery* and *Plastic Surgery Origins and Innovators* unfortunately contain a number of errors relating to Pickerill's career. The reliability of this information is uncertain.
13 H. Schmid. *Henry Percy Pickerill (1879–1956). Inaugural Dissertation. Zur Erlangung der Doctorwürde der Zahnheilkunde der Medizinischen Fakultät der Universität Zürich.* Zürich: Buchdruckerei Schippert, 1960 (p.71–6).

18

1 Sister Josephine, Archivist, Home of Compassion, Island Bay, Wellington.
2 This Register is held in the Photographic Department, Wellington Hospital.
3 H.P. Pickerill. Plastic surgery in the treatment of malignancy. *British Journal of Plastic Surgery* 1: 181–6, October 1948.
4 Agreements with the Wellington Hospital Board, 25 September 1940, 31 July 1942, 29 July 1943, 17 April 1946. Pickerill Papers, Hocken Collections.
5 The Honourable Annette King (Minister of Health). Address to open the International Congress on Vascular Anomalies, Wellington, 23 February 2002.
6 Schmid (*Op.cit.)* lists 20 publications between 1937 and 1954.
7 Pickerill to Hercus, 6 August 1954 (enclosure). Pickerill Letters. *In* Hercus Papers. Hocken Collections MS 1533/35.
8 H.P. Pickerill and C.M. Pickerill. *Babies Nursed by Their Mothers in Hospital.* Undated pamphlet, reprinted from *Health Horizon*, Tavistock House, London. Pickerill Papers, Hocken Collections.
9 Minister of Health to Pickerill, 14 February 1941 and 14 March 1941. Pickerill Papers, Hocken Collections.
10 H. Brew. Paper on hospitalization of young children. Presented at the Annual Conference of the New Zealand Medical Superintendents' Association, 1956. In this paper Helen Brew reviewed the findings of several investigations, including research by H. Bakwin, J. Bowlby, and J. Robertson, showing the serious effects of separation from the mother during traumatic experiences such as can occur during hospitalisation and surgery (Unpublished). Pickerill Papers, Hocken Collections.
11 Domestic Aid – New Regulations – Outpatient Treatment. *Evening Post*, 22 December 1944.
12 Bassam records were deposited, probably after the death of Dame Cecily in 1988, in

the Library of the Wellington School of Medicine, University of Otago; they are now in Dunedin with the Pickerill Papers, Hocken Collections.

13 Post-operative mortalities in cleft palate and infant plastic surgery. (Undated). Pickerill Papers, Hocken Collections.

14 C.M. Pickerill. Hare-lip and cleft palate. A report of seventy consecutive cases. *New Zealand Medical Journal* 41: 121–9, June 1942.

15 Transparencies of many patients treated at Bassam are in the Pickerill Papers, Hocken Collections.

16 C.M. Pickerill and H.P. Pickerill. Elimination of hospital cross-infection in children nursed by the mother. *The Lancet* 425, 27 February 1954.

17 H.P. Pickerill. (Postscript) *In* C. Pickerill. Plastic surgery clinic for babies. *Nursing Mirror and Midwives Journal* 85: ii–iv, 16 August 1947.

18 Operations on infants: the mother's part (Annotation). *The Lancet* 2: 588, 18 October 1947.

19 Cecily Pickerill to E.C. Padgett Jr, Plastic Surgeon's History Project (USA), 14 December 1984.

20 Pickerill to the Director of Medical Services, 4 September 1939. Included in his military records, Defence Force Headquarters, Wellington, and Pickerill Papers, Hocken Collections.

21 The Right Honourable Peter Fraser (Prime Minister) to the New Zealand Trade Commissioner, Sydney, 5 January 1941. Included in Pickerill's military records, Defence Headquarters, Wellington, and Pickerill Papers, Hocken Collections.

22 The *Rangitane*, sailing to England with 200 crew and 111 passengers, was sunk off New Zealand's East Cape on 27 November 1940. Survivors were taken to Emirau Island in the Bismarck Archipeligo, where they landed on 21 December. They embarked on the steamer *Nellore* on 29 December and arrived in Townsville, Australia on 1 January 1941. S.D. Waters. *German Raiders in the Pacific*. In *Episodes and Studies Vol. I. The Official History of New Zealand in the Second World War*. Wellington: War History Branch, Department of Internal Affairs, 1960.

23 Prime Minister to Pickerill (telegram), 6 January 1941. Included in Pickerill's military records, Defence Headquarters, Wellington, and Pickerill Papers, Hocken Collections.

24 H.P. Pickerill. War injuries to the face (lecture to Dental Officers attending a course at the Army School of Instructions, Trentham, New Zealand, April 1940; Hints on the very early treatment of G.S.W. [gun-shot wounds] of the jaws. Copies held at the Dental Defence Directorate, Wellington, and in the Pickerill Papers, Hocken Collections.

25 Director General of Health to the Pickerills, 11 February 1946. Pickerill Papers, Hocken Collections.

26 D. Scott (Editor). *Middlemore Memories. The First 50 Years of Middlemore Hospital.* Publisher unstated, undated.

27 M. Brown, D. Masters, and B. Smith. *Nurses of Auckland. The History of the General Nursing Programme in the Auckland School of Nursing*. Auckland: author publication, 1998 (p.151).

28 Dr J.H. Peat provided a number of insights into the foundation of the Middlemore Plastic Surgical Unit under William Manchester.

29 Tribute to two doctors' work. *Auckland Star*, 7 November 1950.

30 Founder of plastic surgery clinic proposes 'skin banks'. *The Auckland Star*, 7 November 1950.

31 D. Scott. *Op cit*. (p. 53–4).

32 H.P. Pickerill. *Speech Training for Cleft Palate Patients*. Auckland: Whitcombe and Tombs (undated). Pickerill Papers, Hocken Collections.

33 D. Scott. *Op cit*. (p. 54).
34 J.H. Peat *A History of Orthodontics in New Zealand in the Twentieth Century*. Auckland: private publication, 2002 (p.128–30).
35 J.H. Peat. The dental management of children with clefts of the lip and palate. *NZDJ* 70: 109-17, April 1974.
36 J.H. Peat. *A History of Orthodontics in New Zealand in the Twentieth Century*. *Op. cit*. (p.132).
37 Extensive correspondence between Pickerill, the Medical Superintendent at Wellington Hospital, the Chairman of the Hospital Board, and Hutter covers the events described here is contained in Wellington Hospital Archives: Plastic Surgery, 1951–1952. Archives New Zealand (Wellington) Series 7563, Accession W4990, Item 4.
38 H.P. Pickerill. On the possibility of establishing skin banks. *British Journal of Plastic Surgery* 4: 157–65, October 1951.

19

1 H.P. Pickerill. Anatomical and dental difficulties in cleft palate surgery. *NZDJ* 52: 127–32, July 1956.
2 Pickerill to Editor (F.W. Craddock), 6 August 1956. Pickerill Papers, Hocken Collections.
3 Pickerill to Gillies, 2 December 1955; Pickerill to Gibbs (College Secretary), 16 November 1955; Pickerill to McIndoe, 2 December 1955; Pickerill to Gibbs, 5 December 1955; Pickerill to Gibbs, 16 December 1955. Correspondence 1954–1956: Plastic Surgery Section. Hocken Collections MS–1620–14.
4 Pickerill to Gibbs, 19 April 1956. Pickerill Papers, Hocken Collections, MS–1620–14
5 Extract from the Minutes; Draft Objects and Regulations of the Plastic Surgery Section of the Royal Australasian College of Surgeons (Undated). Pickerill Papers, Hocken Collections.
6 Pickerill to B.K. Rank, 9 March 1956. Pickerill Papers, Hocken Collections.
7 Pickerill to Rank, 7 June 1956. Pickerill Papers, Hocken Collections.
8 Wakefield to Pickerill, 17 May 1956; Brown to Pickerill, 18 May; Rank to Pickerill, 15 June; Wheeler (Secretary, Royal Australasian College of Surgeons) to Pickerill, 6 July 1956. Correspondence 1954–1956: Plastic Surgery Section. Hocken Collections MS–1620–14.
9 E.W. Williams (Association Secretary) to Pickerill, 14 June 1955. Pickerill Papers, Hocken Collections.
10 Pickerill to Williams, 21 June 1955. Pickerill Papers, Hocken Collections.
11 Priestley to Pickerill, 2 June 1955; Pickerill to Priestley, 6 July; Fisher to Pickerill, 5 July; Pickerill to Fisher, 12 July; Tonkin to Pickerill, 14 August. Pickerill Papers, Hocken Collections.
12 Pickerill to Priestley, 24 November 1955. Pickerill Papers, Hocken Collections.
13 White to Pickerill, 27 November 1955. Pickerill Papers, Hocken Collections.
14 Pickerill to Priestley, 29 November 1955. Pickerill Papers, Hocken Collections.
15 Priestley to Pickerill, 9 June 1956; Priestley to Pickerill, 14 June; Priestley to Pickerill, 18 June (telegram). Pickerill Papers, Hocken Collections.
16 Pickerill to Priestley, 21 June, 1956. Pickerill Papers, Hocken Collections.
17 Pickerill to Shroff, 19 July; Shroff to Pickerill, 25 and 26 July 1956. Pickerill Papers. Hocken Collections,
18 Pickerill to Walsh, 29 June 1956. Pickerill Papers, Hocken Collections
19 Pickerill to Stanley Wilson, 17 July 1956. Correspondence 1954–1956: Plastic Surgery Section. H.P. Pickerill Papers, Hocken Collections MS–1620–14.

20 Pickerill to the Chancellor (handwritten undated draft). Pickerill Papers, Hocken Collections.
21 Registrar to Pickerill, 6 August 1956. General File No. 632. Hocken Collections AG–18031/0632.
22 Pickerill to the Registrar, 10 August 1956. General File No. 632. Hocken Collections AG–180–31/0632.
23 *Evening Star*, 11 August 1956. Dental School Clipping Book 1952–1959. Hocken Collections AG–508–10.
24 Registrar to Paul Pickerill, 16 August 1956. General File No.632. Hocken collections AG–180–31/0632.
25 J.P. Walsh. The Fiftieth Anniversary of the University of Otago Dental School. *New Zealand Dental Journal* 52: 170–4, October 1956.
26 *ODT*, 22 August 1956. Dental School Clipping Book, 1952–1959. Hocken Collections AG–508–10.
27 H.P. Pickerill. A message from the late Dr. H.P. Pickerill. *NZDJ* 52: 193–4; (Portrait, page 206), October 1956.
28 Walsh to Cecily Pickerill, 31 August 1956. Pickerill Papers, Hocken Collections.
29 Dental Faculty Minutes. Meeting of 6 November 1956. General File No. 632. Hocken Collections AG–180–31/0632.

20

1 F. Hutter. Henry Percy Pickerill (Obituary). *NZMJ* 55: 413–14, October 1956.
2 D. Robb. Henry Percy Pickerill (Obituary). *NZMJ* 55: 514, December 1956.
3 Dr. H.P. Pickerill (Obituary). *NZDJ* 53: 37, January 1957.
4 Henry Percy Pickerill (Obituary). *The Lancet* 2: 579, 15 September 1956.
5 Pickerill to Vivien Jones, 19 September 1953. Pickerill Papers, Hocken Collections.
6 *Evening Post*, 26 December 1967.
7 T.V. Anson. *The New Zealand Dental Services. Official History of New Zealand in the Second World War*. Wellington: Government Printer, 1960.
8 'Beechdale', a notable garden at Silverstream. *New Zealand Gardener*, 14–15, November 1983.
9 Successful Jersey sale. Cow realises 101 guineas. *ODT*, 1 November 1926.

Index

A number in bold indicates a photograph between pages 144 and 145 and between pages 224 and 225